Yinyang Wuxing Spirit Body & Healing

Rhonda Chang

Published by maninriver press
ABN 81168329539
Bretti, NSW, Australia
www.maninriverpress.com

Disclaimer

The information and formulas provided in this book relate only to the author's own experience as a practitioner of traditional yinyang wuxing healing. It is not suggested nor recommended that readers without appropriate training and qualifications use any of the formulas without prior consultation with a qualified physician of traditional Chinese healing.

Yinyang, Wuxing, Spirit, Body & Healing

Rhonda Chang

))\|
maninriver press

Contents

Introduction

THESE days it's not uncommon to find graduates of Chinese medicine asking the question, why is it that what we learn in college doesn't produce reliable results in the clinic? Often their teachers will give the students the impression that they simply haven't yet learnt enough, and that they needed to remember more ancient formulas and get more experience. On the contrary, I would argue it isn't that they haven't learnt and remembered enough, the problem is what's being taught to them—or more precisely, what's not being taught to them. What students now learn in Chinese medicine schools isn't really traditional Chinese healing, it's a modern Chinese medicine, not a traditional one. If it were a traditional Chinese medicine education, the students would be studying in depth the theories of yinyang and wuxing—but they're not. These days yinyang and wuxing barely get a mention or just enough to say that it's been covered. As Ren Yingqiu, one of the founders of modern Chinese medicine, and also the most important compiler of the national Chinese medicine teaching materials, has stated: "The doctrine of yinyang plays an important role in the physiology and pathology of motherland medicine. But we should not overemphasize it. It cannot be the core theory of Chinese medicine."[1]

So what is the core theory of Chinese medicine, if not yinyang wuxing? Chinese medicine as it is taught and practised these days is a medical system called bianzheng lunzhi that on the one hand uses a biomedical view of the body and illness, but on the other hand attempts to use traditional methods, such as herbs and acupuncture, for the physical treatment of illness. In other words, it uses an-

---

[1] Ren Yingqiu "Regarding the question of whether Chinese medicine has a theory" *Journal of Henan Chinese Medicine College* 1980, 4. Note that Ren doesn't even mention wuxing here.

cient methods but not ancient logic. For example, the Han Dynasty scholar Zhang Zhongjing in the *Cold Damage Treatise* discussed a formula called Wulingsan for treating sicknesses that are caused by the disharmony of the body surface (yang) and the interior of the body (yin) with water passage congestion. However, in the teaching of bianzheng lunzhi the formula Wulingsan has become a standard formula for treating the biomedically diagnosed disease of diabetes. Diabetes is of course a biomedical diagnosis, but once Chinese medicine students begin using biomedical diagnosis then they have already left the field of traditional healing, and there is no way of getting back to traditional healing even with traditional herbal medicines or even acupuncture, because the guiding approach has been transformed to a biomedical one not a traditional Chinese medicine approach based on yinyang and wuxing. In the clinic, when patients are diagnosed as diabetic, doctors will almost invariably use the Wulingsan formula. But the effectiveness of Wulingsan in treating diabetes has never been proven by scientific medicine tests. Nor does traditional Chinese healing have a cure for diabetes, and that is primarily because it's not a traditional diagnosis and because it is outside the framework of yinyang wuxing theory. It is only when the conditions of diabetic patients are reassessed in the framework of yinyang wuxing logic that the traditional healing methods can then be appropriately created for each of the cases.

So why is Wulingsan being used to treat diabetes? Why are a lot of old herbal formulas being used to treat diseases with modern biomedical names? The reason is this, and unfortunately it's another thing we can attribute to the influence of Mao Zedong. In the 1950s, Mao Zedong, who disdained things and ideas that were in any way superstitious, or unscientific, wanted to transform traditional Chinese healing into something that could pass for scientific and respectable. The result was that a group of Chinese medicine doctors got together and compared the symptoms recorded in old Chinese medicine texts with biomedical symptoms of diseases. Whenever the old texts revealed a case of illness that had similar symptoms to a biomedical disease, then the modern researchers arbitrarily decided that since the pathological symptoms had similarity to the disease in modern terms then that indeed was the disease and that the old treatment formula could now then be used to treat the disease, whether it be diabetes, malaria, high blood pressure, etc.

There are, however, many cases that have similar symptoms but which are not exactly the same and have different treatment methods as well, so these scholars then divided the biomedical disease into different yinyang natures, for example, pneumonia has cold, hot, wet or dry different categories, and the different treatments would then be set to treat the different pneumonias. The reorganization of the old medical records then became a new Chinese medical system, which came to be called bianzheng lunzhi (sometimes translated into English as pattern differentiation and treatment determination or syndrome differentiation and therapy determination), whereby physicians could recognize patterns of symptoms and from that apply a traditional formula. In this new system of bianzheng lunzhi, which became the national standard of Chinese medicine education from the late 1970s onwards, physicians were no longer concerned primarily with yinyang wuxing, but with what biomedicine was telling them about the body and illness.

A fundamental problem with this system of bianzheng lunzhi is that modern physicians can match symptoms with old formulas but don't have the theoretical knowledge to formulate their own treatment strategies. Since modern physicians don't have the theoretical understanding of how these old formulas were thought out, the majority of the time they are confronted by symptoms that don't neatly match the modern categories of diseases they are now dealing with. At this point the physicians are faced with a diagnostic and treatment impasse.

Symptoms of illnesses manifest in innumerable forms, even if one could remember every experienced formula recorded in the ancient texts, there is no guarantee that one can find the perfect formula to match the illnesses encountered daily in a busy clinic. Sometimes there is a good result but often there isn't. When the practitioners don't have a reasoning system to understand why their healing methods are not working, and are unable to produce concrete healing effects, many begin to question their own skills and career choices. In China some physicians choose to change profession, some choose not to take it too seriously, because after all, it's a profession with high social status and is still a nice way to make a living, a majority turn to using pharmaceutical drugs and barely use any traditional herbs.

Even the most dedicated physicians are more comfortable prescribing something like antibiotics, but because patients who come to a Chinese medicine clinic are seeking an alternative to western medicine, then the doctors most of the time will also prescribe a simple herbal formula or tablets to appease the patients. At least in China such doctors have a choice. For physicians of Chinese medicine practising in other countries the choices are not as wide. Some will endeavour to make a deeper study of traditional healing and find their way back to yinyang wuxing theories. This book is written for those who are on that path or who are looking for the alternative to what they are now doing. And it reflects, through the cases I describe, some of my own experience. But to make use of that experience, an understanding of yinyang and wuxing theories is the vital component.

So what got me onto this path of more than thirty years? When I was quite young I had on several occasions suffered illnesses that western medicine could not help but which traditional healers fixed as easily as turning over one's hand. So I had a belief and respect for traditional healing and I went on hoping to study it. After graduating from Chinese medicine school, I furthered my study with several old style physicians. These physicians didn't have important titles or occupy high positions, mainly because they didn't have the qualifications in the new Chinese medicine system, nevertheless these doctors were highly regarded by patients. At that time, there were still many such traditional healers around. Perhaps it was because of the political environment, but not one such healer ever told me that I must first have a yinyang wuxing view of the body and that I must learn from the ancient texts. But when I asked the reason for their formulation in treating illnesses, the answers were never the same as what I would have got from the university lecturers. Once I asked a healer how to treat a stubborn cough, he said through nourishing soil to create metal, in other words, through strengthening the spleen soil to nurture the lung metal. And the effect was astonishing. Another time, I asked a healer how to treat the western diagnosed illness of hives, he corrected me by saying it is wind rash, and when the blood is cool, the wind ceases. Wind rash means wind is the reason for the symptom of rash, but blood heat is the cause of the wind, so to treat such a symptom one needs to cool the blood and cease the wind.

There are numerous herbs that can cool blood, so there are endless formulas that can treat wind rash.

Gradually, I trained myself into adopting a yinyang wuxing view of the body and the surrounding environment, and resisted thinking of ancient formulas as treating biomedical diseases, but instead to use ancient formulas as a guide to create my own formulas in order to correct yinyang wuxing disorders. In the clinic, many patients would come to me with a biomedical report, however, I would always try to put out of my mind the biomedical aspects of the disease, and to make my diagnosis and treatment strategies according to yinyang wuxing theory. This has been extremely important for me to make flexible and effective treatments for illnesses, regardless of whether I might have previously seen the condition or whether it was for the first time.

Then, if one knows about a herb or a method to treat some symptoms but doesn't know the theory of yinyang wuxing, can the methods be used? The answer is yes and no. To say yes, when a sickness is not complicated and the treatment is straight forward. For example, during a hot summer people get heat rashes, applying aloe vera topically can achieve almost instant relief. So without yinyang wuxing theory, one certainly can use an experienced method to heal ailments that have seemingly clear causes and symptoms. However, if a sickness has slightly complicated symptoms, without the direction of yinyang wuxing theory, an empirical formula not only proves difficult to achieve an effective result, it can also induce an adverse effect. For example, there was a patient who suffered severe pimples, a Chinese medicine practitioner gave him herbs such as dandelion, viola, scutellaria baicalensis, and coptis to clear heat and detoxify poison. At first the patient felt the pimples had improved, so he persisted taking them for 8 months. At the end of the eight months, the pimples were getting worse each day. In traditional Chinese healing, pimples are blood poisons, and dandelion, viola, scutellaria baicalensis, and coptis are herbs that detoxify poison, and reduce swellings, so it seemed to be the correct approach to formulate the prescription, but there was no positive effect, and whatever caused the blood poison was not treated. The dandelion, viola, scutellaria baicalensis, and coptis all have a cool yinyang nature, but long term use on their own will damage kidney heat. In the wuxing cycle, the kidney nourishes the liver, kidney coldness, causes liver weakness, so the blood poison gets worse as do the symptoms get worse. According to yinyang wuxing theory, one would make the treatment to warm the kidney and clear heat and detoxify poison together. This is also to say that the theory of yinyang wuxing makes it vital for flexible and effective traditional Chinese healing.

When writing this book I had in mind that it should be suitable for a general reader to gain information on a yinyang wuxing perspective of the spirit, body and treating illnesses. It is of course suitable for professional practitioners and anyone who has an interest in the nature of traditional Chinese healing. Understanding yinyang wuxing theory may seem profoundly esoteric but it is in fact no harder to understand than marketing, finance, or motor cycle maintenance. Unfortunately, such knowledge isn't taught through our formal education—not even in China. Although the theory of yinyang wuxing is most closely associated with China, it would be a pity if such knowledge were lost to the world, since the ability to overcome illness and have better health through the use of natural materials is a valuable resource for people all over the world.

This book is structured around an introductory chapter, "Yinyang and Wuxing", which outlines the doctrines of yinyang and wuxing, and how they relate to the human spirit, body, healing, illness, causes, diagnosis and symptoms. The "Yinyang Wuxing" chapter is then followed by individual chapters which cover the five wuxing organs, Kidney water, Liver wood, Heart fire, Spleen soil, and Lung metal. All these chapters introduce the causes of yinyang disorder in relation to the specific wuxing organ, outline symptoms, the tongue, the pulse, the skin, and the principles of treatment, and include a number of case studies[2] to demonstrate the principles of treatment, methods of diagnosis and formulation of herbal formulas/prescriptions. After the wuxing organ chapters I provide a chapter on "Spirit and Body" which outlines the causes of disharmony between spirit and body which lead to illness, followed by case studies which show the

---

[2] A number of the cases studies in this book first appeared in my ebook *Menopause and Symptoms of Kidney Water Heat Loss.*

methods of treatment in such cases. The penultimate chapter discusses some difficult cases, which go to emphasize the importance of the yinyang wuxing approach in traditional Chinese healing. Then a short chapter on "Sprains and Bruises", followed by a "Quick Guide" table of the yinyang nature of the spirit, body, signs of illness, & principles for treatment. Finally, some information of decocting/cooking herbal formulas and how to take them. There is also a Glossary of terms and Indexes to Treatments, Formulas[3], and Herbs.

In this book there are some clinical cases where the reader might conclude that the description approximates to a certain biomedical disease. For reasons already outlined above, I have in most cases avoided using the biomedical names of diseases. In addition, adopting biomedicine disease names will unavoidably catch one into an anatomical view of the body and the pathological recognition of diseases. Unless one can portray the body and illnesses from the yinyang wuxing perspective it is impossible to form a treatment strategy in a yinyang wuxing way, and theory and practice are never going to match in this way. Attempting an anatomical diagnosis of disease, while treating the same illness with ancient formulas can only rely on luck and guessing. Thus the effect is unpredictable, and when it fails there is no reasoning system to work out why, this is precisely the fault of modern Chinese medicine and the reason that I am passionate about putting this book forward.

I hope that after reading this book the reader will be better informed and knowledgeable about traditional Chinese healing, and that such knowledge will continue to be passed on.

---

[3]The majority of the formulas used in this book have been created by myself, some I have adopted and modified.

Yinyang & Wuxing

Yinyang wuxing is a theory that elaborates the cycle of life and death. While the doctrine of yinyang explains the inter-dependency of yin and yang, the doctrine of wuxing further interprets the regulation of the changes between yin and yang that manifest different things and phenomena. Although it is common to think of yinyang and wuxing as separate theories, without the concept of wuxing the theory of yinyang is merely a fixed and static idea that has no theoretical purpose in directing any practical activities. In addition, if the concept of wuxing is separated from the concept of yinyang then the theory of wuxing also becomes just another quaint enigma.

The Doctrine of Yinyang

Yin is the base of all things and phenomena that are dark, downward moving and passive by nature. The moon, a dark night, stillness, cold, sinking, stability, adherence, gathering, soft and resisting are yin. Yang is the base of all things and phenomena that are bright, upward moving and active by nature. The sun, a bright day, mobility, hot, rising, fluctuating, loose, separating, upright and opposing are yang.

Yin and yang are the two opposite sides of one thing, but the two opposing sides are not in anyway antagonistic to each other. On the contrary, the yinyang doctrine is about the attraction, reliance and the interdependence of yin and yang. Only when the two sides of yin and yang become intimate do life then emerge and continue. For example, when one calms down and sleeps at night (calm and sleep are yin activities), then one can be energetic and animated during the day (energetic and animated are yang qualities). Water is cold (yin), when it receives heat (yang) it moves and brings up other life.

The incorporation of yin and yang is the doctrine of yinyang. Laozi in the *Dao De Jing* states: "existence [yin] and non-existence [yang] work together to create each other, difficulty [yin] and ease [yang] are coordinates; long [yang] and short [yin] are devoted to each other; height [yang] and depth [yin] lean together; mute [yin] and voice [yang] are congruence; forward [yang] and backward [yin] are accompanying." Existence begins with non-existence; knowing is easy, the unknown is difficult, but knowing comes out of unknowing, ease comes from difficulty; without the short there is no long; height relies on a foundation, a foundation can be seen from a height; a voice can be heard because of the quiet, backward exists because of forward. Between heaven and earth, all things are the phenomena of yin and yang incorporation.

On the other hand, yinyang is in a constant state of movement. When yin reaches its furthermost extent it will be replaced by the emergence of yang; when yang reaches its furthermost extent it will be replaced by the emergence of yin. For example, when the day reaches its warmest point, it will become cooler and darker; when the moon reaches its fullest, it will wane; a high tide will be followed by low tide. Everything rises and falls following the regulation of the rise and fall of yin and yang. For example, owls are yang in nature, they need the night yin in order to be active. Humans are yin in nature and need the daylight yang. During the day people can see things, feel energetic and need to be active, but at night, the eyes are hard to keep open, the body wants to lie down and rest until daylight appears again. Yin and yang are like two sides of a mountain, in the morning the western side is yin and dark and the eastern side is yang and bright, by the afternoon the western side becomes yang and bright and the eastern side becomes yin and dark. The changes are not material but due to the positional change of the sun relative to the earth. During the night, people are less active, but this doesn't mean that the yang disappears, rather at this time the yang hides inside of yin. Similarly, during the day, when people are active doesn't mean that there is no yin, at this time the yin is inside and anchoring the yang, so that yang can rise but not dissipate. The yang motivates the yin, and the yin bears the yang. The doctrine of yinyang elaborates the coordinated rises and falls of yin and yang. The degree of yin, such as heaviness, softness, moistness, gathering, stickiness etc. or the degree of yang such as lightness, straightness, dryness, scattered, looseness etc. all have different levels of quality, and qi is the measure of the quality of yin and yang. The term qi is commonly translated in English as power, force, breath or air. A very heavy thing can be said to have a strong yin qi; a very light thing has a very strong yang qi.

The Doctrine of Wuxing

The doctrine of wuxing consists of the dynamic between wood, fire, soil, metal and water. The interdependency and exchangeability of yin and yang have a fixed pattern. For example, water is cold, moves downward, and coagulates, so it is yin. Water needs yang heat to flow, and create wood. Wood has an upward, growing and straight nature, so it is yang and needs yin water to grow and retain flexibility. When the yang in wood reaches its highest, it will turn to fire. Fire has a floating nature and is extreme yang. Fire needs grounding wood to last. The extreme heat of fire will ultimately fall and become soil. Soil has a nature of adherence, so it is yin and needs yang heat to be loose. The stickiness of soil concentrates to create stones, the loose nature of soil purifies stones to metal. Metal has a nature of being solid, concentrated, and gathering that which is moist, so it is yin and likes to be alone (unmixed with other things), so it is pure. Metal gathers dampness and separates fresh from turbid, and creates water. Hence, water creates wood, wood creates fire, fire creates soil, soil creates metal, and metal creates water in a never ending wuxing cycle.

Within this cycle there is also a controlling cycle. While wood creates fire, it also binds soil to stop soil from being eroded away. While fire creates soil, it also loosens the soil to stop excessive metal. While soil creates metal, it also binds water to stop flooding. While metal creates water, it also stabilizes wood. While water creates wood it also controls fire. Thus, wood, fire, soil, metal and water form a rigorous chain that create one another and at the same time limit one another. (See diagram below).

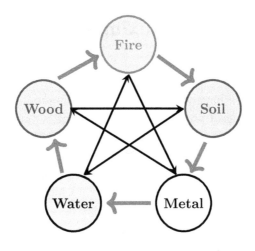

Wuxing

In this wuxing cycle, soil is the central pivot. Water is below soil, and fire is above. The yang heat of fire goes down to water through soil; water receives heat and raises moisture through soil to the atmosphere. Wood through soil absorbs water, and metal is created by soil. So soil connects metal, water, wood, and fire together with itself, but needs to be loose so that nothing will be stuck or trapped within it.

Wuxing concerns not the materiality of things but the yinyang quality of things. The fire in wuxing is not the inflammation and burning, but its active and upward nature. Soil is not the mineral and micro-organism content but a calm, bearing, transforming and charitable nature. Metal is not the mineral structure but a nature of collectivity, and the ability to separate fresh and turbid. Water is not H_2O, but its nature of softness while at the same time its strength, its downwardness, and the ability to maintain heat. Wood is not the fibre but its flexible and protracting nature. The doctrine of wuxing is the purpose of the doctrine of yinyang, yinyang is the foundation of wuxing, omitting wuxing is to ignore the regulatory role of change in yin and yang. Below I outline how yinyang and wuxing theory combine to make them the guide to healing practice.

The Yinyang Wuxing of Human Life

Heaven and earth have yinyang, so too does human life have yinyang. Life is the joining of yin and yang. The spirit is yang and the body is yin. The joining of the spirit and the body is life. The spirit is the qi of heaven, and manifests in five forms of zhi (志)[4]. The five zhi consist of the striving zhi, the aspiring zhi, the reasoning zhi, the lofty zhi and the enduring zhi (see the chapter Spirit and Body for greater detail). A person's spirit is the extension of heavenly qi and remains in connection with heaven. The spirit is invisible, untouchable, immaterial, and active, so it is yang. The body of a human life is conceived from the parents; it is solid, material, and internal, so it is yin.

When the spirit is embodied, the five zhi of the spirit can be exercised and made apparent. The connection of the spirit with the heaven and earth enables the human body's yinyang transformation to be coherent with heaven and earth, that is, a person wakes when the sun rises and sleeps when the sun is down. The connection of the spirit with heaven and earth also makes a person cognisant of his or her surroundings, for example, an appreciation of a brilliant sunset, or an apprehension of darkness. The spirit is the motive force of people's activities, so the connection of a spirit with other spirits is affected by what is happening in their surroundings. For example, a person will fight against an injustice that happens to another, or feel sympathy for the plight of others.

When a spirit joins with a body from conception, the interaction of the yang spirit and the yin body falls into a wood, fire, soil, metal, and water transformation cycle of the human body which collectively become the wuxing organs. That is to say, it is the yang spirit and yin body joined together that create the wuxing organs.

The wuxing organs

In the human body wood is the organ of the liver, fire is the organ of the heart, soil is the organ of the spleen, metal is the organ of the

---

[4]Zhi may be translated into English as will, but I have decided to keep to zhi as will becomes at times clumsy in English.

lung, water is the organ of the kidney, and these together are the wuxing organs. As there is a creative cycle in wuxing, there is also a creative cycle among the wuxing organs.

The lung is a metal organ. Metal has a nature of solidity, convergence, and purity. Metal gathers moisture, then filters what is turbid and creates clean water. Lung metal gathers qi and moisture. It separates turbidity and freshness; it stores all of the body's qi, and makes the body ample and fresh. Lung metal has a nature of absorbing, which makes it a yin dominant organ. But within yin there is also yang, and the yang of lung metal separates—that is, it separates what can be fresh from what is turbid to create fresh kidney water.

The kidney is a water organ. Water has a nature of coldness, coagulating, moving downwards, moistening and nurturing all things, and retains yang heat. Kidney water has a cold, stagnant nature, it is the storage of the body's water, it moistens the body and reserves body heat. Kidney water makes the body able to endure cold or heat, handle heavy work loads and enables the body's growth and reproduction. Kidney water has a cold and coagulating nature which makes it a yin dominant organ. But within yin there is also yang, and the yang of kidney water makes water flow. When kidney water has yang, it is warm and creates liver wood.

The liver is a wood organ. Wood has a nature of being erect, spreading, dissolving decay, and is supple when there is sufficient water. Liver wood has a nature of being upright and able to bend. Liver wood keeps the body straight and flexible. Liver wood stores and supplies blood to the body. Blood is the aggregation of the yinyang essence of the wuxing organs. Blood nurtures the body, clears decay, removes congestion, and keeps the body clean. Liver wood has an erect nature, and is a yang dominant organ. Within yang there is yin, and the yin of liver wood makes it supple. With kidney water moisture, liver wood grows. When its growth is at its extremity, it loses its yin water, and becomes heart fire.

The heart is a fire organ. Fire has a nature of burning heat, it goes upward and is active, and when there is sufficient material (yin), it is grounded and stable. Heart fire is the house of the spirit. The spirit enables people to be active. When the heart fire heat is grounded, the spirit can rest and the person is quiet. Heart fire has a floating nature, and is a yang dominant organ. Within yang there is

13

yin, and heart fire yin sustains the yang heat. When heart fire gains grounding wood, it burns, and creates spleen soil.

The spleen is a soil organ. Soil is by nature viscous, and permeable. It creates and transforms. Soil is the pivot of wuxing, it is the connecting link between fire, wood, metal, and water. Spleen soil has an adhesive nature, it receives and stores food, accommodates the other wuxing organs and their yinyang needs, and is a yin dominant organ. The extreme adhesiveness of spleen soil consolidates stones and metal, and creates lung metal. Within yin there is yang, and the yang of spleen soil maintains the permeability of spleen soil which enables spleen soil to transform food for the yinyang needs of the wuxing organs. The loosening of the spleen soil allows liver wood to get through to absorb moisture from kidney water, allows heart fire to get through to store its yang heat in the kidney water, and allows kidney water to get through to be replenished by lung metal.

While the wuxing organs have a creative cycle, they also have a controlling cycle. Lung metal is softened by heart fire to breathe smoothly. When heart fire cannot control lung metal, the breathing of the person is raspy. Kidney water is controlled by spleen soil to flow along a certain route. When spleen soil cannot control kidney water, there is flooding (oedema). Liver wood needs lung metal to be stable, when lung metal cannot control liver wood, the person is unable to stand straight. Heart fire needs kidney water to be controlled, when kidney water cannot control heart fire, a person suffers palpitations. Spleen soil needs liver wood to have a controlled appetite, when liver wood cannot control spleen soil, food cannot alleviate hunger.

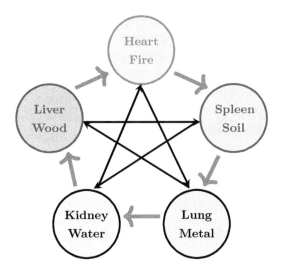

Wuxing Organs

The human body is interlaced by the wuxing organs. The wuxing organs are like trees, the organs are the roots of the trees, the rest of the body are the stems, branches and leaves of the wuxing organs. The leaves of each wuxing organ are all connected. So wuxing organs are interconnected and interdependent with each other. Within each wuxing organ there are also wuxing organs. Within the lung metal, there is heart fire to be smooth; there is spleen soil to be sustained; there is kidney water to be moist; there is liver wood to upkeep the qi passages. Within the kidney water, there is heart fire to keep water warm; there is spleen soil to prevent flooding; there is lung metal to replenish fresh water; there is liver wood to keep water flow without hesitation. Within the liver wood, there is heart fire to be erect; there is spleen soil to be solid; there is lung metal to be brisk; there is kidney water to be flexible. Within the heart fire, there is spleen soil so the fire is grounded; there is lung metal to provide ventilation; there is kidney water to store heat; there is liver wood to be burned upon. Within spleen soil, there is heart fire to enrich; there is lung metal to be permeable; there is kidney water to be adhesive; there is liver wood to be stable.

The interlinking of the wuxing organs through various passages takes the spirit, sustenance, qi, water, and blood all over the body. The heart fire not only hosts the spirit in its root organ, but provides a resting place all over the body for the spirit. Spleen soil stores and transforms food not only in its root organ, but stores and transforms food all over the body. Lung metal not only stores qi in its root organ, but stores qi in every part of the body. Kidney water stores water and reserves body heat not only in its root organ but by its extensions around the whole body. Similarly, liver wood hosts blood not only inside its root organ, but reserves and supplies blood in every part of the body. Therefore, the spirit, food, qi, water, and blood passages follow each of their hosting wuxing organs and interlace the entire body.

Each of the wuxing organs is inter-penetrated with other wuxing organs, but the most important connection of the wuxing organs is the connection with heaven and earth. The yinyang transformations of all the wuxing organs is regulated and maintained by heaven and earth. When the yinyang transformation of any part of the human body is not coherent with heaven and earth, there will be a suffocation of that part and illness occurs. Every part of the human body must breathe freely with heaven and earth at all times to be healthy. Breathing from nose to throat and to the lungs is common knowledge, if it is blocked anywhere along the way, life quickly ceases. In fact, every part of the body must breathe freely to survive. Here the breathing is not the inhalation of air and the exhalation of carbon dioxide but the connection of yin and yang between the body and heaven and earth.

The way that people can be vibrant and active during the day is driven by the light and heat of yang qi from the daytime surroundings; the way that people feel tired and sleepy at night is driven by the darkness and coldness of yin qi from one's nightime surroundings. The breathing of wuxing organs with heaven and earth has a certain channel and order. The description of such channels and order is the doctrine of Jingluo.

Jingluo

The yinyang qi of heaven and earth passes through the human body along certain routes which are called jingluo. Jingluo in English is often translated as meridian. Jingluo is a generic term for jingmai and luomai. Jing means a passage, mai means a mountain range. Luo means net. Jingmai are the large passages that yinyang qi from heaven and earth travel through in the human body and which go up and down like a shuttle back and forth on a mountain range; so it is called jingmai. Luomai is like a small mountain range that nets or connects jingmai together; so it is called luomai.

The yinyang transformation of heaven and earth has twelve periods, for example, a year has a twelve month cycle, a day is in a twelve timing cycle. In ancient China, the twelve periods were named: zǐ (子), chǒu (丑), yín (寅), mǎo (卯), chén (辰), sì (巳), wǔ (午), wèi (未), shēn (申), yǒu (酉), xū (戌), hài (亥). The human body has twelve jingmai that respond according to the particular time within the cycle: foot taiyang urine bladder meridian (足太阳膀胱经), foot shaoyang gall bladder meridian (足少阳胆经), foot yangming stomach meridian (足阳明胃经), foot shaoyin kidney meridian (足少阴肾经), foot jueyin liver meridian (足厥阴肝经), foot taiyin spleen meridian (足太阴脾经), hand taiyang small intestine meridian (手太阳小肠经), hand shaoyang sanjiao meridian (手少阳三焦经), hand yangming large intestine meridian (手阳明大肠经), hand shaoyin heart meridian (手少阴心经), hand jueyin heart-sac meridian (手厥阴心包经) and hand taiyin lung meridian (手太阴肺经).

Of the human body's yinyang cycle that responds to heaven and earth, the *Yellow Emperor's Inner Canon*, states in the chapter "Lingshu Jingshui":

> the foot taiyang meridian responds externally to the river Qing, internally pertains to the urine bladder, which connects with the body's water passage. The foot shaoyang meridian responds externally to the Wei River, internally pertains to the gall bladder. The foot yangming meridian responds externally to the ocean, internally pertains to the stomach. The foot taiyin meridian responds externally to the Hu River, internally pertains to the spleen. The foot shaoyin meridian responds externally to Ru River, internally pertains to the kidney. The foot jueyin meridian responds externally to the Sheng River, internally pertains to the liver. The hand taiyang meridian responds externally to Huai River, internally pertains to the small intestine where the body's water passage begins. The hand shaoyang meridian responds externally to the Lei River, internally pertains to the sanjiao. The hand yangming meridian responds externally to the Jiang River, internally

17

pertains to the large intestine. The hand taiyin meridian responds externally to the He River, internally pertains to the lungs. The hand shaoyin meridian responds to the Ji River, internally pertains to the heart. The hand jueyin meridian responds to the Zhang River, internally pertains to the heart-sac. Of the five zang [wuxing organs] and six fu [the externals of wuxing organs] form twelve meridians, every meridian has an external source and internal roots, so internal and external are well connected, like a circle without end. The human meridians are this way.

The significance is that the human body is not an independent or discrete entity, it is intimately connected with the world outside the body like a waterway. Water can be separated by embankment or land, but its yinyang momentum cannot be barraged by any material. For example, no matter where a person is situated, the yinyang momentum of his or her foot yangming stomach meridian is always responsive to the momentum of the ocean waves.

Along the jingmai and luomai there are many openings like doors and windows to allow the body to breathe with the outside and respond immediately to the yinyang transformations of heaven and earth. These doors and windows are like caves that yin and yang flow in and out of, so these doors and windows are called xue wei. Xue means cave, wei means position. Because xue wei are the places where yin and yang qi go in and out of the body, so they are also called qi xue (qi positions). The practices of inserting needles into the qi xue and the use of moxa sticks to heat the qi xue in order to have them connected with heaven and earth are acupuncture and moxibustion. So the points of xue wei are also called acupuncture and moxibustion positions/points (zhenjiu xue wei).

There are 365 main acupuncture points that respond to a year of yinyang transformations. As the *Inner Canon* explains: "there are three hundred and sixty-five qi xue that exist to respond to a year of the earth's yinyang cycle." The human body is a yinyang aura, yinyang constantly transforms from one to the other, so at any different point along a meridian, the order of yin and yang qi is different. So each qi xue has its own identity and name, and needling a different qi xue regulates different yin and yang orders.

Under normal conditions, the opening and closing of xue wei follows the yinyang transformation of heaven and earth, which dominate people's movements. For example, on a hot day the whole body responds to the yinyang condition of heaven and earth; a person may spread his or her arms, perspire, feel thirsty, drink more liquid, eat cooler food, discard layers of clothing. On a very cold day, the pores of our body close, we hunch our shoulders, eat warm food, and wrap up with layers of clothing, etc. When the yinyang order of the human body is coherent with heaven and earth, the yinyang qi can pass through the body freely, people feel light and jaunty, and have no feelings of being pushed by the yinyang qi of heaven and earth. However, when a person's yinyang qi is incoherent with heaven and earth, the person will feel the impact of the yinyang qi of heaven and earth. For instance, if on a hot day, a person's pores are not open or on a cold day the pores are not closed, the person would be restless and suffer sickness.

The twelve meridians are the passages which the wuxing organs connect with heaven and earth. The passages whether they are free or congested are the core of a healthy or an ill body. Blockage causes pain, where there is pain there is illness. Nevertheless, every blockage of the body is caused by the yinyang disorder of the wuxing organs, in other words, every illness of the body is no more than the yinyang disorder of the wuxing organs.

Yinyang Wuxing Healing

In yinyang wuxing healing, good health is when the body is interconnected with heaven and earth, and the body's yinyang transformations respond appropriately to heaven and earth. Sickness is when a person's connections with heaven and earth encounter obstructions. These obstructions in the yinyang passages are like cars congested on a road that block free movement. When a person's yinyang transformation is unresponsive to the yinyang transformation of heaven and earth, illness invariably arises. The yinyang qi of heaven and earth must not be impeded in any way. But when the yinyang qi of heaven and earth is unable to pass through the body freely through the yinyang passages because of an obstruction, then, in a sense, the body receives a forceful battering from the yinyang qi of heaven and earth. And this is when we are prone to illness.

Illness

In Chinese, the term for illness is jíbìng 疾病, the characters jí 疾 and bìng 病 both have the radical of nè 疒; ne is a symbol of losing balance and leaning on something for support. Within the character of jí 疾 is another character shǐ 矢; shǐ is a character for an arrow. So the word jí means falling after being struck. Bìng is a word for all kinds of imbalance. Jíbìng means losing balance through being struck. The balance is the balance of yinyang cooperation, that is, when yang is high, yin is below and grounding the yang; when yin is great, yang is underneath to provide support. Balance does not mean half yang and half yin, but is a smooth transition between yin and yang following the regulation of wuxing. When yin qi is rising but yang qi is not supporting it; or when yang is above but yin qi is not grounding, a person will not be able maintain balance and will become ill, which is like when a person's left and right feet aren't coordinated and their dance becomes ungainly.

The singular aim of yinyang wuxing healing is to "open" the person to heaven and earth. When a person is open to heaven and earth, there is no illness—all illness happens because of a bodily disconnection with heaven and earth. The pathway between a person and heaven and earth is the pathway of yinyang. When heaven and earth is dominated by yang qi, the human body's yang passages are open; when the heaven and earth is dominated by yin qi, the human body's yin passages are open; fire burns with fire, water flows congruently with water, the flow is free and open. If heaven and earth is dominated by yang qi, but the body is dominated by yin qi, the body will neither be able to rest nor to be active, because the external yang qi will exhaust the yin qi of the body, so it is difficult to rest. On the other hand, the external yang qi cannot go through the body, so the body doesn't receive the yang energy from heaven and earth, so the person is weak. In the same way, if heaven and earth is dominated by yin qi, but a person has his or her yang passages open, then the body will be tired but unable to rest. Because the yin qi from heaven and earth exhausts the body's yang qi and causes tiredness, the yin passages of the body do not receive yin qi from heaven and earth so the body feels unrested. Therefore, all kinds of body unease are forms of illness, and all illnesses are signs of a body unresponsive to the yinyang regulation of heaven and earth.

Causes of obstruction

In the first chapter of the *Inner Canon* we find the principle for good health and long life: "Whoever understands the Dao, will obey the law of yinyang and its regulation of change. Eating and drinking must be moderate, daily routine must be regular, never be exhausted by sexual desire. Thus, the body and spirit can cooperate together and a life can last to its natural age of over a hundred years." Thus one should never overeat or eat at irregular times. In the morning between 6am to 7am, yang qi is rising and surrounds people, so people should rise. At night 9pm to 10pm, yin qi begins to dominate our surrounding environment, so people should go to sleep. Sex exhausts both yin and yang qi, so it should never be over indulged.

In modern industrial societies, excessive eating, drinking, and over exhaustion are still common causes of illnesses, but there are now also a multitude of other factors that inhibit or affect good health. Food additives in processed foods; water, land and air pollution; excessive noise levels in cities; chemicals and gases in our built environment; not forgetting all kinds of radiation and electrical, radio, magnetic rays, waves, and forces, as well as the jobs and everyday stresses of modern living can affect our health while we are barely able to discern them. Many of these factors that deplete our energies and health were not in existence not so long ago, nevertheless, in terms of traditional Chinese concepts of health, all things that disrupt our yinyang wuxing balance cause ill health, the abovementioned factors are no exception to this idea. To the same extent we treat all illness through rebalancing yinyang wuxing.

The most important factor that causes the body to lose its connection with heaven and earth is the disharmony of the spirit with the body. When a zhi of the spirit becomes overwhelmingly strong, it exhausts the yinyang qi of the body, which in turn leads to a yinyang disorder that causes symptoms of illness. For example, when the yang qi of the enduring zhi of the spirit becomes excessively strong, it forces the body to over work, which exhausts kidney water heat and leads to the yinyang disorder of kidney water, and causes people to suffer symptoms such as fatigue. When kidney water loses

21

its yang qi, it limits the exercise of the yang qi of the enduring zhi of the spirit, which will then cause damage to the spirit and show emotional symptoms such as fear. In life, there are many negative factors challenging the zhi of the spirit. When the spirit and body don't work intimately together to deal with the challenges, the zhi of the spirit will be damaged and cause emotional unease. When the zhi of the spirit are damaged, they will inevitably lose their intimate cooperation and cause the body to lose its yinyang order. Hence, people will suffer not only emotional disorders but also physical discomfort. For example, being in an intimidating environment, the yin of the striving zhi of the spirit is challenged, and if the liver wood yin qi has been exhausted through prolonged bending to the challenges, it will no longer support the yin qi of the striving zhi, then the spirit loses its suppleness, and becomes angry. Anger in turn further exhausts the yin qi of liver wood, which causes people to suffer from symptoms such as body tightness and aches.

Diagnosing illnesses

Yinyang disorders of the wuxing organs will present with symptoms; and will also show on the tongue, pulse and skin. Analysing the symptoms, examining the tongue and skin, and taking the pulse are all methods of diagnosing illnesses in traditional Chinese healing. Sometimes, the symptoms, or the tongue, pulse, or skin alone would provide sufficient evidence for diagnosing an illness, other times, all the methods are needed to determine the levels of yinyang disorders, especially when there is more than one wuxing organ that is disordered.

The spirit interacts with the wuxing organs to exercise its zhi. When wuxing organs lose their regular yinyang order to the extent that it is limiting their ability to fulfil the spirit's zhi, then the spirit would be damaged and cause emotional disorders. For example, liver wood yin deficiency would cause the striving will of the spirit to be inflexible and show symptoms of anger. Therefore symptoms of emotional discomfort also provide clues for the diagnosis of yinyang disorders of the wuxing organs.

Symptoms

Symptoms are the uncomfortable signs of yinyang disorder. The reason that yinyang disorders can cause body discomfort is because the disordered yinyang transformation creates blockages between the yinyang passages of the body and heaven and earth. When the blocked yinyang passages encounter heaven and earth's yinyang flow, as the body's passage are not open, the yinyang flow of heaven and earth will strike the body, which causes pain or other uncomfortable symptoms. As each wuxing organ has its own functions, whenever struck by the yinyang qi of heaven and earth the wuxing organ will show its own particular dysfunctions. For example, liver wood is the storage of blood, liver wood yang makes the blood passages erect, so blood will not be congested or decay, that is, to develop puss. Liver wood yin keeps the blood passages flexible, so blood flows smoothly which keeps blood cool. When there are symptoms of blood heat, or decay, these are signs of liver wood yinyang disorders.

As discussed above, a damaged spirit can cause body yinyang disorder, and a yinyang disorder of the body can damage the spirit. For example, a person who is always impatient may indicate damage to their spirit, which may show as tightness in the body, around the neck and shoulders; on the other hand if one has been overworking this may cause kidney water heat loss, which will in turn fail to nourish liver wood yin, and this may also lead to a person feeling impatient.

The tongue

Every part of the human body has yinyang and wuxing, the tongue also has yinyang wuxing. In examining the tongue we look at the texture of the tongue, the coating of tongue, the moisture of the tongue, the shape of the tongue and the colour of the tongue. The texture of the tongue is heart fire; the coating of the tongue is spleen soil; the moisture of the tongue is lung metal; the shape of the tongue is kidney water; the colour of the tongue is liver wood (See the wuxing organ chapters, i.e kidney, liver, etc. for further details of the tongue).

The pulse

Human life is the joining of the spirit and body. Taking the pulse examines the liveliness of the spirit. The body is the host of the spirit, and the spirit is the impetus of the body. A healthy body allows the spirit to make full use of the body. The spirit shows in the pulse as smooth, steady and strong. Any yinyang disorder of the body will affect its ability to respond to the demands of the spirit, so the spirit will react to it and show a pulse that may be wiry, slippery, erratic or rough.

Taking the pulse is like playing with a balloon. In a healthy person, the skin of the balloon is smooth, thin, and elastic; the balloon is full, and bouncy. The floor where the balloon lands is flat and firm. The space where the balloon bounces has no roof and no obstruction. Thus, the pulse shows that the spirit is well connected with heaven and grounded in the body, and the body is free of obstructions.

The most common place for taking the pulse is at the anterior wrist. To take the pulse, the index finger, middle finger and ring finger are placed on the pulse with the index finger closest to the heel of the palm.

Pressing lightly on the skin reveals the surface pulse. The surface pulse is heaven. When the surface pulse is steady and bouncy it indicates that the spirit is well connected with heaven. When pressing down to the floor of the pulse we feel the deep pulse. The deep pulse is the earth. When the deep pulse is steady and bouncy, it indicates that the spirit is well grounded in the body. Between surface pulse and deep pulse is the middle pulse. The middle pulse, between heaven and earth, is where the spirit and body interact and when the middle pulse is smooth and full, the spirit and body are intimate.

The pulse taken by the index finger is called the cun pulse, the middle finger takes the guan pulse and the ring finger feels the chi pulse. Each of the cun, guan and chi pulses reflect the yinyang orders of a wuxing organ. Both left and right wrist have distinct pulse indications. The left cun pulse reflects the heart fire; the right cun pulse reflects the lung metal; the left guan pulse reflects the liver wood. The right guan pulse reflects the spleen soil; the left chi pulse reflects the kidney water; while the right chi pulse also reflects the kidney heat reservoir called mingmen (life gate). Because heat is the life force, the right kidney is the place that processes the heat deposits and withdrawals, so it is called life gate.

Pregnancy pulse

When women become pregnant, it shows clearly on their pulse. From the date of conception to the tenth day, the pulse is like a line of small firm and smooth beads rolling inside a big pulse. The reason for the pulse within another pulse is that there is a new spirit and body gathering inside the pregnant woman's body, which is the baby's pulse. When the spirit and body of the new life are intimate, the pulse within the pulse is firm, smooth and lively. If the baby is a boy, the pregnancy pulse starts to show on the left hand pulse. If the baby is a girl, the pregnancy pulse starts to show on the right hand pulse. Therefore, within ten days of the pregnancy it is easier to check the sex of the baby. A month into pregnancy, both sides of the pulse will have a pregnancy pulse and it is harder to differentiate the sex of the baby. If a pregnant woman has a history of dampness accumulating in her system, her pulse would be muddy and slippery, which makes it less obvious to detect as a pregnancy pulse.

Skin

The yinyang disorder of wuxing organs can be seen on the skin. Heart fire is the host of the spirit, when the yinyang of heart fire is in regular order, the spirit settles in the body. The spirit brings heaven's qi to the body which presents as light, so the brightness or glow of the skin shows the condition of heart fire yinyang order. Spleen soil is the transportation and transformation junction of the wuxing organs, it controls the opening and closing of the skin. For example, spleen soil governs the skin's responsiveness with heaven and earth so on a hot day the skin is open, on a cold day the skin is closed. Lung metal gathers moisture and qi, and separates turbidity and freshness, and is responsible for the freshness and moistness of the skin. The kidney water stores the yang heat of the entire body, is responsible for the growth and reproduction of the body, and the elasticity of the skin. Liver wood stores blood, when the liver wood is in regular yinyang order, the blood is fresh, as blood cleanses the body and the skin, then the skin will appear clean. When the yinyang of liver wood is disordered, the skin will be discoloured or have rashes.

Principles for treating illnesses

Treating yin organs when lacking yang is to strengthen the yang. Treating yang organs when lacking yin is to nourish the yin. But when treating yin organs that lack yin, while nourishing the yin it must also be remembered to strengthen the yang. Treating yang organs when lacking yang, while strengthening the yang it must be remembered to nourish the yin.

As kidney water is a yin organ, which often lacks yang heat, then treating kidney water yang deficiency is to warm kidney water and to ground heart fire heat into kidney water. When treating kidney water yin deficiency, it is to create water. But in longer cases of kidney water yin deficiency, one must not forget to maintain the kidney water heat.

Liver wood is a yang organ, which often lacks yin and becomes hot and dry. Treating liver wood yin deficiency is to clear heat, cool blood and increase water. When treating liver wood yang deficiency, while clearing dampness, detoxifying poison, invigorating blood to restore the straightness of liver wood, one must not forget to cool blood.

Heart fire is a yang organ, which often lacks yin and becomes floating. Treating heart fire yin deficiency is to ground heart fire, raise kidney water, and moisten liver wood. When treating heart fire yang deficiency, while strengthening the yang heat, one must not forget to ground the heat.

Spleen soil is a yin organ, which often lacks yang and loses its permeability. Treating spleen soil yang deficiency is to warm and loosen the spleen soil. Treating spleen soil yin deficiency, while nourishing spleen soil yin, one must not forget to loosen the spleen soil.

Lung metal is a yin organ, which often lacks yang and is unable to separate turbidity and freshness, and then accumulates dampness and mucus. Treating yang deficiency of lung metal is to clear dampness and dissolve mucus. When treating lung metal yin deficiency, while clearing heat, moistening the lung metal, one must not forget to maintain lung metal yang so that dampness and mucus don't develop.

One additional principle in treating illness is that cooling herbs can't be taken on their own over a long period without the accompanying of warming herbs. Because yang heat is the power of life, the long term taking of cooling herbs will damage a person's life force.

Methods of treating illnesses

The central aim of yinyang wuxing healing is to correct disordered yinyang transformation, and re-establish the coherence of the regular yinyang changes of the body with heaven and earth, which is to "open" the yinyang passages. There are many approaches to yinyang wuxing healing, such as shamanism, praying to spirits, qigong, acupuncture, moxibustion, tuina (massage), cupping, oil scraping, and herbal remedies. Among these many methods, there is only one theory, which is yinyang wuxing, with the singular aim of opening the passages. In this book I concern myself primarily with herbal remedies and to some extent acupuncture.

Acupuncture is the insertion of needles into xuewei (acupuncture points) to regulate the body's yinyang order in response to heaven and earth. Moxibustion is using wormwood sticks to cauterize the xuewei to regulate the yinyang order in response to heaven and earth. A healthy person means that his or her body and spirit are well connected with heaven and earth. As acupuncture and moxibustion can free the passages of the body with heaven and earth, so these methods alone can treat all kinds of illnesses. Each meridian has wood, fire, soil, metal and water wuxing points which are called wuxing shu points. The wood shu point is called jǐng 井, the fire shu point is called yíng 荥, the soil shu is called shū 腧, the metal shu is called jīng 经, and the water shu is called hé 合. The selection of needling points are guided by yinyang wuxing theory. As the *Canon On Acupuncture According to Meridian Flow* 《子午流注针经》 states: "Treating a hollow condition (虚), nourish the mother, treating a solid condition (实), sedate the son. For example, the liver is ill, in the solid condition, sedate the yíng shu point. The yíng shu point is fire, it is the son of wood in the wuxing cycle. In a hollow condition, nourish the hé shu point of the liver meridian. The hé shu point is water, it is the mother of wood in the wuxing cycle." To interpret the paragraph, liver wood is a yang organ, when the liver wood is too hot, it is a solid condition. According to wuxing theory, to sedate the son will weaken the mother. The yíng shu is the fire shu point, in the wuxing cycle, it is the son of wood. So needling the yíng shu point of the liver wood meridian with a sedating technique can lower the heat of liver wood. The lack of liver wood growth is a hollow condition, to treat a hollow condition nourish the mother. The hé shu point is water, water makes wood grow, so needling the hé shu point of the liver wood meridian with a nourishing technique will strengthen the liver wood growth.

Tuina is often translated into English as massage. It is a healing technique that literally pushes and pulls a person's skin and muscles to loosen the blockages of yinyang passage.

Cupping is a technique that applies vacuum cups onto a person's skin to suck out the sandy build up of stagnation to the surface of the body, so that the yinyang passages can be loosened and allowed to flow freely again. The technique is like solving traffic congestion by taking some cars off the road onto the footpath to make room for the traffic to flow. Pulling the accumulated sandy stagnations to the surface of the body will loosen the congestion of the yinyang passages to achieve healing effects.

The technique of oil scraping, guasha 刮痧, uses a small piece of smooth wood, bone, or a spoon to scrape the accumulated sandy stagnation to the surface of the skin to open the yinyang passages and heal illnesses. To prevent skin damage, oil is applied to the skin, so it is called oil scraping in English, but the Chinese characters guā means to scrape, while shā is made up of the radical nè 疒 and within the character is the character sha 沙, meaning sand.

Heaven and earth have yinyang wuxing, people have yinyang wuxing, plants, animals, stones, metals, and soil all have yinyang wuxing. By utilizing the yinyang quality of everything between heaven and earth to correct the disordered yinyang wuxing of a person is the traditional approach of Chinese herbal healing.

A major reason for eating is to maintain a person's yinyang transformation needs. For example, on a hot dry day, people will drink more liquids to maintain their yin qi, and on a cold day, people might have a hot soup to maintain the body's yang qi. Some food has more yang qualities and others have more yin qualities. For example, ginger has a warm nature, which means it has a more yang quality. Cucumber has a cool nature, which is a more yin quality. Grain foods are normally warmer than green vegetables, and meat is normally warmer than grains. Eating is the basic way that people and animals use to protect their bodily yinyang harmonies. However, most of the food we normally eat has either a mild yin or yang nature and such food may maintain a body's yinyang quality. But when the yinyang regulation of wuxing organs has already become disordered and causes symptoms of illness, then we need to reach a broader variety of food to maintain yinyang balance. We can then resort to those foods that may be unpalatable, but which also have stronger yin or yang qualities. We tend to call these foods herbs. But, in fact, all foods have healing effects.

Herbs that have strong yinyang natures can effectively correct yinyang disorders and their symptoms, but if taken incorrectly, they can damage a body's yinyang order and cause further illness. For example, aloe vera has a cold and dry yinyang nature; it can quickly clear a heat rash and relieve constipation. But taken for too long, aloe vera will damage kidney water heat. Aconite, as another example, has an extreme dry and hot nature, it can treat joint pains caused by cold and dampness, but it must be cooked for at least two hours to render it safe for consumption otherwise it can cause acute life threatening yinyang disorder. Therefore aconite is considered a poisonous herb. Nevertheless, with proper preparation[5] and cooking, at the appropriate quantity, and for the right body yinyang condition, aconite is a beneficial and safe herb.

The right herbs for right condition means the yinyang nature of herbs must coincide with the needs of the body's yinyang condition. For example, a person may feel cold, regardless of how much clothing is worn and how much hot food has been eaten. In such a situation, if the person takes aconite, the person will assuredly become comfortably warm. So the aconite has the right yinyang quality for the condition of the person's yinyang disorder.

Nature of herbs and pertaining meridians

Yin attracts yang, and yang attracts yin. Herbs with a yang nature grow in a yin environment, herbs with a yin nature grow in a yang environment. Knowing the habitat and growing conditions of a herb provides clues to the nature of the herb. For example, aloe vera grows in warm places, and grows fast when there is water, which indicates

---

[5] Aconite that is purchased from a dispensary has normally been through a process to lessen its poison, nevertheless it still must be cooked for a minimum of two hours before consumption.

that aloe vera is a herb that has cold and dry properties, and is able to clear heat, and dry dampness. By contrast, ginseng grows in cold damp forests, so ginseng has a warm nature, and the ability to warm kidney water and free water flow. Lotus grows in the mud and has a refreshing nature and ability to clear dampness.

The taste of herbs also reveals their yinyang nature. When the herbs get into the body, they go into the wuxing organs that have the same yinyang nature. Things that have a sour taste have a soft nature, in wuxing it is the yin of wood and therefore sour tasting herbs nurture the liver wood yin. Something that has an astringent taste has a dry and hard nature, in wuxing it is the yang of wood and therefore astringent tasting herbs support the liver wood yang.

A bitter taste has a cold nature, in wuxing it is the yin of fire, so bitter tasting herbs support the heart yin and grounds the heart fire yang. A hot taste has a nature of burning heat, in wuxing it is the fire yang; so hot tasting herbs add yang heat to heart fire.

A sweet taste has a sticky nature, in wuxing it is the yin of soil, therefore sweet tasting herbs nurture spleen soil yin. Fragrant things have a nature of divergence, in wuxing it is the yang of soil, so fragrant tasting herbs support the loosening nature of the spleen soil yang.

An oily taste has a rich thickening nature, in wuxing it is the yin of metal, therefore oily tasting herbs lubricate the yin of lung metal. For example, if someone suffers a dry throat, a rich chicken soup can nurture the yin of lung metal and soothe the throat. A pungent taste, such as garlic, has a nature of penetrating and dividing, in wuxing it is the yang of metal. Pungent tasting herbs therefore support lung metal yang.

A salty taste has a nature of upward moving, in wuxing it is the yang of water, therefore, salty tasting herbs, such as Concha ostreae (muli 牡蛎), support kidney water yang. A bland taste or something that is tasteless has a nature of moving downward, and in wuxing it is the yin of water, and so bland herbs support kidney water yin.

It is commonly regarded that sea salt has a cold yinyang nature, it cools blood, detoxifies poison, and clears heat. In fact, the detoxifying poison effects are due to the ability to support liver wood yang, and clear damp poison in the blood, rather than cooling blood effects. For example, when a person perspires profusely it damages the yin and yang of kidney water. If only plain water is replenished, the yang of kidney water is deficient, which makes kidney water unable to rise, and water is not held in the body, so even though drinking plenty of water, it is difficult to quench the thirst. Furthermore, when there is kidney water yang deficiency, water does not rise to moisten the liver wood, and causes liver wood yin deficiency, which would cause tight muscles and sinews, even spasms. Also when a person is lacking salt, there is no strength as a result of lack of kidney water yang heat reserve. Therefore, sea salt, having a salty taste, has an upward moving yinyang nature, rather than a cold yinyang nature.

The yinyang nature of a herb can be multiple, and they are revealed through tastes, growing environment, and their appearances. So the taste and other yinyang natures maybe different, but they are all part of the yinyang nature of a herb.

Different herbs get into the body through the meridians that have the same yinyang nature. Therefore, from the nature of a herb one can have a basic idea of its pertaining meridians. Ginger is hot, has a nature of scattering; spleen soil yang has a nature of looseness, so ginger goes into the spleen soil meridian. Watermelon has a moistening nature, lung metal yin has a nature of gathering moisture, so watermelon goes into the lung meridian. Aconite has a dry and hot nature, it is attracted to what is moist and cool; kidney water has a nature of cold and moist, and kidney water attracts dry heat, so aconite goes into kidney meridian. Fish skin has a flexible nature, liver wood yin has a nature of suppleness, so fish skin goes into liver wood meridian. Oyster shell has an unsmooth and grounding nature; and heart fire yin has a grounding nature, so oyster shell goes into the heart fire meridian. On the other hand, a herb may have more than one yinyang nature, so it can travel through more than one meridian.

One formula to treat different illnesses and different formulas to treat one illness

Symptoms of illnesses come in all forms, but the root cause of illness is never the exception to yinyang wuxing disorders. A wuxing organ's yinyang disorder can show up in all kinds of symptoms depending on the condition of the person and the different levels of the yinyang disorders. A person with kidney water yin loss due to lack of water, may have symptoms of thirstiness, headache, irritability, or fatigue, even to the degree of losing conciousness. Although some people may suffer from slight discomfort, for others it may be more serious, but they can all be treated by giving water to drink. This is the so called one formula for treating different illnesses. Applying the same formula for treating different illnesses requires caution in recognizing the root of the yinyang disorder of the symptoms. The different symptoms in the above example have the same yinyang disorder root cause. If a person suffers from headache, it may be for a reason other than lack of water or loss of yin qi in the kidney, without knowing the root cause of the symptom, yet to give someone a drink of water according to previous experience to treat the headache, the illness won't improve.

At the same time, there are many foods and herbs that can relieve ones thirst. For instance, eating watermelon, lemon, or radish can all quench one's thirst. This is called different formulas for treating one illness. But first, the different food/herb has to have the same yinyang quality, moistening the yin in this case; secondly, the same symptom has to be the same cause of yinyang disorder. If someone suffers thirst but the root cause was not lack of water but kidney water heat loss inhibiting water to rise, then drinking water, eating watermelon, lemon or radish will not be sufficient to quench the thirst.

Thus, the principle in selecting herbs to treat illness is to determine first the nature of the yinyang disorder of the wuxing organs. Different symptoms with the same yinyang disorder can have the same formula; one wuxing organ's yinyang disorder is not limited to one treatment method or formula.

Kidney Water

The human body's development, fertility and water supply are maintained by the yin and yang of kidney water. Kidney water has a cold and downward moving nature, it stores body fluid, and is a yin organ. Kidney water yin retains water to moisten the body. As yin attracts yang, then the cold nature of kidney water attracts heat, and so kidney water reserves the body's heat, which is the yang of kidney water. Kidney water yang moves water to prevent water retention and keeps the body warm. Yang heat is the power of the body, when kidney water reserves have sufficient yang heat, a person is energetic. Water is the foundation of growth and reproduction, but only when water acquires yang heat.

As kidney water stores body strength, and the endurance to bear pressure, the spirit interacts with kidney water to exercise its enduring zhi—i.e. the desire to handle large tasks, whether physical or mental. When the spirit and kidney water are in harmonious cooperation, a person feels confident and imperturbable.

Overall, kidney water is the reservoir of water and the body's yang heat. It is responsible for growth, and fertility. It provides the body with strength and lubrication. Yinyang disorders of kidney water affect people in three main ways: growth and reproduction, water supply, and emotional discomfort.

Causes of kidney water yinyang disorder

Exhaustion, staying up late at night, and bad diet are the common factors that cause kidney water yang deficiency. Activities demand yang heat, overwork exhausts yang heat and causes kidney water yang deficiency. Staying up late forces the yang meridians to open to the yin qi of heaven and earth, and its yang qi to be drained by the yin qi of heaven and earth. Bad diet, such as eating refined sugar, damages kidney water yang qi. If one drinks a cup of dissolved refined sugar, he/she will shortly need to pass urine, and while the quantity of urine may not be great it will be hot, because refined sugar drains kidney water heat. Neglecting to drink water, especially after perspiring heavily, depletes kidney water yin qi and leads to the slowing of water flow, which in turn allows dampness and mucus to accumulate and obstruct the water passages.

Symptoms

Kidney water yang deficiency is heat loss, where water has difficulty in moving upwards, which will cause symptoms such as thirstiness, dry throat, and dry eyes. Insufficient heat in the kidney water also makes a person feel cold. Heat is the yang energy for body movement, growth, and reproduction, which all rely on kidney water heat storage. When kidney water yang heat is low, a person has no physical strength, this also causes growth, development, and reproductive disorders. When there is kidney water heat loss, there is insufficient yang heat to undertake the yang qi of the enduring zhi, and the spirit feels fear.

Kidney water yin deficiency causes an inhibition of water flow, which further causes dampness, mucus growth, and creates congestion and damp heat in the water passages; in such cases, a person will suffer symptoms such as meagre, frequent, urgent, or painful urination. Dampness and mucus damage the blood passages, and may also cause blood in the urine. When there is kidney water yin deficiency, the yin qi of the enduring zhi of the spirit is undermined and the spirit is impatient.

Overall, symptoms relating to growth/development, fertility and water supply disorders are kidney water yinyang disorders.

Tongue

The kidney is a water organ, it retains the body's yang heat. The yin of kidney water fills the tongue, the yang of kidney water holds the tongue. When the yinyang of kidney water is in normal order, the shape of the tongue is round and smooth, it stretches and contracts freely. When kidney water loses heat, the tongue is difficult to contract, appears big and floppy with teeth marks. When the kidney water yin is deficient, the tongue is thin and short.

Pulse

The yin of kidney water lubricates, the yang of kidney water strengthens, when the yinyang of kidney water is normal, the pulse is smooth and strong. Kidney water heat loss will lead to obstructions to water flow, causing water retention, so the pulse is slippery. In severe cases, the pulse is like water passing by without bounce. As each of the wuxing organs exists within as well as extend to the other wuxing organs, so the kidney water heat loss will extend to the other wuxing organs. At first, the heat loss is isolated to kidney water, so the left chi pulse is slippery. Then, when the kidney water heat loss affects the heart fire organ, the left cun pulse is slippery. When kidney water heat loss affects the liver wood organ, the left guan pulse is slippery. When the lung metal organ is affected, the right cun pulse is slippery. When it affects the spleen soil organ, the right guan pulse is slippery. When it affects the kidney reservoir, the life gate, the right chi pulse is slippery. On the other hand, when kidney water yin is insufficient, there is insufficient water, so the body becomes dry, and the pulse is sluggish. When affected by kidney water yin deficiency, the other wuxing organs will have the same sluggish pulse.

The right chi pulse is the mingmen. Mingmen is the interior of the kidney water, it is the reservoir of the body's yin and yang. When there is insufficient yang, water is retained, and the pulse appears slippery. When the yin is deficient, the reservoir is dry, and the pulse is sluggish.

Skin

The kidney water moistens and strengthens the skin. When the yinyang of kidney water is in regular order, the skin is soft and elastic. When the yang of kidney water is damaged, the skin sags and is without tone. When the yin of kidney water is damaged, the skin becomes rough.

Principles for treating kidney water yinyang disorder

The principal treatment for kidney water heat loss is to warm kidney water and ground heart fire into kidney water. Kidney water yin deficiency is often accompanied by dampness and mucus congesting the water passages. In such cases, the principal treatment is to remove dampness and create water. However, as kidney water is a yin organ, with prolonged kidney water yin damage, while nourishing its yin, it must be remembered to maintain its warmth. For kidney water yinyang disorders caused by spirit discomfort, when kidney water yinyang is regulated, the symptoms of spirit discomfort will recover without further treatment.

The remainder of this chapter relates to various clinical cases. The cases recount the patient symptoms, the interpretation of the symptoms from the yinyang wuxing perspective, the treatment strategies, the formulas used, the progression and treatment outcomes. They are cases from my own clinical practice and are related here as examples of how to approach the treatment of illness with yinyang wuxing as the theoretical guide.

Treating kidney water heat loss during menopause

Menopause is a time when women around the age of 50 go through a transition period towards which they stop menstruating. It is the same as when a young girl hasn't yet begun menstruating to the time when she begins menstruating. It is a normal progression in a woman's life and by no means an illness. However, these days many women when they go through menopause have a series of health problems, for example, hot flushes, night sweats, dry mouth, fatigue, sleep loss, and anxiety. As a result, menopause has become a modern day illness. In fact, hot flushes, night sweats, sleep loss, and anxiety are symptoms that anyone at any time can suffer, whether as a child, youth, male or elderly person. In clinical practice I have seen many 18 or 19 year-old young women who have lost their periods and have hot flushes, night sweats and such clinical symptoms. Regardless of what age or sex, people exhibiting these symptoms all indicate abnormal health.

When women experience hot flushes, night sweats, sleep loss, and mood swings during menopause it is because, according to Chinese traditional healing, the kidney water isn't sufficiently warm, and whether one is female, male, old or young, if the kidney water isn't warm they will all experience similar symptoms. According to the extent to which kidney water is not warm, clinical symptoms may be greater or fewer. If a person's kidney water is sufficiently warm, when they reach menopause they are unlikely to have any symptoms.

I once had a 60-year-old Chinese female patient consult with me; she said her periods had just finished and that her Western doctor advised her to take hormone replacements. Because she was worried about the side effects of taking hormones, she wanted to know what alternative Chinese medicine could offer. I asked her what feelings of discomfort she had and she replied that she had none whatsoever. She had entered a definite time of menopause, but she was full of energy, her complexion was glowing, and she had absolutely no sign of any so called "menopausal symptoms".

If a man or young woman has hot flushes, night sweats, and sleep loss, it is accepted that there is an illness, but for a 50 year old woman with these symptoms it's considered just a normal part of going through menopause. However, actually, these are symptoms that are more specific to kidney water heat loss rather than any special link to do with a certain age and gender.

Women during menopause most often have symptoms of kidney water heat insufficiency, but the kidney water heat loss doesn't begin with the onset of menopause, it is accumulated from years of exhaustion but appears more in the period of menopause. During menopause the body is going through a transformation from a time of prime centred on reproduction to a senior time centred on preservation. During this transformation, all the hidden corners of stagnation will be revealed and show symptoms. However, the occurrence of these symptoms shouldn't be a cause for worry. In fact, there are many Chinese herbs that one can use to alleviate these symptoms so that a person will be refreshed while entering into a new period of life.

Nevertheless, if one could take care of one's health at all times, menopause wouldn't be a trouble at all. To mention it again, the reason that many women during menopause show symptoms of kidney water insufficient heat is because they didn't pay enough attention to their bodily needs during menstruation and after giving birth. Although periodical bleeding and giving birth are normal aspects of women's lives, giving special care during menstruation and during the first month of the post-natal period are the normal requirements for women as well. Women begin to menstruate from around 12 to 14 and most women stop menstruating in their 50s. During menstruation a woman's energy reserve is drained with the blood loss, and if she doesn't rest enough the body heat reserve in the kidney water will gradually be exhausted. Also, in general, when we have a cold drink, our stomach and skin will immediately contract, which is to prevent cold water going into the blood and causing blood stagnating, at the same time, the kidney releases its reserved heat to warm the stomach, therefore, frequently having cold drinks would consume the kidney heat reserve. For women, drinking cold drinks around the time of their menses, if their kidney heat reserves are low, will tend to result in painful periods.

Pregnancy is energy demanding, if a woman doesn't rest adequately she will easily drain the kidney heat reserve, but more harm will occur if she doesn't rest after giving birth. While giving birth, the mother's pelvic joints loosen to deliver the baby, but it is not only the pelvic joint that loosens, the entire body's joints are loosened. After delivering the baby, the joints take at least one month to tighten up again. If during this time the woman moves too much, the recovery of the joints will be affected causing back pain, joint pains and altering the body shape. Moreover, when the joints were loosened, the body heat is not as well protected at this moment, and if she is in the wind and cold conditions the kidney heat reserve is easily lost and much effort is required to replenish it again.

Women in their 50s who have symptoms of hot flushes, night sweats, fatigue, fear, panic, loss of sleep, and thirst are most likely to have kidney water heat loss. Some women may have only one or two symptoms, others may have even more symptoms such as headaches and a burning red face etc., but so long as the cause is kidney water heat loss the treatment is more or less the same.

With kidney water heat loss, liver wood isn't moistened, so liver wood becomes hot and dry, and is unable to contain blood in its root organ. The hot blood will then rush along the blood passages causing body heat, and hot flushes. The spleen soil opens pores to release body heat, so there is the symptom of perspiration. The yang heat is further lost with the sweating, so a person is tired. When there is kidney water heat loss, the spirit is unable to exercise its yang qi of the enduring zhi, so the spirit is in fear. Kidney water heat loss and liver wood dryness causes heart fire yang qi to float, and then the spirit is unable to rest, so there is a symptom of sleeplessness. Kidney water heat loss means water flows up with difficulty, so there is a symptom of thirstiness. Again, with kidney water heat loss and liver wood dryness, blood rushes along blood passages, and a person suffers from a red face. The rushing hot blood creates wind, fast wind pushes on meridians causing headaches. Also with liver wood dryness, the heart fire is unable to be grounded and the yang qi of the aspiring zhi is unable to be exercised, so there are symptoms of panic.

The Erxian formula is what I use most to treat kidney water heat loss.

Erxian formula:

Epimedium brevicornum (yinyanghuo) 30g
Curculiginis orchioides (xianmao) 15g
Morindae officinalis (bajitian) 15g
Polygala tenufola (yuanzhi) 10g
Angelica sinensis (danggui) 20g
Anemarrhena asphodeloides (zhimu) 10g
Phellodendri chinensis (huangbai) 10g

Gentiana scabra (longdancao) 30g
Polygoni multiflori (yejiaoteng) 30g
Zizyphus jujube (fried) (chao suanzaoren) 15g
Concha margaritifera (zhenzhumu) 30g
Concha haliotidis (shijueming) 30g
Concha ostreae (muli) 30g
Ossa draconis (longgu) 30g

Erxian Formula in Chinese 二仙汤:

淫羊藿 30g 仙茅15g 巴戟天15g 远志10g 当归20g 知母10g 黄柏10g 龙胆草30g 夜交藤30g 炒酸枣仁15g 珍珠母 30g 石决明30g 牡蛎30g 龙骨30g。

Epimedium brevicornum (yinyanghuo 淫羊藿) has a sweet taste and warm yinyang nature, it goes into the kidney and liver meridians, it warms kidney water, moistens and clears liver wood, so it is an important herb of the formula.

Curculiginis orchioides (xianmao 仙茅) has a pungent taste and a warm yinyang nature, it goes into the kidney and liver meridians, it moves kidney water. It is a general kidney water warming herb.

Morindae officinalis (bajitian 巴戟天) has a pungent taste, and slight warming yinyang nature, it goes into the kidney, liver and lung meridians. The pungent taste supports the lung metal to calm the liver wood, and its warming nature goes to the kidney and pushes kidney water up.

Polygala tenufola (yuanzhi 远志) has a bitter taste, and warm yinyang nature. It goes into the heart and kidney meridians. It raises kidney water to control excessive heart fire and lowers heart fire warmth down to kidney water.

Angelica sinensis (danggui 当归) has a sweet taste and warm yinyang nature. It goes into the heart, liver and kidney meridians. It nourishes heart fire, softens liver wood, loosens spleen soil, harmonizes all wuxing organs and nurtures both the body and spirit. Angelica sinensis is one of the most favourable herbs for harmonizing all wuxing organs.

The above five herbs have a warming nature, however, hot flushes, night sweats, mood swings, thirstiness and loss of sleep are all symptoms of excessive heat. Kidney water warming herbs entering the body, however, will also make liver wood hot and dry. In my clinical practice, sometimes I had Chinese patients who knew a little about herbs and as soon as they saw the warming herbs in their formulas, they would warn me that they were weak but couldn't take tonics. In other words, what they were saying was that their kidney water is cold, but if they took the kidney warming herbs, they would get symptoms of excessive heat, for example, pimples or ulcers. These patients often took cooling herbs. Cooling herbs can relieve some heat symptoms such as dry mouth, and ulcers temporarily, but the more they took of cooling herbs, the cooler the kidney water becomes and the hotter their liver wood. If the cause of the symptoms is cold kidney water then the warming kidney herbs are the best for it. As for the excessive heat symptoms, it just needs to be accompanied with liver wood clearing and cooling herbs plus the heart fire grounding herbs.

Therefore, in the Erxian formula, apart from the above kidney warming herbs there is another group of herbs that have cold to cool, and moist yinyang natures which are: Anemarrhena asphodeloides (zhimu), Cortex Phellodendri chinensis (huangbai), Gentiana scabra (longdancao), Polygoni multiflori (yejiaoteng), and fried Zizyphus jujube (suanzaoren).

Anemarrhena asphodeloides (zhimu 知母) has a bitter taste and cold yinyang nature. It goes into the lung, kidney and liver meridians. It clears dampness in the lung metal; attracts kidney water up to lung metal then spreads water down and moistens the liver wood. So it is used to moisten liver wood.

Cortex Phellodendri chinensis (huangbai 黄柏) has a bitter taste and cold yinyang nature. It goes into the kidney, liver and urine bladder meridians, it clears trapped heat in all wuxing organs. It is used to clear liver wood heat.

Gentiana scabra (longdancao 龙胆草) has a very bitter taste and very cold yinyang nature; it goes into the heart, kidney, liver, and gall bladder meridians. It clears heat and dries dampness. It treats a damp heat kind of jaundice but not a cold damp kind of jaundice. It clears liver wood heat to support liver wood yin, and at the same time dries dampness to support liver wood yang. It also grounds heart fire into kidney water, so it is an excellent herb for floating heart fire, and kidney water heat loss.

Polygoni multiflori (yejiaoteng 夜交藤) has a slightly bitter taste and a mild yin yang nature; it goes into the heart and liver meridians. It is like fine rain gently moistening liver wood and calming the heart fire.

Zizyphus jujube (fried) (chao suanzaoren 炒酸枣仁) has a sour taste and mild yin yang nature. It goes into the heart and liver meridians. The sourness of Zizyphus jujube soothes the dryness of liver wood and eases the rising heart fire.

The last group of herbs Concha margaritifera (zhenzhumu), Concha haliotidis (shijueming), Concha ostreae (muli) and Ossa draconis (longgu) have a salty taste and heavy yinyang nature. Their heaviness grounds the heart fire heat into the kidney water, and their saltiness raises the kidney water to the heart fire.

Concha margaritifera (zhenzhumu 珍珠母) has a salty taste and mild yinyang nature; it goes into heart, liver, and kidney meridians. It raises kidney water, grounds heart fire heat and clears the liver wood yinyang passages.

Concha haliotidis (shijueming 石决明) has a salty taste and mild yinyang nature; it goes into liver, kidney and heart meridians. It raises kidney water, grounds heart fire heat, and clears liver wood passages.

Concha ostreae (muli 牡蛎) has a salty taste and mild yinyang nature; it goes into liver, kidney, heart meridians. It raises kidney water, grounds heart fire, and clears the liver wood passages.

Ossa draconis (longgu 龙骨) has an astringent taste and mild yinyang nature; it goes into heart, kidney, liver meridians. It raises kidney water, grounds heart fire, softens liver wood, and absorbs dampness.

Generally, if women over the age of 50 begin to have period irregularities with symptoms of hot flushes, night sweats and sleeping difficulties but without other symptoms, then the symptoms should improve within seven days of beginning the Erxian formula. Some may not need further treatment. Sometimes after stopping the herbs for a month or two, the symptoms might return but after taking a few weeks of herbs again, symptoms will disappear again. There are also some cases where patients repeatedly took the herbs every now and then for a year or two and eventually the symptoms did not reoccur. These cases indicate that the kidney water heat reserve of the patient was low and unable to get through the menopause transition period. The initial treatment gave a little help but a longer period of treatment was needed. The herbs in the Erxian formula do not harm the body in any way, so after the symptoms disappear, it is better to continue for a month or two then take five packets every month for six months. Passing through menopause will then be very much less debilitating. The Erxian formula is also useful to maintain the body's vitality while under stress, such as when children go through school exams, working late nights, and after a woman has given birth without feelings of illness.

Treating kidney water heat loss in young women with symptoms of hot flushes, insomnia and mood swings

Menstruation is an obvious sign of the regulation of women's fertility cycle. When there is kidney water heat loss, the fertility cycle is obstructed, so the menstruation becomes irregular. The symptoms of hot flushes, night sweats, and irregular periods can happen to women long before actual menopause. I have met numerous cases of women in their 20s and 30s with such symptoms.

I had a patient in her early 30s who came for a consultation because of night sweats, insomnia, and mood swings as well as her period having stopped for three months. After taking seven packets of the Erxian formula, she had a few drops of dark blood for three days, and the night sweats stopped. She slept better but her moods were still low. After taking another 30 days of herbs, she had a normal period with the normal blood quantity and colour. She then stopped taking the herbs for three months, the symptoms all came back and her period was late by ten days. She took another two days of the Erxian formula and her period arrived and the symptoms disappeared. She stopped taking herbs for six months and found that before and after her periods she always had sleeping difficulties and mood swings. So I asked her to take seven days of the herbs beginning three days before her period was due. She did this for a year and no more symptoms of period problems occurred. Ten years later, she came back for a consultation for pimples on her face, occasional night sweats and period delays. After taking another 30 days of the Erxian formula all symptoms cleared.

A 34-year-old woman consulted with me for palpitations and insomnia. She told me that two years after giving birth to her third child, she began to feel very depressed, had mood swings and insomnia every month a week before her period came. This is a classic case of having exhausted the kidney water heat after giving birth, then causing liver wood dryness, heart fire to over burn and disturbing the spirit. The Erxian formula was used to treat this case, and after taking the herbs for a month the patient felt all the symptoms were improved. Over a period of six months she continued to take the herbs for seven days just a week before each period. At the end of the six months, all the symptoms disappeared. Thereafter, for more than ten years, the patient would occasionally come to our clinic asking for three to seven days of the Erxian formula whenever she felt tired or was going through difficult times.

Another 38-year-old female patient came for a consultation suffering from hot flushes, night sweats, insomnia and irregular periods for about two years. Apart from these symptoms she also suffered symptoms such as body aches, swollen lymph glands in her neck, tiredness, and felt emotionally over-sensitive. She had three children who at that time were from the ages of five to eight who were all conceived through IVF. The Western medical advice was that she was having an early menopause due to the IVF procedures. She had taken some hormone therapies but they did not seem to help her.

In the wuxing cycle, kidney water creates liver wood. With kidney water heat loss the liver wood becomes stunted, so there is yin and yang deficiency in the liver wood. The yang of liver wood erects and keeps blood passages open. The yang deficiency of liver wood leads to the blood passages congestion, and allows dampness and mucus to grow in the blood passages, therefore the patient suffered swollen glands in her neck. Kidney water heat deficiency caused the patient to feel tired. Liver wood yin damage undermined the yin qi of the striving zhi of the spirit, which caused the striving zhi to lack flexibility, so the patient was over-sensitive.

After taking three days of the Erxian formula, her period, which was ten days late, finally came. She slept well and all the pains improved. She continued the herbs for three more weeks, and felt normal so she stopped the herbs. After another week, all the symptoms returned, and her period did not arrive on the due date. Another two weeks later, she began to take the herbs again for 30 days and the symptoms subsequently disappeared. But two days before the period was due, all the symptoms returned. Nevertheless, the period arrived on time and once the period began to flow the symptoms disappeared. She continued taking the herbs for another 30 days, and six months later she informed me that she was totally well.

Treating kidney water heat loss in women post-menopause

As I have discussed earlier, the symptoms exhibited among women during menopause are not the normal phenomena of women going through menopause, rather they are signs of kidney water heat loss which makes the menopause transition become difficult. So age is not the major factor of these symptom occurrences. For example, a 65-year-old woman hadn't had her periods for 20 years and had suffered from hot flushes, night sweats and insomnia for 30 years. After she took three days of the Erxian formula, she could sleep but woke up at around 3am because of night sweats, and could not get back to sleep. After taking another seven days of the Erxian formula, there were no signs of night sweats and she could sleep throughout the night until daybreak. But during the day, she would still have a few hot flushes. She took the herbs for another three months and found that most nights she slept well but one or two nights of the week getting into sleep was difficult, and occasionally she had hot flushes and night sweats. She continued the herbs for another three months, and during this time she slept well, had good energy and spirits. Occasionally there were slight hot flushes but these did not affect her daily life, so she stopped the treatment. Four years later, she came back as she felt tired, anxious and forgetful. Lack of energy is a sign of kidney water heat loss, and the body could not be held erect. Because of her kidney reserve was low, she felt panicky. Forgetfulness is not a problem of memory, but rather insufficient energy to pay attention to everything. The treatment for her new symptoms was the same as for her hot flushes and sleeping problems. After taking three days of the herbs, she had good energy again; her moods were calmer and her forgetfulness was no longer a problem.

Treating heavy bleeding menses

The kidney is a water organ, and water creates wood. Liver is a wood organ and a blood reservoir. When kidney water is cold, liver wood can be too dry and hot so that the blood reserve rushes out causing period overflow. On the other hand, when kidney water is cold, reproduction fails to function, so the period stops. Therefore, both no blood and too much blood can all be treated with the warming kidney water formula with the addition of moving blood or stopping bleeding herbs accordingly.

A 49-year-old woman came for a consultation complaining that for almost a year she had had heavy bleeding during her period, sometimes she bled so much that she fainted. She was at the usual age for menopause but her period had no sign of stopping. Instead, every 21 days she would suffer heavy bleeding which lasted for up to ten days and she was exhausted. This was a case of kidney water heat loss, and liver wood dryness, which could not reserve blood. I prescribed the Erxian Xueyu formula which is the Erxian formula plus human hair charcoal and Cyrtomium fortunei charcoal (guanzhong tan). The Erxian formula warms kidney water, soothes the dry liver wood and grounds heart fire; the additional two herbs would nurture blood and stop excessive bleeding.

The patient began taking the herbs when her period was on the seventh day, after one dose of the herbs, her blood flow immediately reduced but still dragged to the tenth day. She continued taking the herbs and by her next period, on the 30th day from the time that her previous period began, the quantity of her blood flow was much reduced. After another three months of taking the herbs, her period was delayed for ten days, and that was her last period and she finished her menopause transition.

Erxian Xueyu formula:

Epimedium brevicornum (yinyanghuo) 30g

Curculiginis orchioides (xianmao) 15g

Morindae officinalis (bajitian) 15g

Polygala tenufola (yuanzhi) 10g

Angelica sinensis (danggui) 20g

Anemarrhena asphodeloides (zhimu) 10g

Phellodendri chinensis (huangbai) 10g

Gentiana scabra (longdancao) 30g

Polygoni multiflori (yejiaoteng) 30g

Zizyphus jujube (fried) (chao suanzaoren) 15g

Concha margaritifera (zhenzhumu) 30g

Concha haliotidis (shijueming) 30g

Concha ostreae (muli) 30g

Ossa draconis (longgu) 30g

Human hair charcoal (xueyutan) 10g

Cyrtomium fortunei charcoal (guanzhong tan) 10g

Erxian Xueyu formula in Chinese 二仙血余汤:

淫羊藿30g 仙茅15g 巴戟天15g 远志10g 当归20g 知母10g 黄柏10g 龙胆草30g 夜交藤30g 炒酸枣仁15g 珍珠母30g 石决明30g 牡蛎30g 龙骨30g 血余炭10g 贯众炭10g.

Human hair charcoal (xueyutan 血余炭) has a bitter taste, and mild yinyang nature, it goes into the liver and stomach meridians. It nurtures blood and stops excessive bleeding.

Cyrtomium fortunei charcoal (guanzhong tan 贯众炭) has a bitter taste and mild yinyang nature. It goes into the liver and stomach meridians. It stops excessive bleeding especially for a woman's flooding period.

Generally, if women in their 50s had increased blood flow during the menses instead of a reduction, after taking three months of the Erxian Xueyu formula, the period would become less and less or totally disappear. If women are in their 30s and 40s, having excessive bleeding during their menses indicates their kidney water heat loss is more serious than those women during menopause, so it is most likely that they will need longer treatment. However, in most cases, patients will stop treatment as soon as their symptoms improve. Then often the symptoms would return two to three months after stopping the herbs, then they would retake the herbs. In many cases the patients would take the herbs on and off until their periods completely stopped. The better way to treat the symptoms is to take the herbs continuously for a year, even when without symptoms. Subsequently the patient could then take seven days of the herbs each time their periods commenced. This way they can avoid the intermittent symptoms, and it also makes the kidney stronger for the next stage of their lives.

Treating kidney water heat loss with symptoms of constant menstrual dripping

In my 30 years of herbal medicine practice, I have seldom met young women who suffered from heavy menstrual bleeding, but I have met many who suffered from constant leaking of blood. For example, I had a 22-year-old patient whose periods began when she was 14 years of age. When she turned 18, she began to drip old blood between menses. She also complained of restless sleep, had many dreams, was very tired during the day and felt unhappy all the time. Her symptoms indicated that not only was her kidney water heat insufficient but that she had pockets of dampness. Often this kind of condition is due to consuming unhealthy food such as refined white sugar. The patient then must avoid eating all food and drinks containing refined white sugar. For herbs, I used the Erxian Putan formula.

The patient reduced her sugar intake and after taking the herbs for a month, the patient's next period cleared on the 10th day. After taking another month of herbs, the period cleared on the 6th day. She then stopped the herbs for a month and the dripping blood returned. She recommenced the herbs for six months, and there were two months which were clean then two other months of dripping, then two months which were clean. The patient took another four months of the herbs and the dripping stopped. After stopping the herbs for a year, there were no further signs of dripping blood, she also gained more energy, slept well, and was happier.

Erxian Putan formula:

Epimedium brevicornum (yinyanghuo) 30g
Curculiginis orchioides (xianmao) 15g
Morindae officinalis (bajitian) 15g
Polygala tenufola (yuanzhi) 10g
Angelica sinensis (danggui) 20g
Anemarrhena asphodeloides (zhimu) 10g
Phellodendri chinensis (huangbai) 10g
Gentiana scabra (longdancao) 30g
Polygoni multiflori (yejiaoteng) 30g
Zizyphus jujube (fried) (chao suanzaoren) 15g
Concha margaritifera (zhenzhumu) 30g
Concha haliotidis (shijueming) 30g
Concha ostreae (muli) 30g
Ossa draconis (longgu) 30g
Taraxacum officinale (pugongying) 30g
Eupatorium japonicum (zelan) 10g
Paeonia lactiflora (chishao) 15g
Sanguisorba officinalis (diyu) 10g
Typha angustifolia L. (charred) (puhuangtan) 10g
Cyrtomium fortunei (charcoal) (guanzhong tan) 10g

Erxian Putan formula in Chinese 二仙蒲炭汤:

淫羊藿30g 仙茅15g 巴戟天15g 远志10g 当归20g 知母10g 黄柏10g
龙胆草30g 夜交藤30g 炒枣仁15g 珍珠母30g 石决明30g 牡蛎30g 龙
骨30g 蒲公英30g 泽兰10g 赤芍15g 地榆10g 蒲黄炭10g 贯众炭10g.

The Erxian Putan formula is the Erxian formula with the addition of Taraxacum officinale (pugongying), Eupatorium japonicum (zelan), Paeonia lactiflora (chishao), Sanguisorba officinalis (diyu); charred typha angustifolia L. (puhuang tan), and charcoal of Cyrtomium fortunei (guanzhong tan). These herbs can be used with the Erxian formula to clear dampness, detoxify poison, and stop bleeding.

Taraxacum officinale (pugongying 蒲公英) has a sweet and slightly bitter taste, and a cold yinyang nature. It goes into the kidney meridian. It clears heat and detoxifies poison, removes dampness and heals ulcers and carbuncles.

Eupatorium japonicum (zelan 泽兰) has a bitter taste and slightly warm yinyang nature. It goes into the liver and spleen meridians. It dissolves stagnant blood, clears dampness and detoxifies poison, promotes regeneration of muscles.

Paeonia lactiflora (chishao 赤芍) has a bitter taste and cold yinyang nature. It goes into liver meridian. It removes masses, disperses blood stagnation and breaks down intestinal swellings.

Sanguisorba officinalis (diyu 地榆) has a bitter taste, and cool yinyang nature. It goes into liver and kidney meridians. It cools the blood, and removes dampness and poison.

Charred typha angustifolia (puhuang tan 蒲黄炭) has a bitter taste and mild yinyang nature. It goes into spleen meridian. It stops bleeding; removes blood stagnation, and drains dampness.

Cyrtomium fortunei (guanzhong tan 贯众炭) stops bleeding.

Treating kidney water heat loss in young women suffering from period loss

Women in their reproductive years who lose their period cycle is a sign of kidney water heat loss, and the fertility cycle is arrested. One of my patients was a 22-year-old woman whose period was a month late. She also had many pimples on her face and back, had palpitations, insomnia and night sweats.

Kidney water heat loss, slows the menstrual cycle, so there is period delay. Liver wood yang damage and damp poison in the blood passages cause pimples. Liver wood yin deficiency fails to store blood in its root. Hot blood stagnates in the blood passages, so there are night sweats. Liver wood yin deficiency causes the heart fire to float, so there are symptoms of palpitations and insomnia. The treatment is to warm kidney water, clear liver wood heat, ground heart fire and add herbs to invigorate blood and remove damp poison with the Erxian Mabian formula.

After taking the first packet of the herbs, the patient's period arrived the same night and she slept well through the night. After taking the herbs for seven days, all the symptoms disappeared. However, thereafter, for six months she would have palpitations, pimples and sometimes hot flushes just before her periods arrived. Therefore I asked her to take more of the same herbs for seven days before her period was due to come. After taking the herbs this way for a year, the symptoms gradually disappeared all together and she no longer needed to take the herbs.

Erxian Mabian formula:

Epimedium brevicornum (yinyanghuo) 30g
Curculiginis orchioides (xianmao) 15g
Morindae officinalis (bajitian) 15g
Polygala tenufola (yuanzhi) 10g
Angelica sinensis (danggui) 20g
Anemarrhena asphodeloides (zhimu) 10g
Phellodendri chinensis (huangbai) 10g
Gentiana scabra (longdancao) 30g

Polygoni multiflori (yejiaoteng) 30g
Zizyphus jujube (fried) (chao suanzaoren) 15g
Concha margaritifera (zhenzhumu) 30g
Concha haliotidis (shijueming) 30g
Concha ostreae (muli) 30g
Ossa draconis (longgu) 30g
Verbena officinalis (mabiancao) 10g
Leonurus japonicas (yimucao) 10g

Erxian Mabian Formula in Chinese 二仙马鞭汤:

淫羊藿30g 仙茅15g 巴戟天15g 远志10g 当归20g 知母10g 黄柏10g 龙胆草30g 夜交藤30g 炒枣仁15g 珍珠母30g 石决明30g 牡蛎30g 龙骨30g 马鞭草10g 益母草10g.

The Erxian Mabian formula is the Erxian formula with the addition of Verbena officinalis (mabiancao) and Leonurus japonicas (yimucao) to promote the flow of the menses and invigorate blood.

Verbena officinalis (mabiancao 马鞭草) has a bitter taste and slightly cold yinyang nature. It goes into the liver and spleen meridians. It promotes blood flow, invigorates blood, improves blood flow in women's menses, and promotes urination.

Leonurus japonicas (yimucao 益母草) has a pungent, slightly bitter taste and cool yinyang nature. It goes into the liver and kidney meridians. It invigorates blood, clears blood blockages, and detoxifies poison.

Another case was a 20-year-old woman whose period was late by two weeks. She also suffered with severe lower abdominal pain. After taking the above formula for three days, her period came and the abdominal pains were reduced. After taking another two months of the herbs, her period regained its usual regularity and there were no more abdominal pains.

Treating kidney water heat loss with symptoms of infertility

The kidney is a water organ, water can maintain heat. Only when kidney water is warm can there be life. Generally, infertility is a sign of kidney water having insufficient heat. I had a 27-year-old female patient who came to me after six years of trying to have a child, but without success. Six times she had undergone IVF, but also without success. My treatment for her was to warm kidney water with the Erxian formula. After taking three months of the Erxian formula, she became pregnant and later had her first son. A year later she tried to have a second child, for six months with no success and she then came back for more herbs. After taking six months of herbs she was pregnant again and later had her second son. Two years later she had her daughter without the help of herbs.

Although this patient did not have any other signs of kidney problem, her infertility itself was an important sign of kidney water heat loss, so the treatment was directed at warming the kidney water. But if only warm herbs were used, the heat may cause liver wood dryness. Moreover, the liver is a reservoir for blood storage, the cooling and moistening liver wood herbs in the Erxian formula can smooth the blood flow which is beneficial for fertility. The heart fire grounding herbs in the Erxian formula on the one hand leads the yang heat of the heart fire into the kidney water which warms the kidney water; and on the other hand they prevent the hot herbs stimulating the heart fire to float. Therefore, the treatment for infertility uses the same formula as treating symptoms of menopause.

Another case was a 49-year-old woman who wanted to have a child. The quantity of blood during her periods wasn't very much, and emotionally she was quite tense. At the age of 49, it was already the time for menopause, but since she was still having her periods, warming her kidney water, clearing liver wood, and grounding heart fire would provide a better chance for getting pregnant. I prescribed the Erxian formula and after taking a year of the Erxian formula, she lost her period. Considering her age, she thought menopause had arrived and gave up the treatment. But after 5 months she realized that she was pregnant and later gave birth to a boy.

In my 30 years of clinical practice, I have not encountered many infertility cases that needed several months or up to a year of treatment, most cases after taking a month of the Erxian formula would fall pregnant. I had a 40-year-old woman who already had a 12-year-old son and wanted to have a second child. After a year of unsuccessful trying, she came for help. After taking three weeks of the Erxian formula, she came and complained that she had missed her period and wondered if the herbs had brought on her early menopause. I took her pulse; it was obviously a pregnant pulse. But she argued that her husband was away, how could she get pregnant? Two months later she came back and said she was pregnant. When asked how she had fallen pregnant without her husband she laughed and said that before her husband went away for work, they had tried that night which was the day that her period had just cleared. She thought that was a safe period, and didn't imagine that the herbs could work so quickly so her first thought was that she had early menopause. In the end she had a baby daughter.

Treating kidney water heat loss with symptoms of miscarriage

Miscarriage is a sign of insufficient kidney water heat which causes water flow congestion that creates dampness that suffocates the foetus. I had a 40 year old woman who came for help to get pregnant. The woman's first child was delivered at 7 months pregnancy. Later she had miscarriage at five months, and then there was a miscarriage at 40 days of pregnancy. At the first consultation, she had tried over a year but could not conceive again. Her period was sometimes a few days late or early, which indicated very early miscarriage. After each miscarriage, the kidney water heat would be drained with the foetus delivered. Often people become more anxious about pregnancy and would try more frequently. But this would not only lead to more frequent miscarriages but also further damage to the kidney water heat. So I asked the patient to take three months of herbs before trying to fall pregnant again. The treatment was focused on warming kidney water, freeing the water passage, strengthening spleen soil to let water pass through and stop growing dampness. The Ejiao Duzhong formula was used to treat this case.

After taking three months of the herbs, the patient fell pregnant. She continued to take the herbs during the entire pregnancy and had a normal childbirth.

Ejiao Duzhong formula:

Radix dipsaci (xuduan) 25g
Eucommia ulmoides (duzhong) 15g
Angelica sinensis (danggui) 24g
Colla corii asini (ejiao) 10g
Rehmannia glutinosa (shudi) 10g
Paeoniae Alba (baishao) 24g
Stigma Maydis (yumixu) 10g
Atractylodis macrocephalae (chao baizhu) 24g
Poria Cocos (fuling) 24g
Fructus amomi (sharen) 10g
Pericarpium citri reticulatae (chenpi) 10g
Scutellaria baicalensis (huangqin) 10g

Ejiao Duzhong formula in Chinese 阿胶杜仲汤:

续断25g 杜仲15g 当归24g 阿胶10g 熟地10g 白芍24g 玉米须10g 炒白术24g 茯苓24g 砂仁10g 陈皮10g 黄芩10g.

Radix dipsaci (xuduan 续断) has a slight bitter taste and slight warm yinyang nature, it goes into the liver and kidney meridians. It clears blood passages, invigorates blood, nurtures blood, and removes damp poison in the blood. It treats excessive discharge, irregular period cycle, backache during pregnancy or after giving birth.

Eucommia ulmoides (duzhong 杜仲) has a sweet taste, and a warm yinyang nature. It goes into the liver and kidney meridians. It warms kidney water, clears dampness, strengthens sinews and bones. It also warms the uterus, and calms the foetus.

Angelica sinensis (danggui 当归) nurtures blood, soothes liver wood, strengthens spleen soil, and harmonizes wuxing organs. It improves both yin and yang qi of all the wuxing organs and calms the foetus.

Colla corii asini, Donkey-hide gelatin (ejiao 阿胶) has a sweet taste and mild yinyang nature. It goes into the heart, liver, and kidney meridians. It nurtures blood, and strengthens the yin of all wuxing organs, and clears dampness. It is used to treat all kinds of poisons and wind in the blood.

Rehmannia glutinosa (shudi 熟地) has a sweet taste and cool yinyang nature. It goes into the liver and kidney meridians. It nurtures blood, frees blood passages, breaks down the dampness and poison in the blood.

Paeoniae alba (baishao 白芍) has a sour taste and mild yinyang nature. It goes into the liver, spleen meridians. It frees blood passages, and dissolves swellings.

Stigma maydis (yumixu 玉米须) has a sweet taste and slightly warm yinyang nature. It goes into the kidney meridian. It opens water passages and removes dampness.

Atractylodis macrocephalae (fried) (chao baizhu 炒白术) has a sweet taste and warm yinyang nature. It goes into the lung, spleen, and stomach meridians. It eliminates wind in the head, consolidates the body surface, and removes dampness and mucus.

Poria Cocos (fuling 茯苓) has a sweet taste and mild yinyang nature. It goes into lung, spleen and stomach meridians. It strengthens spleen soil yang, filters water from dampness; improves digestion, and calms the spirit.

Fructus amomi (sharen 砂仁) has a pungent taste and warm yinyang nature. It goes into the spleen meridian. It strengthens spleen soil yang, promotes qi flow, improves digestion, and calms the foetus.

Pericarpium citri reticulatae (chenpi 陈皮) has a pungent taste, and a warm yinyang nature. It goes into the spleen meridian. It frees qi flow, dissipates dampness, strengthens spleen soil yang, and improves digestion.

Scutellaria baicalensis (huangqin 黄芩) has a bitter taste and cool yinyang nature. It goes into the lung, spleen, large intestine, and gall bladder meridians. It disperses wind, clears heat, removes dampness, detoxifies poison, and eliminates swelling.

Within the formula, Radix dipsaci (xuduan), Eucommia ulmoides (duzhong), Angelica sinensis (danggui) these three herbs are used to warm kidney water, remove dampness, and free blood passages. Colla corii asini (ejiao), Rehmannia glutinosa (shudi), and Paeoniae alba (baishao) are used to nurture blood, and remove dampness and poison in the blood. Stigma maybis (yumixu) is used to remove dampness and open water passages. Atractylodis macrocephalae (chao baizhu), Poria cocos (fuling), Fructus amomi (sharen), Pericarpium citri reticulatae (chenpi) are used to strengthen spleen soil yang, promote qi flow, which follows the wuxing control cycle that builds soil to control water flow. Scutellaria baicalensis (huangqin) is used to clear heat, remove dampness and calm the foetus.

Another case was a 32-year-old woman who had a number of miscarriages over a period of four years. Each pregnancy lasted two months before there was a miscarriage. At the first consultation, she was 36 days pregnant, she was suffering from dizziness, lower back pain, her tongue had a thick white coating and her pulse was very slippery. Back pain, dizziness and slippery pulse during pregnancy indicates kidney water heat loss and that the water passages were congested. There was also accumulated dampness, the thick coating on the tongue also confirmed the wet damp condition inside her body. The treatment was to warm kidney water, strengthen spleen soil to manage water passage, and calm the foetus. I used the above Ejiao

Duzhong formula. After taking 7 days of the herbs, all the symptoms quickly disappeared. She stopped the herbs but a few weeks later, the symptoms came back then she took another seven packets of the same herbs and the symptoms disappeared. In the next five months, she had twice suffered slight dizziness, and after taking the same herbs for 2 days, the dizziness disappeared. Thereafter she was well and had a normal childbirth.

Treating kidney water heat loss with symptoms of impotence

The kidney is a water organ, when water is warm it creates and maintains good health. Therefore, the reproduction capabilities of men and women are affected by the kidney water heat reserve, and the treatment is similar. I had a 30-year-old male patient who complained of extreme tiredness, and many mouth ulcers. He felt his chest was hot, he could not have an erection, and for a year he and his wife tried to start a family without success. He said he drank a lot of Chrysanthemum (juhua 菊花) and Prunella (xiakucao 夏枯草) tea. After taking the tea he felt cool but quickly felt dry and hot in the chest again. Chrysanthemum (juhua) and Prunella (xiakucao) are liver wood cooling herbs, so he felt comfortable after taking them. However, his original problem was kidney water heat loss, and long term use of cooling herbs alone can only mitigate his surface symptoms but not solve the root problem. On the contrary, the cooling herbs had further cooled the kidney water and caused the liver wood to be drier, so the symptoms persisted and affected his reproduction. The Erxian formula was used to warm his kidney water, clear liver wood and ground heart fire. After taking two months of the herbs, he no longer felt heat in the chest, and the ulcers disappeared, his erections also improved and his wife gave birth to a son a year later.

Treating kidney water yin damage with symptoms of impotence

A 29-year-old man came for a consultation as his biomedical test showed his live sperm count was very low. The patient could not have a strong erection, nor could it last very long. His urine was always a deep yellow colour, it smelt strong and he frequently went to urinate. Kidney water yin damage causes water passages to dry and the flow to be congested, which encourages damp and heat to flourish, so there are symptoms of dark yellow smelly and frequent urination. Kidney water yin damage, dampness blocking its yinyang passages also causes the symptoms of weak and short lasting erection. Treatment for this case was to clear damp heat, and free the water passages. I used the Erze formula for this purpose.

The patient and his wife had also attempted IVF several times to conceive but without success. Although the wife did not have any symptoms, having taken hormone treatment to produce more eggs would have drained the kidney yin and yang. So at the same time as treating her husband, I prescribed the Erxian Ejiao formula for the wife to take. The Erxian Ejiao formula is the Erxian formula with the addition of 10g of ejiao. While the Erxian formula warms the kidney water, ejiao would nurture the blood and kidney water yin.

The male patient took ten packets of the Erze formula, and his erection improved. He took the same herbs for a month, his wife fell pregnant and they had a healthy baby daughter thereafter.

Erze formula:

Talcum (huashi) 20g
Euphorbia helioscopia (Zeqi) 10g
Alisma orientalis (Zexie) 10g
Typha angustifolia (puhuang) 10g
Lygodium japonicum (haijinsha) 10g
Plantago asiatica (cheqiancao) 10g
Dioscorea septemloba (bixie) 10g
Dianthus superbus (jumai) 10g
Taraxacum mongolicum (pugongying) 10g
Viola yedoensis makino (zihuadiding) 10g
Phellodendri chinensis (huangbai) 10g
Smilax glabra (tufuling) 10g
Radix rehmanniae (cooked) (shudi) 10g
Radix rehmanniae (raw) (shengdi) 10g
Colla corii asini (ejiao) 10g
Leonurus japonicas (yimucao) 10g
Paeoniae lactiflora (chishao) 10g
Angelica sinensis (danggui) 10g
Glycyrrhiza uralensis radix (gancao) 10g.

Erze formula in Chinese 二泽汤:

滑石20g 泽漆10g 泽泻10g 蒲黄10g 海金沙10g 车前草10g 萆薢10g 瞿麦10g 蒲公英10g 紫花地丁10g 黄柏10g 土茯苓10g 熟地10g 生地10g 阿胶10g 益母草10g 赤芍10g 当归10g 甘草10g.

Talcum (huashi 滑石) has a sweet taste and cold yinyang nature. It goes into stomach and urine bladder meridians. It separates fresh water from turbidity; clears heat; dissolves mucus.

Euphorbia helioscopia (Zeqi 泽漆) has a bitter taste and slightly cold yinyang nature. It goes into the spleen and kidney meridians. It nurtures yin, promotes water flow, dissolves mucus, brings down a fever, and detoxifies poison.

Alisma orientalis (Zexie 泽泻) has a sweet taste and cold yinyang nature. It goes into the kidney and urine bladder meridians. It removes stale water and nurtures fresh water, frees urine flow, reduces water retention, drains dampness, and quenches thirst.

Typha angustifolia (puhuang 蒲黄) has a sweet taste and mild yinyang nature. It goes into the spleen meridian. It clears cold or heat abnormal qi in the chest, stomach, or urine bladder. It frees urine flow, and removes stagnant blood.

Lygodium japonicum (haijinsha 海金沙) has a sweet taste and mild yinyang nature. It goes into the spleen and kidney meridians. It drains damp heat, reduces swelling; it is a spleen and stomach yang tonic herb.

Plantago asiatica(cheqiancao 车前草) has a sweet taste and cold yinyang nature. It goes into the kidney and urine bladder meridians. It clears heat, frees urine flow, cools blood, detoxifies poison.

Dioscorea septemloba (bixie 萆薢) has a bitter taste and mild yinyang nature. It goes into the urine bladder and lung meridians. It clears heat, drains dampness, open meridians, and frees urine flow.

Dianthus superbus (jumai 瞿麦) has a bitter taste and cold yinyang nature. It goes into the kidney, small intestine, and urine bladder meridians. It clears heat, promotes water flow, and opens blood passages.

Taraxacum mongolicum (pugongying 蒲公英) clears heat, detoxifies poison, removes dampness, and heals ulcerative carbuncles.

Viola yedoensis makino (zihuadiding 紫花地丁) has a bitter taste and cold yinyang nature. It clears heat, detoxifies poison, reduces swelling, and strengthens liver wood yang.

Phellodendri chinensis (huangbai 黄柏) clears heat and dries dampness.

Smilax glabra (tufuling 土茯苓) has a mild taste and yinyang nature. It goes into the liver and spleen meridians. It strengthens the spleen soil yang; opens meridians, disperses dampness, removes pus, strengthens liver wood yang, detoxifies poison, and heals severe sores.

Rehmannia glutinosa (cooked) (shudi 熟地) and Radix rehmannia glutinosa (raw) (shengdi 生地) both have a sweet taste and cool yinyang nature. Both go into the liver and kidney meridians. They open blood passages; strengthen liver wood yang, break down damp poison in the blood. Raw rehmannia is cooler than cooked rehmannia and better in cooling blood. Cooked rehmannia is better in nurturing blood and opening blood passages.

Colla corii asini (ejiao 阿胶) eliminates wind, and detoxifies blood poison.

Leonurus japonicas (yimucao 益母草) invigorates blood, breaks down stagnant blood, and detoxifies poison.

Paeoniae lactiflora (chishao 赤芍) cools blood, removes masses and swelling, it breaks down blood stagnation.

Angelica sinensis (danggui 当归) harmonizes and strengthens both the yin and yang of all wuxing organs.

Glycyrrhiza uralensis radix (gancao 甘草) has a sweet taste and mild yinyang nature. It goes into the lung, stomach, spleen meridians. It detoxifies cold and hot poisonous qi in all the wuxing organs.

In the Erze formula, Talcum (huashi) is used to isolate poisons and remove dampness. Euphorbia helioscopia (Zeqi), Alisma orientalis (Zexie), Typha angustifolia (puhuang), Lygodium japonicum (haijinsha), Plantago asiatica (cheqiancao), Dioscorea septemloba (bixie), Dianthus superbus (jumai) are used to clear heat and remove dampness, detoxify poison, and free urine flow. Taraxacum mongolicum (pugongying), Viola yedoensis makino (zihuadiding), Phellodendri chinensis (huangbai), Smilax glabra (tufuling) are used to add more weight on clearing heat and detoxifying poison. Radix rehmanniae (cooked) (shudi), Radix rehmanniae (raw) (shengdi), Colla corii asini (ejiao), Leonurus japonicas (yimucao), Paeoniae lactiflora (chishao) are used to detoxify blood poison. Angelica sinensis

59

(danggui) nurtures both the yin and yang of kidney water, and together with Glycyrrhiza (gancao) harmonizes the wuxing organs.

Treating kidney water yin and yang damage with symptoms of painful swollen testicle

I had a 29-year-old male patient, whose left testicle had been surgically removed as his western physician suspected that it was cancerous. Two years later, his right testicle was swollen and painful, and since he did not want to lose the testicle he wanted to try an alternative treatment. The patient also felt hot, was easily angry, thirsty, and perspired a lot. Asked about his sex life, he said that he had sex two to three times a day without problems.

The sperm of men are the essence of kidney water yin and yang. Excessive sex exhausts kidney water yin and yang. When the kidney water yang is weak, water doesn't rise, so he is thirsty. When kidney water is weak it causes liver wood to be undernourished. Liver wood yin deficiency fails to store blood in its root, and hot blood rushes in the blood passage, so the patient is hot and sweaty. Liver wood yang deficiency causes blood stagnation and decay, which occurred in his testicle because the ejaculations have been drawing blood to rush there, so his testicle was swollen and painful. With liver wood yin being undernourished this deprives the yin qi of the striving zhi of the spirit to be exercised, so he was restless and easily angry. The treatment was to warm the kidney water, clear liver wood heat and ground heart fire, plus detoxify poison, cool blood, and support kidney yin with the Erxian Gongying formula.

A precondition for the treatment, however, was that the patient had to refrain from sex during the treatment. When this 1.9 metre tall young man heard that he had to refrain from sex he suddenly stood up towering over me. He put his hands on his hips and said: "You're joking! My normal doctor said that this has nothing to do with sex. Plus if you don't have sex for too long you'll forget how." I told him that I didn't think anyone could forget how to have sex, but if he didn't stop having sex so often he might lose his only testicle, and then he really would forget about sex. Fortunately, he listened to my advice and didn't have sex for a week and drank his seven packets of herbs. The symptoms then all disappeared. The young man was surprised that he did not miss the sex and he even felt more comfortable without it for a while.

Erxian Gongying formula:

Epimedium brevicornum (yinyanghuo) 30g
Curculiginis orchioides (xianmao) 15g
Morindae officinalis (bajitian) 15g
Polygala tenufola (yuanzhi) 10g
Angelica sinensis (danggui) 20g
Anemarrhena asphodeloides (zhimu) 10g
Phellodendri chinensis (huangbai) 10g
Gentiana scabra (longdancao) 30g
Polygoni multiflori (yejiaoteng) 30g

Zizyphus jujube (fried) (chao suanzaoren) 15g
Concha margaritifera (zhenzhumu) 30g
Concha haliotidis (shijueming) 30g
Concha ostreae (muli) 30g
Ossa draconis (longgu) 30g
Paeonia lactiflora (chishao) 15g
Taraxacum officinale (pugongying) 30g
Viola yedoensis (zihuadiding) 30g
Rheum officinale (dahuang) 10g
Coptis chinensis (huanglian) 10g

Erxian Gongying formula in Chinese 二仙公英汤:

淫羊藿30g 仙茅15g 巴戟天15g 远志10g 当归20g 知母10g 黄柏10g 龙胆草30g 夜交藤30g 炒枣仁15g 珍珠母30g 石决明30g 牡蛎30g 龙骨30g 赤芍15g 蒲公英30g 紫花地丁30g 大黄10g 黄连10.

The Erxian Gongying formula is Erxian formula with the addition of Paeonia lactiflora (chishao), Taraxacum officinale (pugongying), Viola yedoensis (zihuadiding), Rheum officinale (dahuang), and Coptis chinensis (huanglian).

Paeonia lactiflora (chisao 赤芍) cools the blood, and disperses blood stagnation.
Taraxacum officinale (pugongying 蒲公英) cools heat and disperses stagnation.
Viola yedoensis (zihuadiding 紫花地丁) cools heat, strengthens liver wood yang, detoxifies poison and reduces swelling.

Rheum officinale (dahuang 大黄) has a bitter taste, and cold yinyang nature. It goes into the spleen, stomach and large intestine meridians. It cools blood, detoxifies poison, clears heat, breaks down stagnation, removes dampness, and opens bowel motion.

Coptis chinensis (huanglian 黄连) has a bitter taste and cold yinyang nature. It goes into liver, spleen, and large intestine meridians. It extinguishes fire; detoxifies poison, dries dampness, and cools blood.

While the Erxian formula warms kidney water, clears liver wood, and grounds heart fire, Paeonia lactiflora (chishao), Taraxacum officinale (pugongying), Viola yedoensis (zihuadiding) and Rheum officinale (dahuang) and Coptis chinensis (huanglian) cool blood, clear heat, and support kidney water yin.

Treating kidney water heat loss with growth problems

An 18-year-old woman came for a consultation. She looked only 13 years old. She was very thin and her height was about 1.3 metres. I asked whether her mother was coming, and she said: "My mother is at work." Her voice sounded more mature than she looked and after looking at her information form, I realized that she was 18 years old. She told me that since she was 12, she had stopped growing. She didn't have a strong appetite and had difficulties to open her bowels and up to the age of 18, she had yet to have a period.

Growth cannot be without water, kidney water with insufficient heat was the main reason which caused her underdevelopment. Because of low reserves in heat her spleen soil organ was not fertile for digestion, thus she had no appetite for food. In the abovementioned cases of young women losing their periods, the women had previously had normal periods but as their kidney water heat became damaged then their periods became obstructed, so in addition to the basic kidney warming formula I added herbs to promote blood flow. In this case, however, because of the kidney heat was low, the patient's reproductive function had not yet developed, so there was no need to add blood moving herbs to her treatment so I gave her only the basic Erxian formula. The patient took five to seven packets of the herbs every month for three years. In that time her periods began and gradually became regular. Her appetite improved and her bowel motions also became normal. Eight years after the initial consultation she came for a consultation and I could hardly recognize her. Her height was 165cm, and she looked strong and healthy.

Treating kidney water yang damage with alcohol addiction

A 36-year-old man came for a consultation for a solid to touch, bloated, and painful upper stomach. The patient had been a heavy alcohol drinker for many years, and before he came to me, he had been told by western doctors that he had late stage liver cirrhosis and a liver transplant was his only option for treatment. At the first consultation, the patient also complained of feeling physically weak, having body tightness and aches, as well as feeling fearful, panicky, and easily angry. The only way that he could get into sleep he believed was to get drunk.

Alcohol drains out kidney water heat, and kidney water heat damage causes the symptom of bodily weakness. Kidney water heat loss limits the exercise of the yang qi of the enduring zhi, which sustains the confidence of the spirit. When the spirit loses confidence, it becomes to degrees fearful. When kidney water heat is low it fails to nurture the liver wood and causes liver wood yin and yang deficiency. Liver wood yin sustains the flexibility of people, when liver wood yin is deficient, there is the symptom of tightness and aching body. When liver wood loses its flexibility, it deprives the exercise of the striving zhi of the spirit. The yin of the striving zhi of the spirit supports the suppleness of the spirit qi, when it is unable to be exercised, the spirit is easily angry. Liver wood is the blood reservoir, the yang of liver wood makes erect the blood passages, so blood flow is unrestricted and fresh. The root of the liver wood sits in the upper stomach, when its yang is damaged, the blood passages collapse and blood stagnates which allows mucus and dampness to stick in the liver wood root, so the upper stomach in this case is solid to touch.

When kidney water heat is insufficient, the spleen soil becomes cold and hardened and loses its permeability, as a result the qi passages are obstructed and this causes stomach bloating and pain. On the other hand, the yin deficiency of liver wood agitates the heart fire yang heat to float, which then prevents the spirit from resting in its chamber, so the patient cannot sleep without first getting drunk.

However a state of drunkenness is not the same as the spirit resting, it is a sign that the heart fire is unable to be grounded, and pushes the spirit out of the body. It is a state of unconsciousness.

The yin qi of the aspiring zhi of the spirit provides calmness to the spirit qi. When the heart fire is ungrounded, it obstructs the exercise of the aspiring zhi yin qi of the spirit, so the spirit is panicky. The treatment is to warm kidney water, nurture liver wood, invigorate blood, soften and dissolve hard mucus, and smooth qi flow with Erxian Rulian formula.

After taking the herbs for a month, the patient didn't have the uncontrollable desire for alcohol any more. Then he felt calmer, slept better, and his stomach was softer. He continuously took the herbs for six months, all the symptoms disappeared and he completed the treatment. But 10 years later, he came back to me for another consultation as he had fallen back into drinking alcohol. This time, his liver was swollen and painful. I gave him the same treatment as the previous time and after taking the herbs for two months, he was able to control the addiction again. He took another 4 months of the herbs, and all the symptoms disappeared again. Seven years later, however, he was drinking again, his face was grey, he had a swollen stomach, liver pain, and no appetite. Again he took the herbs and was able to stop drinking alcohol.

Preparation and drinking the herbs: One packet of the herbs with 3 litres of cold water was boiled for 2 hours so that the liquid was reduced to 1 litre. The decoction was poured into a large flask. At any time that the patient felt the onset of a mood swing, or a desire to drink alcohol, he would have 100-200 ml of the liquid which would calm him down. He drunk multiple times a day to finish the entire litre in a day.

Erxian Rulian formula:

Epimedium brevicornum (yinyanghuo) 30g	15g
Curculiginis orchioides (xianmao) 15g	Polygala tenufola (yuanzhi) 10g
Morindae officinalis (bajitian)	Angelica sinensis (danggui) 20g
	Anemarrhena asphodeloides (zhimu) 10g

Phellodendri chinensis (huangbai) 10g
Gentiana scabra (longdancao) 30g
Polygoni multiflori (yejiaoteng) 30g
Zizyphus jujube (fried) (chao suanzaoren) 15g
Concha margaritifera (zhenzhumu) 30g
Concha haliotidis (shijueming) 30g

Concha ostreae (muli) 30g
Ossa draconis (longgu) 30g
Olibanum (ruxiang) 5g
Myrrh (moyao) 5g
Curcuma zedoaria (ezhu)10g
Concha arcae (walengzi) 30g
Cyperus rotundus (xiangfu) 10g
Toosendan fructus (chuanlianzi) 10g
Areca catechu (dafupi) 10g
Fructus aurantii (zhiqiao) 10g

Erxian Rulian formula in Chinese 二仙乳棟汤:

淫羊藿30g 仙茅15g 巴戟天15g 远志10g 当归20g 知母10g 黄柏10g 龙胆草30g 夜交藤30g 炒枣仁15g 珍珠母30g 石决明30g 牡蛎30g 龙骨30g 乳香10g 没药10g 莪术10g 瓦楞子30g 香附10g 川楝子10g 大腹皮10g 枳壳10g

The Erxian Rulian formula is the Erxian formula with the addition of Olibanum (ruxiang), Myrrh (moyao), Curcuma zedoaria (ezhu), Concha Arcae (walengzi), Cyperi rotundi (xiangfu), Toosendan fructus (chuanlianzi), Areca catechu (dafupi) and Fructus aurantii (zhiqiao).

Olibanum (ruxiang 乳香) has a slightly bitter and astringent taste, and warm yinyang nature, it goes into the liver meridian. It invigorates blood; eliminates abscesses, ulcers and poisonous swellings, and removes dampness in the blood.

Myrrh (moyao 没药) has a slightly bitter and astringent taste, and even yinyang nature, it goes into the liver meridian. It invigorates blood, breaks down nodules and stagnant blood, disperses swellings, and removes damp poison.

Curcuma zedoaria (ezhu 莪术) has a bitter and pungent taste, and warm yinyang nature. It goes into the liver and spleen meridians. It breaks down qi and blood stagnation, disperses nodules, and eases pain.

Concha arcae (walengzi 瓦楞子) has a salty taste, and mild yinyang nature. It goes into the liver and spleen meridians. It breaks down abdominal masses and nodules; it also dissolves stagnations of mucus, blood and qi.

Cyperus rotundus (xiangfu 香附) has a pungent taste, and slightly warm yinyang nature. It goes into liver, spleen, stomach, and lung meridians. It opens meridians, eases qi flow, strengthens spleen soil yang qi, and relieves oppression.

Toosendan fructus (chuanlianzi 川楝子) has a bitter taste and cold yinyang nature. It goes into the spleen, and stomach meridians. It removes gas, clears liver wood fire, and stops all abdominal pain.

Areca catechu (dafupi 大腹皮) has a pungent taste and slightly warm yinyang nature. It goes into the spleen and lung meridians. It moves gas downward and out, drains dampness, chases out wind, and relaxes the intestine.

Aurantii fructus (zhiqiao 枳壳) has a pungent and bitter taste, and slightly cool yinyang nature. It goes into lung, spleen, stomach, and large intestine meridians. It breaks down stagnated qi, dissolves mucus, and eliminates food stagnation.

Within the Erxian Rulian formula, the Erxian formula is used to warm kidney water, nurture liver wood, and ground heart fire yang qi. Olibanum (ruxiang), Myrrh (moyao) are used to invigorate blood, and remove the dampness and mucus in the liver wood. Curcuma zedoaria (ezhu), Concha Arcae (walengzi) are used to soften and dissolve the hardened mucus, and Cyperus rotundus (xiangfu), Toosendan fructus (chuanlianzi), Areca catechu (dafupi) and Fructus aurantii (zhiqiao) are used to smooth qi flow and stop the stomach pain.

Another alcohol addiction case was a 50-year-old patient. Before he came to me, he had been addicted to alcohol for about 4 years which had caused him to lose his well-paid job and damaged his family life. The patient came for help to stop the addiction. He said when the craving for alcohol occurred, he felt very fearful, panicky to the point it made him shake, and he could not sit or stand comfortably. Sometimes, when he didn't have money to buy proper alcohol, he would resort to methylated industrial alcohol which would cause bleeding from the skin.

As alcohol had damaged his kidney water yang qi, it was unable to support the enduring zhi to exercise its yang qi, which made the spirit fearful. When kidney water yang is deficient and fails to moisten the liver wood the result is liver wood dryness. As liver wood is the blood reservoir, when it is dry, blood cannot stay in its root but rushes into the blood passages which causes heat and wind. The wind then causes the symptoms of shaking, and the inability to stand or sit still. The yin qi of the aspiring zhi sustains the prudency of the spirit, but when liver wood is too dry, it stimulates the heart fire yang to float. The ungrounded heart fire is unable to permit the yin qi of the aspiring zhi to be exercised, which then causes the spirit to panic. The treatment was to warm kidney water, cool and soften liver wood, and ground heart fire with the Erxian formula.

The patient boiled each of the packets of herbs with 3 litres of cold water for 2 hours to reduce the liquid down to 1.5 litres. He drunk a large mouthful of the decoction whenever he felt an urge to drink alcohol. At first, a large mouthful could hold back the desire for alcohol for an hour or so, then gradually he didn't feel the desire as often or as strong, so he continued to drink the herbs in this manner. He did this for three months, and during that time he didn't have any alcohol. After taking the herbs for five months, he no longer had that uncontrollable desire for alcohol, and could resist drinking alcohol even without herbs.

Treating kidney water heat loss with symptoms of dry eyes

A fifty-year-old woman came for help for dry, sticky, painful eyes, and blurred vision. For a year, the patient's period had become less and less but still regular. At the age of 50, she was in the menopausal transition period. In the cycle of human life, people progress through a period of physical growth, a period of reproductive maturity, and then a period of preservation, at the periods of change, kidney water heat is demanded to pass through the transitions. Therefore, illnesses that occur at these points most often are related to kidney water heat loss. As for this case, the kidney water heat loss slows the water flow which delays the gathering of moisture of lung metal and causes the yin deficiency of lung metal, so there is the symptom of dry eyes. The yin deficiency of lung metal causes yinyang disharmony which further causes the yang damage of lung metal. When there is lung metal yang damage it fails to separate turbidities and to create fresh water, so there are symptoms of sticky eyes and blurring eyesight. With kidney water heat loss the liver wood becomes dry and hot and fails to store blood. Hot blood stuck in the blood passages in the area of the eyes results in sore eyes. The treatment is to warm kidney water, clear liver wood, ground heart fire, clear lung metal, and brighten the eyes. The Erxian Shihu Qinghao formula was used.

At the same times as taking the Erxian Shihu Qinghao formula, I also asked the patient to apply a hot towel to the eyelids and gently massage the eyeballs 2-3 times a day. The eye massage is also effective for correcting both short or long eyesight.

After taking seven packets of the herbs, the patient's eyes were less dry, and no longer painful. She took another 30 packets of the same herbs, and her eyes were no longer dry, nor painful, and her eyesight was improved.

Erxian Shihu Qinghao Formula:

Epimedium brevicornum (yinyanghuo) 30g
Curculiginis orchioides (xianmao) 15g
Morindae officinalis (bajitian) 15g
Polygala tenufola (yuanzhi) 10g
Angelica sinensis (danggui) 20g
Anemarrhena asphodeloides (zhimu) 10g
Phellodendri chinensis (huangbai) 10g
Gentiana scabra (longdancao) 30g

Polygoni multiflori (yejiaoteng) 30g
Ziziphus jujube (fried) (suanzaoren) 15g
Concha margaritifera (zhenzhumu) 30g
Concha haliotidis (shijueming) 30g
Concha ostreae (muli) 30g
Ossa draconis (longgu) 30g
Artemisia apiacea (qinghao) 5g
Dendrobium nobile (shihu) 40g
Flos Chrysanthemi Indici (yejuhua) 10g

Erxian Shihu formula in Chinese 二仙石斛青蒿汤:

淫羊藿30g 仙茅15g 巴戟天15g 远志10g 当归20g 知母10g 黄柏10g 龙胆草30g 夜交藤30g 炒枣仁15g 珍珠母30g 石决明30g 牡蛎30g 龙骨30g 青蒿5g 石斛40g 野菊花10g

The Erxian Shihu Qinghao formula is the Erxian formula with the addition of Artemisia apiacea (qinghao), Dendrobium nobile (shihu), Flos Chrysanthemi Indici (yejuhua). These three herbs not only clear lung metal heat and brighten eyesight, but also concentrate the effects of the herbs to the eyes.

Artemisia apiacea (qinghao 青蒿) has a bitter taste, very cold yinyang nature. It goes into the lung, liver, and kidney meridians. It removes dampness, clears heat, dissolves mucus, stops regular fever, and brightens eyesight.

Dendrobium nobile (shihu 石斛) has a sweet taste and mild yinyang nature. It goes into the lung, kidney meridians. It strengthens water yin, brightening eyesight, and consolidates the yinyang order of all wuxing organs.

Flos chrysanthemi indici (yejuhua 野菊花) has a bitter taste and cool yinyang nature. It goes into the lung, and liver meridians. It eliminates wind, clears heat, brightens eyesight, reduces swelling, and detoxifies poison.

Treating kidney water heat loss with symptoms of flushing red face

A 54-year-old woman who suffered from a flushing red face came to me for a consultation. In the previous six months her menses came every two months, and the flushing red face would get worse just before her menses. That the red face occurred around the time of her period indicated that the problem was related to her reproductive cycles. When liver wood becomes dry because of kidney water heat loss, blood stores in the blood passage rather than in the root of liver wood, so there is a symptom of flushing red face. Treatment was to warm the kidney water, cool and clear liver wood heat, ground the heart fire, and cool the blood. I used the Erxian Shihuang formula.

After taking 7 packets of herbs the symptoms seemed to be better but not obviously so. She took another 14 days of the herbs and her face began to cool and there was less redness. She stopped the herbs for two weeks, her period came, and her face got red again. Then she took the herbs again for two weeks, and the redness of the face became less obvious. She then stopped the herbs again for six months, the face got red again but not as red as previously. Then the patient started to take the herbs again, on and off for about a year, her period gradually stopped and the flushing red face didn't recur.

Erxian Shihuang formula:

Epimedium brevicornum (yinyanghuo) 30g
Curculiginis orchioides (xianmao) 15g
Morindae officinalis (bajitian) 15g
Polygala tenufola (yuanzhi) 10g
Angelica sinensis (danggui) 20g
Anemarrhena asphodeloides (zhimu) 10g
Phellodendri chinensis (huangbai) 10g
Gentiana scabra (longdancao) 30g
Polygoni multiflori (yejiaoteng) 30g
Zizyphus jujube (fried) (chao suanzaoren) 15g
Concha margaritifera (zhenzhumu) 30g
Concha haliotidis (shijueming) 30g
Concha ostreae (muli) 30g
Ossa draconis (longgu) 30g
Paeonia lactiflora (chishao) 30g
Coptis chinensis (huanglian) 10g
Gypsum (shigao) 20g
Rheum officinale (dahuang)10g

Erxian Shihuang formula in Chinese 二仙石黄汤:

淫羊藿30g 仙茅15g 巴戟天15g 远志10g 当归20g 知母10g 黄柏10g 龙胆草30g 夜交藤30g 炒枣仁15g 珍珠母30g 石决明30g 牡蛎30g 龙骨30g 赤芍30g 黄连10g 石膏20g 大黄10g

The Erxian Shihuang formula is the Erxian formula with the addition of Paeonia lactiflora (chishao), Coptis chinensis (huanglian), gypsum (shigao), and Rheum officinale (dahuang).

Paeonia lactiflora (chishao 赤芍) cools blood.
Coptis chinensis (huanglian 黄连) extinguishes fire heat; detoxifies poison, dries dampness, and cools blood.
Gypsum (shigao 石膏) has a mild sweet and plain taste and slightly cold nature. It goes into the lung, and stomach meridians. It moistens lung metal, clears heat, cools blood, disperses disordered yin qi, calms restlessness, separates fresh water from turbidity, and dissolves mucus.

Rheum officinale (dahuang 大黄) cools blood, detoxifies poison.

In the Erxian Shihuang formula, the Erxian formula warms kidney water, clears liver wood, grounds heart fire. By adding Paeonia lactiflora (chishao), Coptis chinensis (huanglian) gypsum (shigao) and Rheum officinale (dahuang) these herbs clear heat and cool the blood to relieve the symptom of flushing red face. But these four cooling herbs used on their own don't have obvious effects for relieving the flushing red face symptom. As a red face is a symptom of kidney water heat loss, liver wood dryness and blood hotness, cooling blood herbs alone will treat the symptom but not the cause. Sometimes, it may give temporary symptom relief, but often it leads to symptoms getting worse later on because cooling herbs can also cool the kidney water making an adverse effect. On the other hand, if I were to prescribe only the basic formula to warm the kidney water, cooling the liver wood and grounding the heart fire, while the red face symptom would eventually disappear it might also take a little longer to get this result.

Another 54-year-old female patient suffered from a flushing red face. The red face first appeared two years beforehand when her periods had stopped. She had hot flushes one or two times a day and night sweats every two to three days. Her mood was good, she slept well but her bowel was dry and difficult to open at times. Heat loss of kidney water slows water flow, which causes the large intestine to lose its lubrication, so she had dry and difficult bowel motions. This case was treated for cold kidney water and dry liver wood with hot blood using the above formula. After taking the herbs for seven days, some days she found the face was not as red but other days would be the same, however, there were fewer hot flushes and night sweats and they were less intense, and her bowels opened freely. She stopped the herbs for a month, and there were no hot flushes and night sweats but the red face came back as bad as before. She took seven days of the same herbs again and the red face was much improved. She continued to take the herbs for another two weeks. The redness of her face was not so obvious any more, so she stopped the herbs. Two months later her face became a bit red again, so she took another seven days of the herbs. One year later, she came to the clinic and told me that she had not had the red face again.

Treating kidney water heat loss with the symptom of dry mouth

A 70-year-old man had suffered from dry mouth, frequent urination, difficulty in opening his bowels, because it was hard and dry, bloated stomach, fatigue, quick temper, and restless sleep. He did not want to follow his Western doctor's instruction to take insulin treatment, so he came to me for alternative advice.

When kidney water has insufficient heat, water cannot rise, so there is a feeling of dry mouth and thirstiness. But because kidney water hasn't enough heat to hold water, drinking lots of water won't quench the thirst; instead, it merely makes him pass water often. When kidney water loses heat, the large intestine loses its lubrication, so there is a symptom of dry and difficult bowel motion. Kidney water heat loss, and draining spleen soil yang heat can cause spleen soil to lose its permeability, and qi becomes stagnated, so there is a bloated stomach feeling. Kidney water heat loss means its yang qi reserve is low, so there is a symptom of tiredness. With kidney water heat loss, the liver wood gets dry and hot, the yin of the striving zhi of the spirit is hampered, so there is a symptom of quick temper. Dry liver wood causes heart fire to float, and disturbs the spirit's rest, so the patient has restless sleep. The treatment is then focused on warming kidney water, clearing liver wood, and grounding heart fire with the Erxian Fugui Dahuang formula.

The patient also had a sweet tooth and often ate cakes, drank wine and coffee. Because white sugar in the cakes and alcohol, and coffee drained his kidney water heat, the precondition to expect the treatment to be successful was that the patient had to stop consuming white sugar and drinking wine and coffee.

The patient took the herbs for three months, after which he no longer felt constantly thirsty. He also had normal frequency of urination, and by avoiding sweets, wines and coffee, his feelings of bloated stomach became better and his blood sugar reading became normal. As a result, his Western doctor no longer insisted on the insulin treatments. Later he stopped the herbs but continued to avoid sweets, alcohol and coffee, and adopted a non-dairy diet. After a year, he lost 10 kilograms in weight and said he felt ten years younger.

Erxian Fugui Dahuang formula:

Radix aconitum carmichaeli (treated) (zhi fuzi) 10g
Cortex cinnamomi (rougui) 10g
Epimedium brevicornum (yinyanghuo) 30g
Curculiginis orchioides (xianmao) 15g
Morindae officinalis (bajitian) 15g
Polygala tenufola (yuanzhi) 10g
Angelica sinensis (danggui) 20g
Anemarrhena asphodeloides (zhimu) 10g
Phellodendri chinensis (huangbai) 10g
Gentiana scabra (longdancao) 30g
Polygoni multiflori (yejiaoteng) 30g
Zizyphus jujube (fried) (chao suanzaoren) 15g
Concha margaritifera (zhenzhumu) 30g
Concha haliotidis (shijueming) 30g
Concha ostreae (muli) 30g
Ossa draconis (longgu) 30g
Rheum officinale (dahuang) 10g

Erxian Fugui Dahuang formula in Chinese 二仙附桂大黄汤:

制附子10g 肉桂10g 淫羊藿30g 仙茅15g 巴戟天15g 远志10g 当归20g 知母10 g 黄柏10g 龙胆草30g 夜交藤30g 炒枣仁15g 珍珠母30g 石决明30g 牡蛎30g 龙骨30g 大黄10g.

The Erxian Fugui Dahuang formula is the Erxian formula with the addition of Radix aconitum carmichaeli (treated) (zhi fuzi), cortex cinnamomi (rougui) and Rheum officinale (dahuang).

Radix aconitum carmichaeli (zhi fuzi 制附子) has a pungent and hot taste; a dry and hot yinyang nature. It goes into the kidney, mingmen and heart meridians. It fortifies heart fire yang, strengthens the kidney water heat; eliminates wind, cold and dampness. It also breaks down any accumulated masses in the body, and heals cold and dampness that causes knees and lower back pain. **Note:** As Radix aconitum carmichaeli has a strong yinyang nature, it must be boiled for at least two hours in the preparation otherwise it can harm the body, so it is considered a poisonous herb.

Cortex cinnamomi (rougui 肉桂) has a pungent taste and hot yinyang nature. It goes into the heart, spleen, and kidney meridians. It fortifies heart fire yang, warms kidney water, opens blood passages, and advocates all herbs efficacies.

Rheum officinale (dahuang 大黄) cools blood, detoxifies poison, breaks down stagnation, clears dampness, and opens bowel motions.

In the Erxian Fugui Dahuang formula, Radix aconitum carmichaeli (treated) (zhi fuzi) is used for its dry and hot nature to strengthen the warming kidney water effect; cortex cinnamomi (rougui) is used for not only its hot nature to add more heat in the formula but also for its ability to lead heart fire downward to the kidney water. The use of Rheum officinale (dahuang) is to promote bowel motions and detoxify damp poisons to loosen the spleen soil.

Another patient was a 59-year-old woman who had a dry and sticky mouth for three years. At the first consultation, she had a dry mouth, dry skin, and dry sticky eyes. Her vision was unclear; she was tired most of the time but could not sleep well. She drank a lot but could not quench her thirst, and had to run to the toilet within a few minutes. The patient had been seeing Chinese medicine practitioners and had been taking herbs to nourishing the yin, such as raw and cooked Radix rehmanniae (shengdi, shudi), rhizome anemarrhenae (zhimu), radix trichosanthis (tianhuafen), ophiopogon japonicas (maimendong) etc. for a long time. Sometimes, she felt the herbs made her feel better, but overall, the symptoms had persistently remained and progressively became worse.

Nourishing yin herbs can temporarily reduce dry symptoms, but the main reason for the dryness was the kidney water heat loss, if this issue is not dealt with, the symptom would persist. So for this case, the treatment I gave was to warm kidney water, soften liver wood, ground heart fire, and brighten eyesight. The formula was the Erxian Shihu formula. (See "Treating kidney water heat loss with symptoms of dry eyes".)

After taking the herbs for seven days, the patient felt all her symptoms had improved. She continued taking the herbs for three months, as a result she had more restful sleep, no longer felt constantly tired and no longer had dryness of the mouth or eyes.

Treating kidney water heat loss with symptoms of swollen feet

A 62-year-old man came to me for help with swollen feet. For five years the patient would have swollen feet whenever he was on a flight for a few hours, or sleeping very late. Normally after a good rest, the swelling would disappear. However, at the first consultation his feet had been swollen for a week without getting any better. He felt tired, vexed, and had restless sleep. Kidney water heat loss and water flow that is slower causes water retention, so there are symptoms of swollen feet. Kidney water heat loss means the body lacks yang qi, so there is a symptom of tiredness. With kidney water heat loss, liver wood becomes dry and hot, which stimulates the heart fire to float, so there is a symptom of restless sleep. When kidney water heat is low it restricts the exercise of the yang qi of enduring zhi of the spirit, so the spirit is down and depressed. Sleeping late at night allows the yin qi of the heaven and earth to wash out the yang qi of the body causing yang deficiency, so the feet would swell more obviously after a late night sleep. The treatment was to warm kidney water, clear liver wood, ground heart fire, and free the water passages. I used the Erxian Yixu formula.

After taking the herbs for three days, the swelling of the feet abated but the patient still felt tired and vexed. He took seven more days of the herbs, and all the symptoms disappeared. But the fact that he had had swelling of the feet over a period of 5 years meant he had little kidney heat reserve, and this time the symptoms had persisted, which was a sign of overtaxing the energy reserves. I therefore suggested that he take the herbs for another six months. After taking it for 3 months, the patient no longer suffered swollen feet even after an eight to nine-hour flight. He continued to take the herbs for another 3 months and felt energetic and in good spirits.

Erxian Yixu formula:

Coix Lacryma-jobi (yiyiren) 30g
Stigma Maydis (yumixu) 30g
Epimedium brevicornum
(yinyanghuo) 30g

Curculiginis orchioides
(xianmao) 15g
Morindae officinalis (bajitian)
15g

Polygala tenufola (yuanzhi) 10g
Angelica sinensis (danggui) 20g
Anemarrhena asphodeloides (zhimu) 10g
Phellodendri chinensis (huangbai) 10g
Gentiana scabra (longdancao) 30g
Polygoni multiflori (yejiaoteng)

30g
Zizyphus jujube (fried) (suanzaoren)15g
Concha margaritifera (zhenzhumu) 30g
Concha haliotidis (shijueming) 30g
Concha ostreae (muli) 30g
Ossa draconis (longgu) 30g

Erxian Yixu formula in Chinese 二仙薏须汤:

薏苡仁30g 玉米须30g 淫羊藿30g 仙茅15g 巴戟天15g 远志10g 当归20g 知母10 g 黄柏10g 龙胆草30g 夜交藤30g 炒枣仁15g 珍珠母30g 石决明30g 牡蛎30g 龙骨30g.

The Erxian Yixu formula is the Erxian formula with the addition of Coix Lacryma-jobi (yiyiren), and Stigma maydis (yumixu) to open water passages and remove water retention.

Coix Lacryma-jobi (yiyiren 薏苡仁) has a sweet taste and mild yinyang nature. It goes into liver, spleen, and kidney meridians. It frees water flow, and removes dampness.
Stigma Maydis (yumixu 玉米须) has a sweet taste and mild yinyang nature. It goes into liver, spleen, and kidney meridians. It frees water flow, removes dampness, and cools blood.

Treating kidney water yang deficiency with symptoms of mouth ulcers

A 20-year-old woman always suffered mouth ulcers just before her menses began. The patient had been suffering a long time with loss of sleep, restlessness and body tension. When kidney water heat loss fails to nurture liver wood, there is liver wood yang damage, and blood decay, so there are symptoms of mouth ulcers. With kidney water heat loss, the period cycle becomes difficult, obstruction of energy flow is more obvious and ulcers are more pronounced during this time. Kidney water heat loss causes liver wood dryness, heart fire to float and disturb the spirit, so she had loss of sleep. With liver wood dryness, the body loses flexibility, so she felt body tension and restlessness. Treatment was to warm kidney water, soften liver wood, ground heart fire, cool blood, and detoxify poison with the Erxian Chilian formula.

After taking three packets of the herbs, the patient's ulcers healed. Thereafter, for three months, she would have three packets of the herbs one week before her period and she no longer had ulcers.

There are many cases of ulcers that are caused by eating chemically impregnated food, particularly in factory processed food. Once such food is no longer consumed ulcers will usually disappear without treatment, although an external application of toad liquid can accelerate the healing process.

Erxian Chilian formula:

Epimedium brevicornum (yinyanghuo) 30g
Curculiginis orchioides (xianmao) 15g
Morindae officinalis (bajitian) 15g
Polygala tenufola (yuanzhi) 10g
Angelica sinensis (danggui) 20g
Anemarrhena asphodeloides (zhimu) 10g
Phellodendri chinensis (huangbai) 10g
Gentiana scabra (longdancao) 30g
Polygoni multiflori (yejiaoteng) 30g
Zizyphus jujube (fried) (chao suanzaoren) 15g
Concha margaritifera (zhenzhumu) 30g
Concha haliotidis (shijueming) 30g
Concha ostreae (muli) 30g
Ossa draconis (longgu) 30g
Paeonia lactiflora (chishao) 30g
Coptis chinensis (huanglian) 10

Erxian Chilian formula in Chinese 二仙赤连汤:

淫羊藿30g 仙茅15g 巴戟天15g 当归20g 知母10g 黄柏10g 夜交藤30g 远志10g 酸枣仁15g 龙胆草30g 珍珠母30g 石决明30g 龙骨30g 牡蛎3g0 赤芍30 黄连10

The Erxian Chilian formula is the Erxian formula with the addition of Paeonia lactiflora (chishao), and Coptis chinensis (huanglian) to strengthen the cooling blood effect.

Toad liquid preparation:

Begin with 1g of Venenum bufonis (toad) powder (chansufen 蟾酥粉) and mix with 50 ml of 60-70 percent alcohol/spirit and allow to sit for at least three hours. Use a cotton bud to dip into the toad liquid, dab on the ulcer and press it for two seconds. The ulcer pain can stop quickly and normally within a day the ulcer will heal.

Toad powder is derived from the glands secretion of Venenum bufonis. It has a pungent taste and warm yinyang nature. It is poisonous and needs to be handled carefully, making sure not to contact the eyes. Internal use should not be done without professional supervision. However, the toad secretion can break down stagnated blockages of all kinds, it will open meridians, and has strong detoxification effects. It treats all kinds of stubborn sores and skin irritations. For broken sores and skin irritations, the toad secretion can have immediate effect. For unbroken pussy sores, the skin should be broken and then dabbed with the toad liquid. It can also effectively treat swollen and painful throats and nostrils. Toad liquid will make the dabbed area feel numb and painful, but the numbness and pain will disappear within 10 minutes.

Treating kidney water yin & yang deficiency with symptoms of mouth ulcers

For men, the most common cause of both kidney water yin and yang weakness is excessive ejaculation. Sperms are the essence of the kidney water yinyang energy. Over ejaculation forces the kidney to disperse reserved yinyang energy and, as a result, kidney water yin and yang qi are lost. I once had a 30-year-old male patient who came for a consultation complaining that he often felt extremely tired, thirsty, and agitated. But what bothered him the most were mouth ulcers. There were many mouth ulcers at one time, when some got better new ones would already begin to appear. He was in a lot of pain. When I asked him what his sex life was like, he made a long sigh, and said it was a big problem. He felt the desire for sex all the time, and felt bad to trouble his wife too often, so he masturbated frequently. Sometimes even at work he masturbated in the toilet, otherwise he found it hard to control sudden rages, but after masturbating, he would feel very lethargic and difficult to concentrate with his work.

This was a typical case of over ejaculation which caused kidney water yin and yang deficiency. The kidney water is the reservoir of the body's vitality, when it is depleted through excessive ejaculation, so the person feels exhausted; when kidney water yin is exhausted through the excessive ejaculation, so the person has a dry mouth. When kidney water is weak and fails to nourish liver wood this causes liver wood yang deficiency, and blood decay, so there are ulcers. When liver wood is not nourished by kidney water this leads to liver wood yin deficiency and inflexibility, it barricades the yin qi of the striving zhi from being exercised, so he was agitated.

Without prescribing any herbs for this patient I asked him not to ejaculate for one week. One week later he came back for his consultation, his mouth ulcers had mostly healed, his mouth no longer felt dry, and he no longer felt as tired, but instead felt rather happy. Therefore there was no need for other treatment.

Treating kidney water yin deficiency with symptoms of scant, frequent, urgent, and painful urination

A 19-year-old young woman came for help as she had been repeatedly suffering from scant, frequent, urgent, and painful urination (SU). She had had a boyfriend for a year, and from the time they first began to have sex, after each intercourse she tended to have symptoms of SU. She had been taking antibiotics whenever these symptoms occurred, but afterwards she suffered from an itchy vagina and heavy discharge. At the first consultation, she had been having the SU symptoms for a several hours and she also had a slightly feverish feeling.

With kidney water yin deficiency, the water passage is drier and difficult to flow, which encourages dampness and mucus to arise. The gathering of fermenting dampness creates heat, so there are symptoms of scant, frequent, urgent urine. Kidney dampness damages liver wood yang, causing blood decay in the urine bladder, so it was painful to pass urine. For women, this often happens after sex. If a woman has kidney water yin deficiency, water is not plentiful, then

79

if her partner carries dampness in his penis, when having intercourse the dampness gets into the vagina, blocks the water passages, then the symptoms occur. Treatment is to clear heat, remove dampness, cool blood, detoxify poison, and free water flow with the Xiaoji formula.

The method for taking the Xiaoji formula are: cook two packets of the herbs together with 3-4 litres of cold water (sufficient to cover the herbs) and boil down to 1 litre in about 60-90 minutes. Drink 250 ml of the decoction every four hours. If the patient falls asleep, wait till she is awake then drink again.

Each time the patient took a drink of the herbs, her symptoms eased for about four hours, then the pain would start again and she would take the herbs again. After the third cup of herbs, she fell asleep. The next day she kept drinking 250 ml of the herbs every four hours. By the evening of the third day, the symptoms stopped returning. On the fourth day she drank the herbs twice a day and no symptoms occurred and she stopped the herbs on the fifth day. She did not suffer any vagina itch or excessive discharge at the end of the treatment.

Xiaoji formula:

Taraxacum mongolicum (pugongying) 30g
Viola yedoensis makino (zihuadiding) 30g
Scutellaria baicalensis (huangqin) 10g
Coptis chinensis (huanglian) 10g
Phellodendri chinensis (huangbai) 10g
Rheum officinale (dahuang) 10g
Eupolyphaga sinensis (tubiechong) 10g
Scolopendra subspinipes (wugong) 1 piece
Sanguisorba officinalis (diyu) 10g
Paeoniae lactiflora (chishao) 10g
Cirsium setosum (xiaoji) 10g
Cirsium japonicum (daji) 10g
Nelumbo nucifera (oujie) 10g
Plantago asiatica (seeds) (cheqianzi) 10g
Plantago asiatica (whole plant) (cheqiancao) 15g
Dioscorea septemloba (bixie) 10g
Dianthus superbus (jumai) 10g
Typha angustifolia (puhuang) 10g
Cyathula officinalis (chuanniuxi) 10g
Polygonum aviculare (bianxu)

10g
Cremastra appendiculata
(shancigu) 10g
Glycyrrhiza radix (gancao) 10g
Radix rehmanniae (raw)
(shengdi) 10g
Radix rehmanniae (cooked)

(shudi) 10g
Asparagus cochinchinensis
(tianmendong) 10g
Ophiopogon japonicas
(maimendong) 10g
Talcum (huashi) 20g
Paeoniae alba (baishao) 10g

Xiaoji formula in Chinese 小蓟汤

蒲公英30 紫花地丁30 黄芩10 黄连10 黄柏10 大黄10 土鳖虫10 蜈蚣1（只）地榆10 赤芍10 小蓟10 大蓟10 藕节10 车前子10 车前草15草薢10 瞿麦10 蒲黄10 川牛膝10 萹蓄10 山慈菇10 甘草10 生地10 熟地10 天门冬10 麦门冬10 滑石20 白芍10

Taraxacum mongolicum (pugongying 蒲公英) clears heat, detoxifies poison, heals ulcerated carbuncles.
Viola yedoensis makino (zihuadiding 紫花地丁) clears heat, detoxifies poison, and eliminates swelling.
Scutellaria baicalensis (huangqin 黄芩) disperses wind, clears heat, drains dampness, detoxifies poison, and eliminates swelling.
Coptis chinensis (huanglian 黄连) purges intense heat; detoxifies poison, rids dampness, and cools blood.
Phellodendri chinensis (huangbai 黄柏) removes stagnated heat in all wuxing organs; removes dampness, detoxifies poison, and reduces swelling.
Rheum officinale (dahuang 大黄) clears heat, cools blood, opens bowels, and detoxifies poison.
Eupolyphaga sinensis (tubiechong 土鳖虫) has a salty taste and cold yinyang nature. It goes into the liver meridian. It breaks down stagnant blood, eliminates abdominal mass, smooths women's period blood flow, and removes stubborn stagnation.
Scolopendra subspinipes (wugong 蜈蚣) has a pungent taste and warm yinyang nature. It goes into the liver meridian. It breaks down cold or hot stagnation; dissolves damp poison in the blood.
Sanguisorba officinalis (diyu 地榆) has a bitter taste, and cool yinyang nature. It goes into the liver and kidney meridians. It cools blood, eliminates dampness, and removes poison.
Paeoniae lactiflora (chishao 赤芍) removes stagnated masses, dis-

perse blood stagnation, and breaks down intestinal wind and swelling.
Cirsium setosum (xiaoji 小蓟) has a sweet taste, and cool yinyang nature. It goes into the liver and spleen meridians. It cools blood, stops bleeding, detoxifies poison, and eliminates swelling.
Cirsium japonicum (daji 大蓟) has a sweet taste and mild yinyang nature. It goes into the liver, kidney, and urine bladder meridians. It cools blood, detoxifies poison, and removes carbuncles.
Nelumbo nucifera gaertn (oujie 藕节) has a sweet and astringent taste, and a mild yinyang nature. It goes into liver and urine bladder meridians. It drains dampness and dissolves mucus; it also dissolves dampness and mucus in the blood.
Plantago asiatica (Cheqianzi 车前子 seeds; Cheqiancao 车前草 whole plant) all have a sweet taste and cold yinyang nature. They go into the urine bladder meridian. They clear heat, free urine flow, cool blood, and detoxify poison. The seeds have a stronger ability to free urine flow and the whole plant has better ability in clearing heat.
Dioscorea septemloba (bixie 萆薢) clears heat, removes dampness, opens meridians, and promotes urine flow.
Dianthus superbus (jumai 瞿麦) clears heat, promotes water flow, and opens blood passages.
Typha angustifolia (puhuang 蒲黄) clears abnormal heat or cold in the chest, stomach, and urine bladder, promotes urine flow, and removes blood stagnation.
Cyathula officinalis (chuanniuxi 川牛膝) has a slightly bitter taste and mild yinyang nature. It goes into the liver, kidney meridians. It eliminates wind, drains dampness, clears urine and promotes its flow. It also leads other herbs down to the urine bladder.
Polygonum aviculare (bianxu 萹蓄) has a bitter taste and mild yinyang nature. It goes into the stomach and urine bladder meridians. It eliminates parasites, drains dampness, and stops itchiness.
Cremastra appendiculata (shancigu 山慈菇) has a pungent taste and cold yinyang nature. It goes into the lung, stomach, and liver meridians. It clears mucus and detoxifies poisons.
Glycyrrhiza (gancao 甘草) detoxifies poisons in all wuxing organs.
Radix rehmanniae (shengdi 生地 raw, shudi 熟地 cooked) have a sweet taste and cool yinyang nature. They go into the liver and kidney meridians. They open blood passages, break down damp poison

in the blood. Raw rehmanniae is cooler and better in cooling blood; whereas cooked rehmanniae is better in nurturing blood and opening blood passages.

Asparagus cochinchinensis (tianmendong 天门冬) has a sweat taste and cold yinyang nature. It goes into the lung meridian. It nurtures yin, creates water, and clears damp poison.

Ophiopogon japonicas (maimendong 麦门冬) has a sweet taste and mild yinyang nature. It goes into the lung meridian. It nurtures yin, moves water downward, and clears dampness.

Talcum (huashi 滑石) has a sweet taste and cold yinyang nature. It goes into the stomach, urine bladder meridians. It isolates turbidity, clears heat, and removes mucus.

Paeoniae Alba (baishao 白芍) has a sour taste and mild yinyang nature. It goes into the liver and spleen meridians. It opens and smooths blood passages and removes swelling.

In the Xiaoji formula, Taraxacum mongolicum (pugongying), Viola yedoensis makino (zihuadiding), Scutellaria baicalensis (huangqin), Coptis chinensis (huanglian), Phellodendri chinensis (huangbai), and Rheum officinale (dahuang) are used to clear heat and detoxify poison. Eupolyphaga (tubiechong), Scolopendra subspinipes (wugong), Sanguisorba officinalis L (diyu), Paeoniae lactiflora (chishao), Cirsium setosum (xiaoji), Cirsium japonicum (daji) and Nelumbo nucifera Gaertn (oujie) are used to clean the damp poison in the blood. Plantago asiatica seeds and the whole plant (cheqianzi, cheqiancao), Dioscorea septemloba (bixie), Dianthus Superbus (jumai), Typha angustifolia (puhuang), Cyathula officinalis Kuan (chuanniuxi), Polygonum aviculare (bianxu) and Cremastra appendiculata (shancigu) are used to remove dampness and promote urine flow. Glycyrrhiza (gancao) is used to detoxify the wuxing organ's poison, and harmonize the wuxing organs. Both raw and cooked Radix rehmanniae (shengdi, shudi), Asparagus cochinchinensis (tianmendong), Ophiopogon japonicas (maimendong) are used to create water, nurture the yin, and clear dampness. Talcum (huashi) is used to isolate turbidity. Paeoniae Alba (baishao) is used to open the blood passages.

Treating kidney water yin and yang deficiency with symptoms of scant, frequent, urgent and painful urination

A 50-year-old woman who had SU for 20 years, was constantly taking antibiotics to cope with the symptoms. Before she came to consult with me, she had been taking antibiotics everyday for six months but still had SU which made her unable to sleep at night. At the first consultation, the patient had to leave the consultation twice to urinate. The patient not only had painful, urgent and frequent urination but also suffered itching in her vagina.

If bacteria are a kind of damp poison, antibiotics can kill the bacteria and relieve the symptoms, but what makes the bacteria uncontrollable in the body is the blockage between body and heaven and earth. Blockages creates dampness; prolonged dampness will become poisonous mucus. If the yinyang passage between body and heaven and earth is not open, one lot of bacteria will be eliminated but another lot will quickly grow back. In addition, the build-up of antibiotics in the body further blocks the body's yinyang passage and promotes the growth of damp poison and provides beneficial conditions for the bacteria's expansion in the body. The patient was in effect trapped by the antibiotics. If she didn't take antibiotics, the pain was unbearable, but the more she took the worse her condition became. This case had a double source of dampness. One was the body's yinyang disorder that caused the blockage creating dampness, and the other was the blockage caused by antibiotics that created dampness in the body.

With kidney water yin deficiency, the water flow is slow and therefore allows damp mucus to accumulate. Mucus and dampness congest the water passages and ferment to become damp heat so that she has scant, frequent, urgent and painful urination. The patient was 50 years old, which is around the time of the menopause transition, and the kidney water heat is more demanding in order to get through the transition. When kidney water heat is low, the water passages get more congested, so the symptoms are worse at this time. The treatment is to first nurture the kidney water yin, detoxify poison, clear damp heat, free urine flow to relieve the SU symptoms, but it should be followed by kidney water warming, and freeing water flow herbs to relieve the SU symptoms at the same time assist the menopause transition. To nurture kidney water yin, and free urine flow the Xiaoji formula was used. To warm kidney water, and free urine flow the Erxian Gongying formula was used.

The patient took 7 packets of the Xiaoji formula, and was also taking her antibiotics, her pain was reduced. Then she took another 7 packets of the same herbs and the pains stopped. She then stopped the antibiotics and continued to take the Xiaoji formula. Two weeks later, the pain came back and she took one tablet of antibiotics and the pain stopped and her period came. She took another 2 weeks of the Xiaoji formula, she was fine until she had a glass of wine, and the pain returned. She took another tablet of antibiotics and the pain reduced. (These days wine is often produced with the addition of refined sugar, which damages kidney water yang qi and breeds dampness in the body.)

At this point I began to add the Erxian Gongying formula in conjunction with the Xiaoji formula. I asked the patient to alternate between the two prescriptions. In the morning she would have 250 ml of the Xiaoji formula and in the evening she would have 250ml of the Erxian Gongying formula. In the next six months, she had the SU symptoms very occasionally, and when it happened, she took two packets of the Xiaoji formula and the symptoms would be controlled, and she no longer resorted to any antibiotics. Thereafter, I gave her only the Erxian Gongying formula to warm kidney water and support the kidney water yin at the same time. She took it for a year, felt well and stopped the treatment. After stopping the herbs for a year, her period stopped, she had a bit of hot flushing and night sweats and came back for some herbs, and she said that the SU symptoms did not occur again.

Erxian Gongying formula:

Epimedium brevicornum (yinyanghuo) 30g
Curculiginis orchioides (xianmao) 15g
Morindae officinalis (bajitian) 15g

Polygala tenufola (yuanzhi) 10g
Angelica sinensis (danggui) 20g
Anemarrhena asphodeloides (zhimu) 10g
Phellodendri chinensis (huangbai) 10g

Gentiana scabra (longdancao) 30g
Polygoni multiflori (yejiaoteng) 30g
Zizyphus jujube (fried) (chao suanzaoren) 15g
Concha margaritifera (zhenzhumu) 30g
Concha haliotidis (shijueming) 30g
Concha ostreae (muli) 30g
Ossa draconis (longgu) 30g
Paeonia lactiflora (chishao) 15g
Taraxacum officinale (pugongying) 30g
Viola yedoensis (zihuadiding) 30g
Rheum officinale (dahuang) 10g
Coptis chinensis (huanglian) 10g

Erxian Gongying formula in Chinese 二仙公英汤:

淫羊藿30g 仙茅15g 巴戟天15g 远志10g 当归20g 知母10g 黄柏10g 龙胆草30g 夜交藤30g 炒枣仁15g 珍珠母30g 石决明30g 牡蛎30g 龙骨30g 赤芍15g 蒲公英30g 紫花地丁30g 大黄10g 黄连10.

See the Erxian Gongying explanation at "Treating kidney water yin and yang damage with symptoms of pain and swollen testicle."

Treating kidney water yin damage with symptoms of frequent and difficult urination in men

A 35-year-old male patient came for a consultation who had been suffering from frequent, urgent, difficult urination for six months which had forced him to stop work. His urine colour was dark and smelly; he also had problems with weak erections.

For men to suffer from frequent, and obstructed urination is often a result of over ejaculation. Sperm is the essence of the male kidney yin and yang. Over ejaculation depletes kidney water's yin and yang reserve.

In this case, with kidney water yin deficiency the water passage becomes dry, the water flow is congested, which encourages the dampness and mucus to flourish. Dampness and mucus block water passages so there is difficulty passing urine; dampness ferments and creates heat, so there are symptoms of frequent and urgent, smelly, and dark coloured urination. Dampness and mucus blocks the yinyang passages, and the flow of yang qi is restricted, so there is a symptom of weak erections.

The treatment was focused on clearing damp heat, dissolving mucus, dispersing stagnation, detoxifying poison, and freeing the urine passage. During the treatment he was advised not to ejaculate. For treatment I used the Xiaoji Niuxi formula.

After taking ten packets of the herbs he was able to return to work, and afterwards he intermittently took the herbs for three months and completely recovered.

Xiaoji Niuxi formula:

Taraxacum officinale (pugongying) 10g

Viola yedoensis makino (zihuadiding) 10g

Talcum (huashi) 20g

Alisma orientalis (zexie) 10g

Euphorbia helioscopia (zeqi) 10g

Dioscorea septemloba (bixie) 10g

Dianthus superbus (jumai) 10g

Plantago asiatica (cheqiancao) 15g

Cremastra appendiculata (shancigu) 10g

Cirsium setosum (xiaoji) 10g

Cirsium japonicum (daji) 10g

Sanguisorba officinalis (diyu) 10g

Paeoniae lactiflora(chishao) 10g

Paeoniae Alba (baishao) 10g

Colla corii asini (ejiao) 10g

Glycyrrhiza radix (gancao) 10g

Eupolyphaga sinensis (tubiechong) 10g

Leonurus japonicas (yimucao) 15g

Typha angustifolia (puhuang) 10g

Radix rehmanniae (raw) (shengdi) 10g

Radix rehmanniae (cooked) (shudi) 10g

Asparagus cochinchinensis (tianmendong) 10g

Ophiopogon japonicas (maimendong) 10g

Angelica Sinensis (danggui) 20g

Cortex Cinnamomi (rougui) 10g

Achyranthes bidentata (huainiuxi) 10g

Cyathula officinalis (chuanniuxi) 10g.

Xiaoji Niuxi formula in Chinese 小蓟牛膝汤:

蒲公英10g 紫花地丁10g 滑石20g 泽泻10g 泽漆10g 萆薢10g 瞿麦10g 车前草15g 山慈菇10g 小蓟10g 大蓟10g 地榆10g 赤芍10g 白芍10g 阿胶10g 甘草10g 土鳖虫10g 益母草15g 蒲黄10g 生地10g 熟地10g 天门冬10g 麦门冬10g 当归10g 肉桂10g 怀牛膝10g 川牛膝10g

Taraxacum officinale (pugongying 蒲公英) clears heat and detoxifies poison.

Viola yedoensis (zihuadiding 紫花地丁) clears heat, detoxifies poison, and dissolves swelling.

Talcum (huashi 滑石) isolates turbidity, extinguishes fire, and dissolves mucus.

Alisma orientalis (zexie 泽泻) removes stagnant water and creates fresh water, promotes urine flow, dissolves water retention, drains dampness, and quenches thirst.

Euphorbia helioscopia (zeqi 泽漆) promotes water flow, dissolves mucus, and reduces fever.

Dioscorea septemloba (bixie 萆薢) clears heat, removes dampness, and promotes urine flow.

Dianthus superbus (jumai 瞿麦) clears heat, and promotes water flow.

Plantago asiatica (cheqiancao 车前草) opens water passages, clears heat, cools blood, detoxifies poison.

Cremastra appendiculata (shancigu 山慈菇) dissolves mucus and disperses poison.

Cirsium setosum (xiaoji 小蓟) cools blood, stops bleeding, detoxifies poison, and dissolves swelling.

Cirsium japonicum (daji 大蓟) cools blood, detoxifies poison, and dissolves carbuncles.

Sanguisorba officinalis (diyu 地榆) cools blood, drains dampness, and removes poison.

Paeoniae lactiflora (chishao 赤芍) removes build ups, eliminates blood stagnation.

Paeoniae alba (baishao 白芍) opens blood passages, dissolves swelling.

Colla corii asini (ejiao 阿胶) clears wind and poisons in the blood passage.

Glycyrrhiza radix (gancao 甘草) detoxifies poison.

Eupolyphaga sinensis (tubiechong 土鳖虫) breaks down blood stagnation, removes abdominal mass.

Leonurus japonicas (yimucao 益母草) invigorates blood, breaks down blood stagnation, and detoxifies poison.

Typha angustifolia (puhuang 蒲黄) promotes urine flow, dissolves blood stagnation.

Raw and cooked **Radix rehmanniae** (shengdi 生地 and shudi 熟

地) break down damp poison in the blood.

Asparagus cochinchinensis (tianmendong 天门冬) nurtures yin, creates water, and removes damp poison.

Ophiopogon japonicas (maimendong 麦门冬) nurtures yin, moves water downward, clears dampness.

Angelica sinensis (danggui 当归) harmonizes wuxing organs.

Cortex cinnamomi (rougui 肉桂) warms kidney water, opens blood passages, and ignites the effectiveness of all herbs.

Achyranthes bidentata (huainiuxi 怀牛膝) has a sour and bitter taste, and mild yinyang nature. It goes into the liver and kidney meridians. It disperses blood stagnation, reduces swelling, clears urine, and promotes urine flow. It treats cold and dampness that causes aching bones, and leads herbs to move downwards.

Cyathula officinalis (chuanniuxi 川牛膝) has a slightly bitter taste and mild yinyang nature. It goes into the liver and kidney meridians. It disperses wind, drains dampness, cleans urine, and promotes urine flow. It leads herbs to move downwards.

Within the Xiaoji Niuxi formula, Taraxacum officinale (pugongying), Viola yedoensis (zihuadiding) are used to clear heat and detoxify poison. Talcum (huashi) is used to isolate turbidity and remove dampness. Alisma orientalis (zexie), Euphorbia helioscopia (zeqi), Dioscorea septemloba (bixie), Dianthus superbus (jumai), Plantago asiatica (cheqiancao), Cremastra appendiculata (shancigu) are used to dissolve mucus, remove dampness, and free the urine passage. Cirsium setosum (xiaoji), Cirsium japonicum (daji), Sanguisorba officinalis (diyu), Paeoniae lactiflora(chishao), Paeoniae alba (baishao), Colla corii asini (ejiao), Glycyrrhiza (gancao) are used for cooling blood, detoxifying poison, and free blood passages. Eupolyphaga (tubiechong), Leonurus japonicas (yimucao), Typha angustifolia (puhuang) are used to break down stagnant blood. Raw and cooked Radix rehmanniae (shengdi, shudi), Asparagus cochinchinensis (tianmendong) Ophiopogon japonicas (maimendong) are used to nurture kidney water yin, create water, and remove dampness. Angelica sinensis (danggui), cortex cinnamomi (rougui) are used to free blood passages, harmonize wuxing organs, and maintain kidney water warmth. Achyranthes bidentata (huainiuxi) and Cyathula officinalis (chuanniuxi) are used to open the urine passage and lead other herbs downwards to the urine bladder.

Another 45-year-old man had frequent and urgent urine for 5 years. Each night he needed to get up four or five times to pass urine. The quantity of urine was never great, the flow was slow, and the colour was always dark with bubbles. The bubbles were an indication of kidney water yin deficiency and dampness in the urine passage. The treatment was the same as the above case. He took three packets of the Xiaoji Niuxi formula; his urine flow became easier, but he still got up three times a night to pass urine. After taking the herbs for ten days he got up to pass urine two to three times a night. He continued to take the herbs for three more months; by the end of this time he would only get up once a night to pass urine, the quantity was sufficient, and the colour had lightened.

Treating kidney water heat loss with symptoms of mood swings

I had a 65-year-old female patient who complained of anxiety and unhappiness. She said when she was about 50 years of age, she began to have hot flushes, loss of sleep, dry mouth, tiredness, back pain, and on and off feelings of anxiousness. Her anxieties were triggered by her husband's drinking habits. If she drove past a liquor shop her chest would become tight and she would begin to feel anxious. She had asked her husband to stop drinking alcohol, but the husband said that he never got drunk, drank only one bottle of beer a day and didn't see that as a problem. He felt his wife was picking on him, and he said if he stopped drinking she would have found something else to complain about him. The patient was upset that her husband would not help her and cooperate with her healing; so she began to review all the bad times that they had been through, and felt it was difficult to live together any longer. The patient's anxiety were certainly not rooted in her husband's beer drinking, but were symptoms of her own body's illness. I asked the patient not to argue with her husband at this stage, but to concentrate on improving her own health. Once she felt well again, then she would be able to make reasonable judgements about her relationship with her husband.

The kidney is a water organ; water is yin, and likes yang heat. Kidney water yang deficiency results in water not rising, so there is a symptom of dry mouth. Kidney water heat is the strength of life, insufficient heat makes one fatigued, and suffer back pain. When kidney water heat loss fails to moisten liver wood, the liver wood becomes dry. Liver wood is a reservoir of blood, dry liver wood means the blood reservoir is depleted and blood rushes out of the liver wood root. The hot blood fills the blood passages and causes hot flushes and night sweats. Dry liver wood also leads to overheated heart fire which disturbs the spirit's rest, so sleep is disturbed. With kidney water heat loss, the yang qi of the enduring zhi of the spirit has no energy to be carried through, so the spirit is fearful. The principle of treatment is to warm the kidney water, cool and nurture liver wood, and ground the heart fire. Once the body yinyang is in good order, the spirit will be able to make use of the body, and the mood swings will stop. The Erxian formula was used for these purposes.

After taking the herbs for six months, the patient's symptoms gradually subsided. At the end of the treatment, I asked her what she would do about the relationship with her husband and she replied with a little embarrassed smile: "actually, he is not that bad." Which means when the patient's body yinyang becomes in regular order, her thoughts changed and the emotional blockage opens up without needing other treatment.

Treating kidney water heat loss with symptoms of nightmares

Nightmares are reflections of spirit and body disharmony. In the day, spirit and body disharmony will cause people to have emotional discomfort such as sadness, fear, anger, worry or anxiety. At night, these emotions will manifest as unpleasant dreams, for example, if a person dreams of someone close who dies in the dream and wakes up sobbing this would indicate a condition where lung metal and spirit are not in harmony. A dream of a dark room, seeing a ghost and waking up shaking indicates kidney water and spirit are not in harmony. A dream of being bullied or angry is the liver wood and spirit have trouble together. A dream of being in a crowd and unable to find a way out is the spirit disharmony with the spleen soil. When spirit and heart fire are not in harmony, a person will not be able to sleep at all. The spirit and body disharmony can be relieved by regulating the body's yinyang orders to invite the spirit's closeness with the body.

I had a 65-year-old patient who suffered from nightmares and had come for help. The most frequent nightmares she had were about the Second World War, when as a small child she feared hearing bombs and air strikes. For a month or so, she would wake up every night as a result of such dreams and found herself sweating and shaking. The reason that she suddenly began to dream about such experiences after 60 years was because her body was experiencing the same spirit and kidney water disharmony as she had had during the war. During the war, her spirit was shocked and lost its intimacy with kidney water, so she had fear and shaking feelings. The current war dreams also indicated the loss of spirit and kidney water intimacy, but this time the yinyang disorder of kidney water caused the spirit's unease. In the first instance, the spirit and kidney water disharmony is of external cause; the latter one is of the body's yinyang disorder. For the externally caused spirit and body disharmony, once the external conditions change, in most case, people regained normal functioning without treating the body. For internal yinyang disorders that cause spirit and body disharmony, after the body's yinyang order is regulated, the harmony of spirit and body will be restored. For this patient, the treatment was with the Erxian formula to warm kidney water, clear liver wood heat and ground heart fire.

After taking seven days of the Erxian formula, the patient no longer had frightening nightmares.

Liver Wood

The liver is a wood organ, it has a nature of being erect and extending. Liver wood is also a yang organ, and is a storage for blood. As yang attracts yin, liver wood attracts yin water and becomes supple. Therefore, liver wood yang sustains the uprightness and firmness of the body while liver wood yin sustains the suppleness and flexibility of the body.

Liver wood stores blood, which nourishes and cleanses the body, clears away stagnation, and maintains the free flow of the body's yinyang passages. A strong liver wood yang makes the body erect, and holds up the blood passages so that the blood flow is free and fresh. A strong liver wood yin makes the body flexible, the blood passages pliable, and the blood flow gentle and smooth.

Because of the uprightness and supple nature of liver wood, the spirit relies on liver wood to exercise its striving zhi. When the spirit and liver wood are in good cooperation, a person is able to stand tall, shrink down, be straightforward and abiding. In short, liver wood enables a person to be erect and supple, it stores blood, nourishes and cleanses the body, and makes a person audacious.

Causes of liver wood yinyang disorder

Kidney water heat loss is the main reason for liver wood yin deficiency. When water is cold, wood cannot grow; when kidney water is cold and sluggish, it fails to moisten liver wood and causes liver wood dryness. A yin deficiency of liver wood leads to an inability to store blood, therefore blood rushes in the blood passages instead of being calmly stored inside the root of liver wood, and this causes heat in the blood.

Liver wood yang deficiency is mostly caused by eating food that has become spoiled, rancid etc., or which have artificial preservatives, colourings, etc. Rotten and chemically loaded food blocks the body yinyang passages, causes blood decay, and damages liver wood yang qi.

A liver wood yinyang disorder that fails to respond to the striving zhi of the spirit is often the cause of spirit anger or timidity.

Symptoms

Liver wood stores blood, a yin deficiency of liver wood means it is unable to store blood in its root, and hot blood rushes in the blood passages creating excessive body heat. Hot blood creates wind, wind damages or obstructs the blood and yinyang passages, which causes symptoms such as itching, or pain, or loss of balance. Liver wood yin deficiency also causes a person to lose their suppleness, which would exhibit symptoms such as tightness of the joints and muscles, and an inflexibility of movements. When liver wood yin is damaged and inflexible, the yin qi of the striving zhi is unable to be exercised, so it is firm but not gentle, and the spirit exhibits anger.

When there is liver wood yang damage, the blood storage and passages are unable to become full and erect, which congests blood flow, and causes decay and poison in the blood showing symptoms such as pussy swellings, ulcers, and sores. When there is liver wood yang damage, the body is unable to be erect, the yang qi of the striving zhi is deprived of being exercised, so the striving zhi is gentle but not firm, therefore the spirit exhibits timidity.

Overall, illnesses caused by liver wood yinyang disorder fall into three main areas: wind disorders, blood disorders, and spirit disorders.

Tongue

Liver wood contains blood. The yang qi of liver wood governs the erectness of the blood passages, so blood flow is free, which keeps blood fresh. The yin qi of liver wood governs the softness of the blood passages, so blood flow is gentle, and is cool. When the yinyang of the liver wood is in normal order, blood flows calmly and is fresh, so the tongue is pink and reddish. When the liver wood yin is weak, blood flows urgently and becomes hot and the tongue is a deep red. When the liver wood yang is damaged, blood flow is obstructed, and becomes stale, and the tongue is dull in colour.

Pulse

The yang of liver wood keeps erect the blood passages, the yin of liver wood softens the blood passages. When the yinyang of liver wood is in normal order, the pulse is elevated and soft. A yin deficiency of liver wood makes it lose its softness, so the left guan pulse is tight, which is like a balloon changing into a football, the skin of the balloon hardened and inelastic. When liver wood yin deficiency extends to heart fire and kidney water, the left cun, guan, and chi pulses become a tight line, like a string of a violin, which shows the unhappiness of the spirit as if trapped in a solid cage. When the liver wood yin deficiency extends to the lung metal, the right cun pulse is tight; when it extends to the spleen soil, the right guan pulse is tight; when it extends to the mingmen, the right chi pulse is tight. On the other hand, when liver wood yang is weak, the pulse loses its firmness, like a balloon without enough air to provide it with bounce, so the pulse is floppy. When the liver wood yang deficiency affects the other wuxing organs, the relevant pulse will become floppy.

Skin

Liver wood stores blood, when the yinyang of liver wood is in normal order, the blood is fresh, the skin is smooth with no discolouring or bumps. When there is liver wood yin deficiency, hot blood rushes in the blood passages, making the skin a deep red. With liver wood yang deficiency, the blood decays and is stagnant, the skin is discoloured, or jaundiced, and sometimes with rashes or sores.

Principles for treating liver wood yinyang disorder

The principle for treating liver wood yin deficiency is to warm kidney water to moisten and strengthen the liver wood yin, and to cool the blood. The principle for treating liver wood yang deficiency is to invigorate blood, detoxify poison, clear dampness, and remove mucus. It is like reviving an unhealthy tree, trimming out its old branches, stems, and dead leaves to allow the yang qi to spread. Liver wood yang damage is often accompanied with some degree of yin deficiency, so while invigorating blood, it is often necessary to clear dampness, cool blood, or warm kidney water to nurture liver wood.

Treating liver wood yin deficiency with symptoms of spasms

Liver wood is a yang organ; over exhaustion will drain its water yin and make it dry. It is like an overgrown tree where the water becomes insufficient to support it, so the leaves will fall. As such, the air flow becomes harsh and turns into wind. Liver wood is the blood storage; dry liver wood means that blood cannot store in its root but is pushed out into the blood passages, which causes blood heat. Hot blood will create wind, like a fire that attracts cold air and creates wind. Internal wind damages the yinyang passages, which causes a disordering of the transformation of wuxing organs, and makes a person ill.

A 30-year-old female patient often felt anxious and had headaches. When she became too tired or worried, she would suffer convulsions in which her muscles and sinews would tighten and her body shake. She would froth at the mouth and lose consciousness. For over ten years she had been taking pharmaceutical drugs to control the symptoms.

This case was diagnosed as liver wood yin deficiency. Because a lack of yin causes the liver wood to become inflexible, so the muscles and sinews tighten up. The dry liver wood fails to store blood in its root. Hot blood rushing in the blood passages causes wind, so there is a symptom of shaking. Frothing at the mouth is effluent dry blood blown out by wind. Loss of consciousness is a symptom of extreme dryness of liver wood causing the over burning of heart fire forcing the spirit to leave the body. Although the main symptoms are the liver wood yin deficiency, in the wuxing cycle, it is kidney water that nourishes liver wood. Mental and physical exertion both demand yang qi. When kidney water has low yang qi reserves then a person will easily tire. When kidney water heat is further exhausted then liver wood becomes extremely dry and internal wind begins to rise, so convulsions occur. The treatment for this case is to warm kidney water to soften liver wood, at the same time, cool the blood heat, ground heart fire, and calm the spirit. I used the Erxian Hupo formula.

After taking seven packets of the herbs, the patient felt happier. She took another seven packets of the herbs and stopped her pharmaceutical medication without problem. From thereon, she would take three packets of the herbs whenever she felt unwell such as during symptoms of tiredness or headache. On and off she took the herbs for a year without recurrence of the convulsions or loss of consciousness.

Erxian Hupo formula:

Epimedium brevicornum (yinyanghuo) 30g
Rhizoma curculiginis orchioides (xianmao) 15g
Radix morindae officinalis (bajitian) 15g
Polygala tenufola (yuanzhi) 10g
Angelica sinensis (danggui) 20g
Rhizome anemarrhenae (zhimu) 10g
Phellodendri chinensis (huangbai) 10g
Gentiana scabra (longdancao) 30g
Polygoni multiflori (yejiaoteng) 30g
Zizyphus jujube (fried) (chao suanzaoren) 15g
Concha margaritifera (zhenzhumu) 30g
Concha haliotidis (shijueming) 30g
Concha ostreae (muli) 30g
Ossa draconis (longgu) 30g
Amber (hupo) 10g
Panax ginseng (renshen) 30g

Erxian Hupo formula in Chinese二仙琥珀汤:

淫羊藿30g 仙茅15g 巴戟天15g 远志10g 当归20g 知母10g 黄柏10g 龙胆草30g 夜交藤30g 炒枣仁15g 珍珠母30g 石决明30g 牡蛎30g 龙骨30g 琥珀10g 人参30g。

The Erxian Hupo formula is the Erxian formula with the addition of amber and ginseng.

Amber (hupo 琥珀) has a slightly sweet and plain taste, and mild yinyang nature. It goes into the heart and liver meridians. It harmonizes all the wuxing organs, and calms the spirit.

Panax ginseng (renshen 人参) has a sweet taste and warm yinyang nature. It goes into the kidney meridian. It warms kidney water and calms the spirit in all wuxing organs.

Treating liver wood yin deficiency with symptoms of hyperactivity

I had a seven-year-old boy brought to me because of his restlessness. The boy complained that he felt upset, had nightmares and was always thirsty. He was told by the school to leave as he was disturbing the class. The mother said the boy was easily upset, he could not sit or stand still for a minute, he had little appetite and had not been growing. The boy had a heavily coated tongue. When I asked the boy not to drink soft drinks, his mother worried that if he weren't allowed to have soft drinks that the boy might become dehydrated since he never liked to drink water. I told the mother not to worry about the boy being dehydrated, if he didn't want to drink she shouldn't make him drink, after a while when he really became thirsty he would drink water.

This case was diagnosed as liver wood yin deficiency. Because when liver wood yin is deficient, it is dry which means that blood runs out of its storage and rushes in the blood passages, which creates heat and wind. It is like wind blowing around, so he was hyperactive. When liver wood is dry and inflexible, the yin qi of the striving zhi of the spirit is unable to be exercised, and becomes too harsh, so he was easily angry. Although the direct problem is the liver wood yin deficiency, a major factor is that the white sugar in soft drinks causes the kidney water heat loss which in turn fails to moisten liver wood. Because of the kidney water heat loss, the patient's growth was stunted. Also, with kidney water heat loss, water could not rise so he felt thirsty. As there was kidney water heat loss, and the yang qi of the enduring zhi of the spirit was unable to be carried out, so the spirit was afraid, and the boy often had nightmares. White sugar creates dampness and mucus which causes the spleen soil to be impermeable and leads to the symptoms of low appetite and thick coating on the tongue. Treatment was to warm kidney water, soften liver wood, and ground heart fire with the Erxian formula. As for the spleen soil dampness, once the patient stopped the sugar intake, the spleen soil dampness could recover without further treatment.

After taking seven days of the herbs and avoiding sweet drinks and food, the boy said water was sweet and he did not mind drinking it. After six months of taking the herbs on and off, the boy's appetite increased, his general behaviour was better, he was no longer disruptive in class, and the school no longer asked him to leave.

Most of the so-called hyperactive patients I have encountered suffered similar symptoms to the above case, once they stopped consuming white sugar, and took the Erxian formula for a month or two, they all recovered as expected.

Treating liver wood yin deficiency with symptoms of headache

A 48-year-old female patient saw me and complained of severe headaches. Over a period of four months, she would experience headaches a week before her menses and the headaches were persisting longer and getting worse with each month. She was worried that she had developed a brain tumour, and this feeling tended to disrupt her sleep.

This case was diagnosed as liver wood yin deficiency causing headache, because around period time, more blood flows out of liver wood, and if the liver wood is already dry, this means more blood is in the blood passages rather than stored in the root of liver wood. This extra blood that gets into the blood passages would cause the blood to overheat and create wind. Strong wind rushes up to the head then causes severe headache. This is how the headache would be more obvious around the time of her period. Then again, as kidney water governs reproduction, headaches around the time of her menses indicates that kidney water heat is insufficient, and that there are obstructions to the menses cycle. Also kidney water heat loss causes liver wood to lack moistness, which then causes the blood to rush in the blood passages creating wind and headache. Therefore, the direct cause of the headache is the liver wood yin deficiency, but the kidney water heat loss results in liver wood yin deficiency. The treatment then is to warm kidney water, soften liver wood, cease wind, and stop headaches with the Erxian Xiongzhi formula.

After the first dose of herbs the patient's headache stopped immediately. She took another six days of the herbs and as she no longer had headaches she stopped the herbs. A year later she had the headaches again. She took another seven days of the herbs, the headaches ceased, and she didn't have a recurrence of the headaches.

Erxian Xiongzhi formula:

Epimedium brevicornum (yinyanghuo) 30g
Rhizoma curculiginis orchioides (xianmao) 15g
Radix morindae officinalis (bajitian) 15g
Polygala tenufola (yuanzhi) 10g
Angelica sinensis (danggui) 20g
Rhizome anemarrhenae (zhimu) 10g
Phellodendri chinensis (huangbai) 10g
Gentiana scabra (longdancao) 30g
Polygoni multiflori (yejiaoteng)
30g
Zizyphus jujube (fried)(chao suanzaoren) 15g
Concha margaritifera (zhenzhumu) 30g
Concha haliotidis (shijueming) 30g
Concha ostreae (muli) 30g
Ossa draconis (longgu) 30g
Angelica dahurica (baizhi) 15g
Gastrodia elata (tianma) 15g
Uncaria rhynchophylla (gouteng) 15g
Ligusticum wallichii (chuanxiong) 10g

Erxian Xiongzhi formula in Chinese 二仙芎芷汤:

淫羊藿30g 仙茅15g 巴戟天15g 远志10g 当归20g 知母10g 黄柏10g 龙胆草30g 夜交藤30g 酸枣仁15g 珍珠母30g 石决明30g 牡蛎30g 龙骨30g 白芷15g 天麻15g 钩藤15g 川芎10g

The Erxian Xiongzhi formula is based on the Erxian formula with the addition of Angelica dahurica (baizhi), Gastrodia elata (tianma), Uncaria rhynchophylla (gouteng), and Ligusticum wallichii (chuanxiong) to open apertures and lead herbs towards the head to stop headaches.

Angelica dahurica (baizhi 白芷) has a pungent taste and warm yinyang nature. It goes into lung and liver meridians. Its pungent nature goes up to the head. It opens nasal apertures, stops wind and headaches.
Gastrodia elata (tianma 天麻) has a pungent taste and warm yinyang nature. It goes into the liver meridian. It clears liver wood,

stops wind, and leads herbs towards the head.

Uncaria rhynchophylla (gouteng 钩藤) has a sweet taste and slightly cold yinyang nature. It goes into the liver meridian. It clears liver wood, stops wind, and leads herbs upward to the head.

Ligusticum wallichii (chuanxiong 川芎) has a pungent taste and warm yinyang nature. It goes into the liver meridian. It disperses wind, smooths qi flow, clears heat, and leads herbs up to the head.

Sometimes, people suffer persistent headaches without seeming to have other obvious symptoms to help identify which wuxing organs' yinyang disorder is responsible for the cause of headaches, however, the tongue and pulse can always give reliable clues. I treated a 38-year-old man who had headaches for as long as he could remember. In fact, he said he didn't know what it was like to be without a headache. When the pain became unbearable, in order to cope, he would take a painkiller. He could not relate the headaches to anything else. It seemed that apart from headaches he didn't have any other physical complaints. When I felt his pulse, his left hand side pulse was quite tight, and his tongue was red. On the left hand side are the heart, liver and kidney pulses. The tight pulse meant the liver wood was dry and it had already affected the heart fire and kidney water. The red tongue indicated that his liver wood was hot. No other symptoms could mean that his yinyang disorder was at the periphery rather than at the root of the wuxing organ. For treatment I used the above Erxian Xiongzhi formula.

Because the patient didn't know whether he could cope with the taste of the herbs, I gave him only three packets of the herbs to try. Six months later the patient came back and said he hadn't had a headache since he took the three packets of the herbs. But in the previous two days he had the headaches again so I prescribed for him another ten days of the same herbs to ensure the disorder was completely regulated.

Treating liver wood yin & yang damage with symptoms of zhongfeng (struck by wind)

Liver wood is blood storage; the yin deficiency of liver wood causes blood heat and wind; the yang deficiency of liver wood causes damp poison to flourish in the blood. Therefore, blood heat and wind

101

symptoms indicate liver wood yin deficiency; blood poison symptoms anywhere in the body indicate liver wood yang damage. The principles for treating blood heat and wind are to cool blood; the principle to treat blood poison is to invigorate blood, remove dampness, and detoxify poison.

Zhongfeng or "struck by wind" is a condition where liver wood is extremely dry, blood becomes very hot, and strong wind forces blood to flow exceedingly fast out of its passages. One of my patients was a 73-year-old woman who had had an attack by wind (zhongfeng) in her head three years prior to seeing me. The woman had been taking blood pressure tablets for 20 years including one to enlarge the blood vessels, one to drain fluid out of her blood, and one to slow her heart rate; nevertheless, she still suffered a stroke (zhongfeng) while religiously taking the pills. During her first consultation with me, she fell asleep, and her tongue, which was a dull colour, drooped out of her mouth. Her family said that she was constantly sleepy. She suffered from slurred speech, could not walk without someone holding her arm and could not look after herself. Since the attack of zhongfeng, she was on heavier does of the drugs to control her blood pressure.

After the zhongfeng, blood rushed out of the blood passages and liver wood yang qi also leaked out. Liver wood yang governs the body's erectness. The liver wood yang damage affected both her ability to straighten her body and to keep her body balance. Stagnant blood obstructing the blood passages creates dampness and mucus, so her tongue colour was dull and she could not move the tongue freely, which restricted her speech. With kidney water yang heat deficiency, the tongue loses its strength to hold back, so her tongue was big and stretched out. The overload of chemical drugs blocked her spirit and body's interaction, so she was always sleepy.

The treatment was to warm kidney water, soften liver wood, cease wind; also to invigorate blood, remove stagnation, and dissolve mucus. I used the Erxian Rumo formula.

After taking the herbs for three months, all the symptoms improved and she began to reduce her pharmaceutical drugs. After a year of taking the herbs, she stopped all the pharmaceutical drugs and had good energy. She no longer needed help to walk, and could take care of her own household tasks and spoke without slurring.

Erxian Rumo formula:

Epimedium brevicornum (yinyanghuo) 30g
Rhizoma curculiginis orchioides (xianmao) 15g
Radix morindae officinalis (bajitian) 15g
Polygala tenufola (yuanzhi) 10g
Angelica sinensis (danggui) 20g
Rhizome anemarrhenae (zhimu) 10g
Phellodendri chinensis (huangbai) 10g
Gentiana scabra (longdancao) 30g
Polygoni multiflori (yejiaoteng) 30g
Zizyphus jujube (fried) (chao suanzaoren) 15g
Concha margaritifera (zhenzhumu) 30g
Concha haliotidis (shijueming) 30g
Concha ostreae (muli) 30g
Ossa draconis (longgu) 30g
Gastrodia elata (tianma) 10g
Ligusticum wallichi (chuanxiong) 10g
Olibanum (ruxiang) 5g
Myrrh (moyao) 5g
Panax pseudoginseng (sanqi) 10g

Erxian Rumo formula in Chinese 二仙乳没汤:

淫羊藿30g 仙茅15g 巴戟天15g 远志10g 当归20g 知母10g 黄柏10g 龙胆草30g 夜交藤30g 炒枣仁15g 珍珠母30g 石决明30g 牡蛎30g 龙骨30g天麻10g 川芎10g 乳香5g 没药5g 三七粉10

The Erxian Rumo formula is the Erxian formula with the addition of Gastrodia elata (tianma), Ligusticum wallichi (chuanxiong), Olibanum (ruxiang), Myrrh (moyao), and Panax pseudoginseng (sanqi).

Gastrodia elata (tianma 天麻) clears liver wood, stops wind, and leads herbs to the head.
Ligusticum wallichii (chuanxiong 川芎) disperses wind, smooths qi flow, clears heat, and leads herbs up to the head.
Olibanum (ruxiang 乳香) invigorates blood, eliminates carbuncles and boils; it reduces poisonous swellings, and detoxifies damp poison in the blood.
Myrrh (moyao 没药) invigorates blood, disperses blood stasis, breaks down nodules, reduces swelling, eliminates dampness, and detoxifies poison.
Panax pseudoginseng (sanqi 三七) has a sweet and slightly bitter

taste, and a mild yinyang nature. It goes into the liver and stomach meridians. It removes stagnant blood, and regenerates fresh blood.

In the Erxian Rumo formula, while the Erxian formula warms kidney water, clears liver heat, grounds heart fire; Gastrodia elata (tianma), Ligusticum wallichi (chuanxiong) are used to stop wind; Olibanum (ruxiang), Myrrh (moyao) and Panax pseudoginseng (sanqi) are used for invigorating blood and breaking down blood stasis.

Another female patient who was 58 years of age had been taking blood pressure tablets for more than ten years. When she had her first consultation with me, she had, a week earlier, suffered an attack of zhongfeng. She had headaches, the left side of her face was slightly paralysed and her speech was slurred. After taking three months of the Erxian Rumo formula, she no longer had any facial paralysis, nor headaches and her speech was fine.

Treating liver wood yin & yang damage with symptoms of wind rash

A 23-year-old woman came for help with severe skin rashes. At the first consultation, it was the second day that she had had the rash. The patient's whole body was covered with light reddish lumps. The redness disappeared when pressed. Her face was swollen and she could not open her eyes properly. Her feet were swollen and she could not wear her normal shoes. The swelling of the rash was worse between late afternoon to the following morning. During the hours around midday the swelling subsided somewhat. She suffered waves of unbearable itch, loss of appetite and sometimes even vomited. She first experienced the rash after she had taken antibiotics for three months to treat severe diarrhoea. Over the following three years she then frequently had occurrences of such rashes. During those three years she took antihistamines to control the condition, but in the last six months, the rashes had become more frequent and more severe. For the previous two occurrences she even resorted to taking steroids to control the rashes.

Liver wood yang damage causes damp poison in the blood passages, and the long standing dampness would build up to create heat and wind. Damp poison damages liver wood yin, and exacerbates blood heat and wind. Wind causes qi to block the blood passages, so the body had lumps. Wind is naturally unsteady, and wind rashes come and go fitfully. The light colour of the rash indicates the lumps are air stagnation; when the air is pushed aside, then the colour of the rash disappears. During the day yang qi is dominant in the outside environment, which supports the damaged liver wood yang qi, and suppresses the damp poison, so the wind eases, and the rash is less severe. In wuxing cycle, liver wood binds the spleen soil, when liver wood yin and yang are damaged, the spleen soil loses its binding and bearing ability, so it is unable to accept food. It is similar to when hillsides are cleared of trees, which then leads to landslides and damaged soil, which in turn loses the carrying and transforming capabilities. The principle of treatment is to remove damp poison to support liver wood yang, to cool blood to support liver wood yin, and cease wind. For treatment I used the Zijingpi formula.

An hour after taking the first cup of the herbs, the rash had significantly subsided, and the itchiness was improved. Four hours later the patient took the second cup of the herbs, and the rash was further reduced. The following day there were still rash marks, and slight swelling, however the itching had further reduced. The patient felt hungry and enjoyed her meal without vomiting. As expected her bowel motion was loose. After finishing the second packet of herbs, the rash had completely disappeared. When I told the patient to avoid sweets and sugary food, she said that she suffered a sweet tooth, and had been eating a lot of chocolate. Six months later the patient came back for a consultation, she had not been eating chocolate or other sweet food, and she had been completely free of any rashes.

Zijingpi formula:

Schizonepetae herba (jingjie) 15g
Saposhnikouia diuaricata (fangfeng) 15g
Cryptotympana pustulata (chanyi) 15g
Gypsum (shigao) 20g
Paeoniae lactiflora (chishao) 30g
Paeonia suffruticosa (mudanpi) 15g
Lium usitatissimum (humaren) 10g
Cercis chinensis (zijingpi) 15g
Pseudolarix amailis (tujingpi) 5g
Rheum officinale (dahuang) 10g

Zijingpi formula in Chinese 紫荆皮汤:

荆芥15g 防风15g 蝉衣15g 石膏20g 赤芍30g 牡丹皮15g 胡麻仁10g 紫荆皮15g 土荆皮5g 大黄10g

Nepeta cataria (jingjie 荆芥) has a pungent taste and warm yinyang nature. It goes into the lung and liver meridians. It opens the lung breathing passages, breaks down stagnated qi, discharges blood stagnation, removes dampness, and frees joints.

Saposhnikovia divaricate (fangfeng 防风) has a sweet taste and warm yinyang nature. It goes into the lung and spleen meridians. It opens meridians, disperses wind in all wuxing organs.

Periostracum cicadae (chanyi 蝉衣) has a sweet taste and cool yinyang nature. It goes into lung and liver meridians. It cools blood, ceases wind, and draws out poison.

Gypsum (shigao 石膏) isolates turbidity and removes dampness.

Paeonia lactiflora (chishao 赤芍) cools blood, removes nodules, disperses blood stagnation, breaks down wind and swelling in the large intestine.

Paeonia suffruticosa (mudanpi 牡丹皮) has a pungent taste and cold yinyang nature, it goes into the liver and kidney meridians. It cools blood, breaks down nodules, and removes blood stagnation in the stomach and large intestine.

Lium usitatissimum (humaren 胡麻仁) has a sweet taste and mild yinyang nature. It goes into the liver meridian. It cools blood, detoxifies poison, clears turbidity, removes dampness, and opens bowel motions.

Cercis chinensis (zijingpi 紫荆皮) has a bitter taste and mild yinyang nature. It goes into the liver and spleen meridians. It cools blood, dissolves swelling, clears liver wood, detoxifies poison, and opens bowel motions.

Pseudolarix amailis (tujingpi 土荆皮) has a pungent taste and warm yinyang nature. It goes into the spleen and lung meridians. It invigorates blood, eliminates parasites, removes dampness, cleanses mucus, and stops itchiness. It also has a strong effect on opening bowel motions.

Rheum officinale (dahuang 大黄) cools blood, detoxifies poison, breaks down stagnation, opens bowel motions, and removes dampness.

In the Zijingpi formula each herb contributes to removing dampness, cooling blood, and detoxifying poison. The herbs that remove dampness and detoxify poison relieve the symptoms of the rash and itching, but primarily the herbs act to strengthen liver wood yin and yang qi, which in turn deals with the root cause of the condition. Schizonepetae herba (jingjie), Saposhnikouia diuaricata (fangfeng), Cryptotympana pustulata (chanyi) also promote qi flow and stop wind. Gypsum (shigao) also isolates turbidity. Paeoniae lactiflora (chishao), Paeonia suffruticosa (mudanpi), Lium usitatissimum (humaren), Cercis chinensis (zijingpi), Pseudolarix amailis (tujingpi) and Rheum officinale (dahuang) also open bowel motions and expel poisons.

Preparation and taking the herbs:

Place a packet of Zijingpi formula in a pot and add 1 litre (4 cups) of cold water, bring the herbs to boil and keep boiling for an hour until there is around 500 ml (2 cups) of liquid left. Drain the liquid out into a jug/container and discard the dregs. Drink 250 ml (1 cup) of the decoction. This formula is likely to cause loose bowel motions, however, if the loose bowel is too discomforting then the decoction can be reduced, eg., twice each day, but each time only 125 ml.

Another case was a 59-year-old man who had a dry skin rash on his neck for two years. The rash was thick and rough with peeling dry skin, but was only occasionally itchy. A month before his visit, there appeared over the original rash a smaller redder rash with small millet-sized red dots of clear and sticky discharge, it was itchy on and off. When he came for a consultation, for the previous two days, he had been suffering from hives that covered his body, affecting his legs, hips, shoulders, and chest. The colour was light reddish and went away when pressed. The patient was now also suffering from waves of severe itch.

In the beginning, it was liver wood yang damage with dampness in the blood causing skin damage, so the rash appeared. The thick and rough skin indicated the dampness had thickened and had become mucus. Later, the stagnation of dampness and mucus caused heat, and damaged liver wood yin, so there were small red rashes with discharge on the top of the thick skin rash. Heat then caused wind, so a wind rash developed. The treatment aimed to remove mucus, clear dampness, cool blood, and cease wind. The prescription I used was the Tujing Biechong formula.

After taking the first packet of herbs, the patient had ten incidents of watery bowel motions during the day, and slight stomach pains which disappeared after each bowel motion. His rash was slightly improved. After taking two packets of the herbs, all his rashes were significantly improved. The smaller red rash with sticky discharge dried up and the colour of the rashes was lighter. The larger lumpy rash disappeared but returned with some small lumps on and off. After taking the third packets of the herbs, all the rashes disappeared.

Tujing Biechong:

Schizonepetae herba (jingjie) 15g

Saposhnikouia diuaricata (fangfeng) 15g

Cryptotympana pustulata (chanyi) 15g

Gypsum (shigao) 20g

Paeoniae lactiflora (chishao) 30g

Paeonia suffruticosa (mudanpi) 15g

Lium usitatissimum (humaren) 10g

Pseudolarix amailis (tujingpi) 10g

Smilax glabra (tufuling) 20g

Cortex dictamni (baixianpi) 15g

Kochia scoparia (difuzi) 15g

Scolopendra subspinipes (wugong) $\frac{1}{2}$ piece (i.e. 5-6 cm)

Eupolyphaga (tubiechong) 10g

Mesobuthus martensii (quanxie) 10g

Talcum (huashi) 20g

Radix rehmanniae (raw) (shengdi) 10g

Radix rehmanniae (cooked) (shudi) 10g

Ophiopogon japonicas (maimendong) 10g

Asparagus cochinchinensis (tianmendong) 10g

Glycyrrhiza radix (gancao) 10g

Tujing Biechong Formula in Chinese: 土荆鳖虫汤:

荆芥15g 防风15g 蝉衣15g 石膏20g 赤芍30g 牡丹皮15g 胡麻仁10g 土荆皮10g 土茯苓20g 白鲜皮15g 地肤子15g 蜈蚣1/2 土鳖虫10g 全

蝎10g 滑石20g 生地10g 熟地10g 麦冬10g 天冬10g 甘草10g

The Tujing Biechong formula is a modification of Zijingpi formula. This case of wind rash shows more severe evidence of mucus and dampness. Pseudolarix amailis (tujingpi) has a strong effect on removing dampness and mucus, and stops itchiness, so the dosage was increased from 5 grams to 10 grams; the extra 5 grams of Pseudolarix amailis (tujingpi) has more effect on cooling blood than 15 grams of Cercis chinensis (zijingpi), so I removed Cercis chinensis (zijingpi). Pseudolarix amailis (tujingpi) also has a very strong effect on opening bowel motions, 10 grams of it can make one have very loose bowels; and Rheum officinale (dahuang) also has a strong effect on opening bowel motions. To avoid too much discomfort with bowel motions, the Tujing Biechong formula omitted Rheum officinale (dahuang). Then I added Smilax glabra (tufuling) Cortex dictamni (baixianpi) Kochia scoparia (difuzi), Scolopendra subspinipes (wugong), Eupolyphaga (tubiechong), Mesobuthus martensii (quanxie), Talcum (huashi), raw and cooked Radix rehmanniae (shengdi, shudi), Ophiopogon japonicas (maimendong), Asparagus cochinchinensis (tianmendong), Glycyrrhiza radix (gancao).

Smilax glabra (tufuling 土茯苓) opens meridians, removes dampness,clears liver wood, detoxifies poison, heals malignant sores.
Cortex dictamni (baixianpi 白鲜皮) has a salty taste and cold yinyang nature. It goes into the spleen, stomach and urine bladder meridians. It removes dampness, clears heat, ceases wind, clears liver wood, and detoxifies poison.
Kochia scoparia (difuzi 地肤子) has a bitter taste and cold yinyang nature. It goes into the kidney and urine bladder meridians. It clears heat, moistens skin, drains dampness, clears liver wood, and detoxifies poison.
Scolopendra subspinipes (wugong 蜈蚣) has a pungent taste and warm yinyang nature. It goes into the liver meridian. It breaks down cold or hot stagnations, dissolves blood mucus and dampness, clears liver wood, and detoxifies poisons.
Eupolyphaga (tubiechong 土鳖虫) breaks down blood stagnation, eliminates lumps, and dissolves stubborn stagnations.
Mesobuthus martensii (quanxie 全蝎) has a pungent taste and

mild yinyang nature, it goes into the liver meridian. It opens orifices, dissolves mucus, and ceases wind.

Talcum (huashi 滑石) isolates turbidity, clears heat, and dissolves mucus.

Raw and cooked Radix rehmanniae (shengdi 生地, shudi 熟地) refresh liver wood, break down dampness and poison in the blood.

Ophiopogon japonicas (maimendong 麦门冬) has a sweet taste and mild yinyang nature. It goes into the lung meridian. It nurtures yin, creates water, and removes dampness.

Asparagus cochinchinensis (tianmendong 天门冬) has a sweet taste and cold yinyang nature, it goes into the lung meridian. It nurtures yin, cultivates water, drains dampness, clears liver wood, and detoxifies poison.

Glycyrrhiza radix (gancao 甘草) harmonizes the wuxing organs, and detoxifies poison.

Within the Tujing Biechong formula, the Zijingpi formula clears dampness, detoxifies poison, cools blood, and stops wind. By adding Smilax glabra (tufuling), Cortex dictamni (baixianpi), Kochia scoparia (difuzi) the effect of draining dampness is strengthened. Adding Scolopendra subspinipes (wugong), Eupolyphaga (tubiechong) can soften and disperse hard nodules, and remove mucus in the blood. Mesobuthus martensii (quanxie) was added to strengthen the effect of stopping wind. Talcum (huashi) was added to isolate turbidity and make it easier to be removed. Raw and cooked Radix rehmanniae (shengdi, shudi), Ophiopogon japonicas (maimendong), Asparagus cochinchinensis (tianmendong) are used to cultivate water to soften and cleanse mucus. Glycyrrhiza (gancao) was added to harmonize the wuxing organs and detoxify poison.

Treating liver wood yin & yang damage with symptoms of wind pain in the joints

A 56-year-old male patient was woken up by throbbing pain in his right knee. The same day he came for a consultation. At the time, his right knee was obviously swollen, red, and hot to touch. The patient was also experiencing severe throbbing joint pains.

Wind pain in the joints is caused by liver wood yin and yang damage as a result of dampness, mucus, and heat blocking the blood passages. As liver wood stores blood, when the liver wood yin is damaged, blood rushes out of the liver wood and becomes hot, therefore the damaged joint was red and hot to touch. Blood heat creates wind, wind moves fast, therefore, the pain came suddenly. With liver wood yang damage, blood is trapped and allows dampness and mucus to flourish. The dampness and mucus block the flow of blood, the wind strikes the blockages and so there is throbbing pain.

The treatment was to cool blood, cease wind, dissolve dampness and mucus, detoxify poison, and open the meridians with the Magui formula.

After taking one packet of the herbs, the patient reported that the redness, swelling, and pain in his joints were significantly reduced. He took seven packets of the herbs and he recovered completely.

Magui formula:

Gypsum (shigao) 20g
Rhizoma anemarrhenae (zhimu) 10g
Atractylodis lancea (cangzhu) 10g
Atractylodis macrocephalae (baizhu) 10g
Semen coicis (yiyiren) 15g
Scutellaria baicalensis (huangqin) 10g
Coptis chinensis (huanglian) 10g
Cortex phellodendri (huangbai) 10g
Cinnamomum cassia (guizhi) 10g
Ephedra sinica (mahuang) 10g
Caulis Lonicerae japonicae (jinyinhuateng) 30g
Uncaria rhynchophylla (gouteng) 15g
Clematis chinensis (weilingxian) 15g
Morus alba (sangzhi) 10g
Notopterygium incisum (qianghuo) 10g
Angelica pubescentis (duhuo) 10g
Trachelospermum jasminoides (luoshiteng) 30g
Sarcandra glabra (zhongjiefeng) 15g
Tripterygium wilfordii (leigongteng) 10g
Paeoniae lactiflora (chishao) 10g
Radix Paeoniae alba (baishao) 10g
Glycyrrhiza radix (gancao) 10g

Magui formula in Chinese 麻桂汤:

石膏20g 知母10g 苍术10g 白术10g 薏苡仁15g 黄芩10g 黄连10g 黄柏10g 桂枝10g 麻黄10g 金银花藤30g 钩藤15g 威灵仙15g 桑枝10g 羌活10g 独活10g 络石藤30g 肿节风15g 雷公藤10g 赤芍10g 白芍10g 甘草10g

Gypsum (shigao 石膏) clears heat, isolates turbidity, and removes dampness.

Rhizoma anemarrhenae (zhimu 知母) opens the lung breathing passages, drains dampness, and removes turbidity.

Atractylodis lancea (cangzhu 苍术) removes poisonous qi and dissolves mucus and dampness.

Atractylodis macrocephalae (baizhu 白术) removes head wind, guards the body surface, and removes dampness and mucus.

Semen coicis (yiyiren 薏苡仁) has a sweet taste and mild yinyang nature. It goes into the liver, spleen and kidney meridians. It removes dampness, eases water flow, and opens meridians.

Scutellaria baicalensis (huangqin黄芩) disperses wind, clears heat, removes dampness, detoxifies poison, and dissolves swelling.

Coptis chinensis (huanglian 黄连) extinguishes fire heat, detoxifies poison, dries dampness, and cools blood.

Cortex phellodendri (huangbai 黄柏) clears heat, dries dampness, and detoxifies poison.

Cinnamomum cassia (guizhi 桂枝) expels poisonous qi in the skin, relaxes skin and flesh, opens meridians.

Ephedra sinica (mahuang 麻黄) has a pungent taste and warm yinyang nature. It goes into the lung meridian. It relaxes skin and flesh, removes poisonous qi from all the wuxing organs, and opens blood passages.

Caulis Lonicerae japonicae (jinyinhuateng 金银花藤) has a sweet taste and cool yinyang nature. It goes into the lung meridian. It opens the lung breathing passages, eases water flow, disperses wind, removes mucus, and opens meridians.

Uncaria rhynchophylla (gouteng 钩藤) clears liver wood, ceases wind, and opens the meridians.

Clematis chinensis (weilingxian 威灵仙) has a pungent taste and warm yinyang nature. It goes into the urine bladder meridian. It disperses all forms of wind, opens the wuxing organ yinyang passages, disperses cold stagnation, removes dampness, and opens meridians.

Morus alba (sangzhi 桑枝) has a slightly bitter taste and mild yinyang nature. It goes into the liver meridian. It promotes water flow, disperses wind, and frees joints.

Notopterygium incisum (qianghuo 羌活) has a pungent taste and warm yinyang nature. It goes into the urine bladder and liver meridians. It disperses wind, opens meridians, stops headache and joint pain.

Angelica pubescentis (duhuo 独活) has a sweet taste and warm yinyang nature. It goes into the kidney and liver meridians. It disperses wind, removes dampness, scatters cold, and treats wind pain in the joints.

Trachelospermum jasminoides (luoshiteng 络石藤) has a slightly sweet taste and mild yinyang nature. It goes into the liver and kidney meridians. It disperses wind, eases water flow, invigorates blood, and opens meridians.

Sarcandra glabra (zhongjiefeng 肿节风) has a bitter taste and mild yinyang nature. It goes into the heart and liver meridians. It disperses wind, opens meridians, invigorates blood, and dissolves swelling.

Tripterygium wilfordii (leigongteng 雷公藤) has a bitter taste, and cold yinyang nature. It goes into the heart and liver meridians. It disperses wind, invigorates blood, open meridians, dissolves swelling, and stops pain.

Paeoniae Lactiflora (chishao 赤芍) cools blood, disperses wind, removes build ups, and disperses blood stagnation.

Paeoniae alba (baishao 白芍) smooths liver wood tension, opens blood passages, and dissolves swelling.

Glycyrrhiza radix (gancao 甘草) harmonizes the wuxing organs and detoxifies poison.

In the formula, Gypsum (shigao), Rhizoma anemarrhenae (zhimu), Atractylodis lancea (cangzhu), Atractylodis macrocephalae (baizhu), Semen coicis (yiyiren) are used to remove dampness and dissolve turbidity. Scutellaria baicalensis (huangqin), Coptis chinensis (huanglian), Cortex phellodendri (huangbai) are used to clear heat and dry dampness. Cinnamomum cassia (guizhi) , Ephedra sinica (mahuang), Caulis Lonicerae japonicae (jinyinhuateng), Uncaria rhynchophylla (gouteng), Clematis chinensis (weilingxian), Morus alba (sangzhi), Notopterygium incisum (qianghuo), Angelica pubescentis (duhuo) are used to disperse wind, open meridians, free joints; Trachelospermum jasminoides (luoshiteng), Sarcandra glabra (zhongjiefeng), Tripterygium wilfordii (leigongteng), Paeoniae lactiflora (chishao), Paeoniae alba (baishao) are used to open blood passages and disperse wind. Glycyrrhiza (gancao) is used to harmonize the wuxing organs.

The Magui formula is very effective in treating the symptoms of joint wind pains through repairing the damaged liver wood yin and yang. The wind pain is a result of liver wood yin and yang damage, but the damage didn't only happen when the symptoms occurred. The liver wood yin and yang damage has to be an underlying condition. Inadequate food and drink accumulate more damp poison, then the symptoms become obvious. When treating this kind of condition, the herbs should be taken over a period of six months to repair the damaged liver wood yin and yang to prevent the re-occurrence of joint wind pain. Nevertheless, during the treatment, one should avoid taking alcohol, white sugar and other processed products as they may further damage the liver wood yin and yang.

Treating liver wood yin & yang damage with symptoms of wind and damp pain

Wind and damp pain is a result of wind and damp obstructing the joints. A 30-year-old Asian female patient came for a consultation with widespread joint pains. The patient had been seeing biomedical practitioners and was diagnosed with rheumatoid arthritis. She was worried, however, about the side effects of the drugs that she was prescribed, and wanted to try herbs first. At the first consultation, her pain was so severe that she could not walk and was carried into the clinic by her husband. At the time all her joints large and small were red, swollen, and hot to touch. She also had strong pains that shifted from one place to another.

Liver wood yang damage causes damp poison to block the blood passages; liver wood yin damage causes blood heat. The damp poison, and heat joined together stagnate in the joints causing the swelling and pains in the joints. The liver wood yin deficiency creates blood heat, and the heat creates wind. Wind moves fast and strikes the stagnant damp poison and heat, causing the pain to move from place to place. When I asked the patient whether she had experienced any changes in her lifestyle or diet before the illness began, she said that she had given birth six months earlier and following her doctor's instructions, she had been eating a lot of dairy products, which she had never consumed much before. Considering the case could well have been caused by the dairy products that damaged liver wood yang qi, I asked the patient to avoid taking dairy products. The treatment was to remove dampness, disperse wind, and open the meridians with the Qiteng formula.

After taking seven packets of the herbs, the patient reported that her pain was occasionally eased. She took the herbs continuously for eight months, all symptoms subsequently disappeared. She also went back to her biomedical practitioner for a blood test and was told that she no longer had rheumatoid arthritis. Twenty years later, the patient passed by my clinic and reported that she had not had any joint pain since.

Qiteng formula:

Aconitum carmichaeli (fuzi) 10g
Sabia japonica (qingfengteng) 30g
Trachelospermum jasminoides (luoshiteng) 30g
Caulis lonicerae japonicae (jinyinhuateng) 30g
Caulis piperis kadsurae (haifengteng) 30g
Uncaria rhynchophylla (gouteng) 15g
Morus alba (sangzhi) 10g
Tripterygium wilfordii
(leigongteng) 15g
Kadsura interior (jixueteng) 30g
Gypsum (shigao) 20g
Atractylodis lancea (cangzhu) 20g
Atractylodis macrocephalae (baizhu) 20g
Cinnamomum cassia (guizhi) 10g
Ephedra sinica (mahuang) 10g
Paeoniae lactiflora (chishao) 10g
Paeoniae alba (baishao) 10g
Angelica sinensis (danggui) 15g
Glycyrrhiza radix (gancao) 10g

Qiteng formula in Chinese 七藤汤:

附子10g 清风藤30g 络石藤30g 金银花藤30g 海风藤30g 钩藤15g 桑枝10g 雷公藤15g 鸡血藤30g 石膏20g 苍术20g 白术20g 桂枝10g 麻

黄10g 赤芍10g 白芍10g 当归15g 甘草10g

Aconitum carmichaeli (fuzi 附子) expels wind, cold and damp poisonous qi, breaks down stagnation and lumps, treats cold and damp caused back and knee pain.

Sabia japonica (qingfengteng 清风藤) has a bitter taste and mild yinyang nature. It goes into the liver and kidney meridians. It disperses wind, eases water flow, removes dampness, and opens meridians.

Trachelospermum jasminoides (luoshiteng 络石藤) disperses wind, eases water flow, invigorates blood, and opens meridians.

Caulis Lonicerae japonicae (jinyinhuateng 金银花藤) eases water flow, disperses wind, removes mucus, and opens the meridians.

Caulis Piperis kadsurae (haifengteng 海风藤) has a bitter taste and slightly warm yinyang nature. It goes into the heart, and kidney meridians. It clears dampness, disperses wind, opens the meridians, smooths blood passages, and soothes qi flow, and loosens spleen soil.

Uncaria rhynchophylla (gouteng 钩藤) stops wind and opens the meridians.

Morus alba (sangzhi 桑枝) eases water flow, expels wind, and smooths joints.

Tripterygium wilfordii (leigongteng 雷公藤) expels wind, invigorates blood, opens the meridians, dissolves swelling, and stops pain.

Kadsura interior (jixueteng 鸡血藤) has a slightly sweet taste and warm yinyang nature. It goes into the heart and spleen meridians. It invigorates blood, warms the lower back and knees, nurtures spleen soil, and dries dampness.

Gypsum (shigao 石膏) isolates turbidity and removes dampness.

Atractylodis lancea (cangzhu 苍术) removes the poisonous qi of dampness and mucus.

Atractylodis macrocephalae (baizhu 白术) expels wind, drains dampness, and removes mucus.

Cinnamomum cassia (guizhi 桂枝) frees skin to breathe, expels poisonous qi, and harmonizes skin and flesh.

Ephedra sinica (mahuang 麻黄) eases stagnation in the flesh, induces sweating, and removes cold or hot stagnation.

Paeoniae lactiflora (chishao 赤芍) cools blood, removes build ups, and disperses blood stagnation.

Paeoniae alba (baishao 白芍) opens and smooths blood passages, dissolves swelling.

Angelica sinensis (danggui 当归) harmonizes the wuxing organs and nurtures spirit and body.

Glycyrrhiza (gancao甘草) can harmonize the wuxing organs and detoxifies poisons.

In the formula, Aconitum carmichaeli (fuzi) is the leading herb to expel wind, cold, and damp poisonous qi, and frees joint pain. Sabia japonica (qingfengteng), Trachelospermum jasminoides (luoshiteng), Caulis Lonicerae japonicae (jinyinhuateng), Caulis Piperis kadsurae (haifengteng), Uncaria rhynchophylla (gouteng), and Morus alba (sangzhi) are used to add more strength to stop wind and open the meridians. Tripterygium wilfordii (leigongteng), Kadsura interior (jixueteng) are used to invigorate blood and open the meridians. Gypsum (shigao), Atractylodis lancea (cangzhu), Atractylodis macrocephalae (baizhu) are used to expel dampness and turbidity; Cinnamomum cassia (guizhi), Ephedra sinica (mahuang) free stagnation between skin and flesh to expel dampness. Paeoniae lactiflora (chishao) is used to cool blood and stop wind. Paeoniae alba (baishao), Angelica sinensis (danggui) and Glycyrrhiza (gancao) are used to smooth the blood passages.

Note: This formula, because of the aconitum carmichaeli, requires at least two hours of boiling before drinking the decoction.

Another case was a 34-year-old woman who had been feeling body heaviness and lethargy during the day. During the morning she found it difficult to keep her eyes open, but it would get better in the afternoons or when she stayed outdoors. Her neck and shoulders were very tight and painful when pressed. At the first consultation, the patient had had the symptoms for four months. In the morning, the body's yang meridians open, but in this case dampness blocked the yang meridians, and the yang qi could not move freely through the body, so the patient felt the energy encounter from heaven and earth, and therefore she felt sleepy, tired and had neck and shoulder tightness. Being outdoors, or having physical activities, would help to evaporate dampness, open the meridians, and allow the qi of heaven and earth to pass through the body, so her symptoms were less severe.

Treatment is to expel dampness and open the meridians with the above Qiteng formula.

After taking one packet of Qiteng formula, the patient felt she had suddenly woken up. After another two packets of the herbs she felt completely normal and stopped the herbs.

Another 30-year-old woman came for a consultation as she had been trying to have a baby for four years without success. The patient had been taking anti-inflammatory and steroid drugs for a diagnosed rheumatoid arthritis condition for more than 10 years. But her biomedical doctor had told her that the drugs were not affecting her ability to have a child. However, the way that drugs were helping her cope with pain was to block the pain messages. From the yinyang wuxing perspective, the messages of pain are a symptom of blockage in the yinyang passage, while blocking the message the drugs created more blockages in the yinyang passage and disturbed the changing cycle of yinyang wuxing, thus affecting her reproductive ability. So for the purpose of getting pregnant she simply needed to get rid of the drugs. But the patient could not cope with the joint pains, so I prescribed the Qiteng formula to expel dampness, and open the meridians to help her stop the drugs.

After taking one month of the herbs, her joint pain was improved, so she began to reduce her drug intake. After six months of taking the herbs, she managed to stop all the drugs and with no significant joint pains. After stopping the drugs for less than a month, she became pregnant. During her pregnancy she did not have any pain and didn't need to take herbs either. She had a healthy baby boy. After delivering the baby, her pain returned but the patient chose to take the drugs to cope with the pain. Two years later, she wanted to have another baby and came back for herbs. After taking the same herbs for four months, she was able to stop taking the biomedical drugs completely and was able to get pregnant immediately after that. Later she had a healthy baby daughter.

Treating liver wood yin & yang damage with symptoms of chest pain

A 60-year-old male patient came to me for a consultation with chest pains. Prior to seeing me, the patient had been hospitalized for severe chest pain and loss of conciousness. The hospital told him that three of his arteries in his heart were 95 per cent blocked, and he needed to have bypass surgery immediately The patient's family brought him to my practice and hoped that he could avoid the surgery. During the first consultation, the patient suffered frequent stabbing chest pains. He was agitated, his face was red, and he had intermittent headaches.

Liver wood yang damage, dampness and mucus had grown in the blood and blocked the blood passages in the chest, which caused the chest pain. Liver wood yin deficiency fails to store blood in the root but allows blood to rush in the blood passages, which causes the symptoms of red face. Blood heat creates wind, the fast travelling wind causes headaches. The spirit relies on liver wood to exercise its striving zhi, the liver wood yin deficiency prevents the yin qi of the striving zhi from being exercised, so the spirit appears to be agitated. Severe liver wood yin deficiency causes heart fire to float and forces the spirit out of the body, so he passed out. The treatment is to invigorate blood, remove mucus, warm kidney water, soften liver wood, and ground heart fire. I used the Erxian Rumo formula.

The patient took the herbs on and off for a year, at the end of the year, his chest pains and headaches only occurred after drinking alcohol. So he gradually stopped drinking alcohol and continued to take the herbs on and off for five years, within this time, he didn't have chest pains or facial redness, his moods also became calmer, and he rarely had headaches again.

Erxian Rumo formula:

Epimedium brevicornum (yinyanghuo) 30g
Rhizoma curculiginis orchioides (xianmao) 15g
Radix morindae officinalis (bajitian) 15g
Polygala tenufola (yuanzhi) 10g
Angelica sinensis (danggui) 20g
Rhizome anemarrhenae (zhimu) 10g

Phellodendri chinensis (huangbai) 10g
Gentiana scabra (longdancao) 30g
Polygoni multiflori (yejiaoteng) 30g
Fried Zizyphus jujube (chao suanzaoren) 15g
Concha margaritifera (zhenzhumu) 30g

Concha haliotidis (shijueming) 30g

Concha ostreae (muli) 30g

Ossa draconis (longgu) 30g

Gastrodia elata (tianma) 10g

Ligusticum wallichi (chuanxiong) 10g

Olibanum (ruxiang) 5g

Myrrh (moyao) 5g

Pseudoginseng (sanqi) 10g

Erxian Rumo formula in Chinese 二仙乳没汤:

淫羊藿30g 仙茅15g 巴戟天15g 远志10g 当归20g 知母10g 黄柏 10g 龙胆草30g 夜交藤30g 炒酸枣仁15g 珍珠母30g 石决明30g 牡蛎30g 龙骨30g 天麻10g 川芎10g 乳香5g 没药5g 三七粉10g.

For formula explanation see "Treating liver wood yin and yang deficiency with symptoms of zhongfeng (struck by wind)".

Treating liver wood yin and yang damage with symptoms of red, swollen, burning and painful eyes

I had a five-year-old girl brought in for a consultation with red, swollen, hot and painful eyes and with a lot of pussy discharge. The girl had fallen asleep on her toy teddy bear for a few hours and woke up with these problems in her eyes.

Liver wood yin damage causes blood heat; liver wood yang damage causes the blood passages to lose their erectness and allows the external damp poison to reside in the blood passages in the area of the eyes, so she had symptoms such as red, swollen, hot, painful and pussy discharge in her eyes. The treatment was to remove dampness, clear heat, detoxify poison, and brighten the eyes with the Sangcao formula.

Externally I also asked the patient to use cotton wool to dab her eyes with naturally fermented vinegar to allow a small amount of vinegar get into her eyes. Vinegar has a sour taste and is cool in yinyang nature. It goes into the liver meridian. It clears liver wood, dissolves dampness, and detoxifies poison.

The patient followed the instructions drinking the herbs and washing her eyes with vinegar, within 24 hours her red swollen painful eye symptoms had significantly improved. After two packets of the herbs all symptoms disappeared.

Sangcao formula:

Morus alba (sangye) 10g
Chrysanthemum indicum (juhua) 10g
Chrysanthemum Indicum (wild) (yejuhua) 10g
Prunella vulgaris (xiakucao) 10g
Celosia argentea (qingxiangzi) 10g
Eriocaulon buergerianum
(gujingcao) 10g
Lonicera japonica (jinyinhua) 10g
Oldenlandia diffusa (baihuasheshecao) 10g
talcum (huashi) 20g
Gypsum (shigao) 20g
Glycyrrhiza radix 10g

Sangcao formula in Chinese 桑草汤:

桑叶10g 菊花10g 野菊花10g 夏枯草10g 青箱子10g 谷精草10g 金银花10g 白花蛇舌草10g 滑石20g 石膏20g 甘草10g

Morus alba (sangye 桑叶) has a sweet and bitter taste, and cold yinyang nature. It goes into the lung, and liver meridians. It eliminates wind, relieves skin blockages, clears heat, and brightens eyes.

Chrysanthemum morifolium (juhua 菊花) has a sweet and bitter taste, and cold yinyang nature. It goes into the lung and liver meridians. It eliminates wind, clears heat, detoxifies poison, clears liver wood, and brightens eyes.

Chrysanthemum indicum (yejuhua 野菊花) eliminates wind, clears heat, reduces swelling, detoxifies poison, clears liver wood, and brightens eyes.

Prunella vulgaris (xiakucao 夏枯草) has a bitter taste and cold yinyang nature. It goes into the liver and gall bladder meridians. It clears heat, dissolves mucus, eliminates masses, clears liver wood, and detoxifies poison.

Celosia argentea (qingxiangzi 青箱子) has a bitter taste and cool yinyang nature. It goes into the liver meridian. It disperses wind, clears heat, detoxifies poison, and brightens eyes.

Eriocaulon buergerianum (gujingcao 谷精草) has a sweet taste and cool yinyang nature. It goes into the liver and stomach meridians. It disperses wind, scatters heat, clears liver wood, detoxifies poison, and brightens eyes.

Lonicera japonica (jinyinhua 金银花) has a sweet taste and cold yinyang nature. It goes into the lung meridian. It clears heat and liver wood, and detoxifies poison.

Oldenlandia diffusa (baihuasheshecao 白花蛇舌草) clears heat, removes stagnation, eliminates swelling, detoxifies poison, and clears masses in the lungs.

Talcum (huashi 滑石) isolates turbidity, cools heat, and dissolves mucus.

Gypsum (shigao 石膏) isolates turbidity and clears heat.

Glycyrrhiza (gancao 甘草) harmonizes the wuxing organs, and detoxifies poison.

In the Sangcao formula, Morus alba (sangye), chrysanthemum morifolium (juhua), chrysanthemum Indicum (yejuhua), Prunella vulgaris (xiakucao), Celosia argentea (qingxiangzi), Eriocaulon buergerianum (gujingcao) are the herbs to clear liver wood, and heat; they all go to the eyes. Lonicera Japonica (jinyinhua) and oldenlandia diffusa (baihuasheshecao) are used for an added cooling effect. Talcum (huashi), and gypsum (shigao) are used to isolate turbidity to help the removal of mucus. Glycyrrhiza is used to harmonize liver wood.

Treating liver wood yin& yang damage with symptoms of swollen gums and toothache

A 55-year-old male patient had suddenly started to have toothache and within half an hour the pain had become very severe, it throbbed and his face was swollen. He went to a dentist immediately, and the dentist told him to take antibiotics for a week to get the inflammation down then return to take the tooth out. The patient telephoned me asking for options, I told him to ask his dentist to insert a cotton ball saturated with organic eucalyptus oil into the tooth cavity. The dentist at first refused, but after the patient's repeated request, the dentist did so. Before leaving the dentist's surgery, the patient's toothache had already subsided. The patient was also able to avoid having the tooth extracted and instead the dentist gave him a gold filling.

The reason for using eucalyptus oil to relieve the toothache was that swollen red gums with toothache are a symptom of liver wood yin and yang damage, blood heat and damp poison blocking the blood passages. Eucalyptus oil cools blood, detoxifies blood poison and revives liver wood yin and yang qi.

Eucalyptus oil (anshu you 桉树精油) has a pungent taste and cool yinyang nature. It goes into the liver and lung meridians. It clears heat, cools blood, dissolves mucus, expels dampness, invigorates blood, and detoxifies poison.

Every swollen gum with toothache case that I have met after applying eucalyptus oil has recovered from the pain. The method is: clean a sewing needle with boiling water, then use it to separate the affected gum from the tooth until blood clots come out, then drip the eucalyptus oil into the wound. The pain should stop immediately. If not, it means the blood clot has not been totally released, push the flesh of the gum away from the tooth again and drip the eucalyptus oil repeatedly until the pain stops.

Another case was a 47-year-old woman who had long ago lost a tooth. Six months before her visit, a lump had begun to grow where the lost tooth had been. The lump was reddish, as high as a tooth, solid and painful when pressed. She had tried to break it with a sewing needle, it made a little blood ooze out but it seemed to aggravate it more and made it larger. I used Mylabris phalerata (banmao) powder mixed with honey, and applied a pea-sized paste on her cheek externally in the area where the lump was. Within four hours, there was blistering where the paste was applied, the lump became white and soft. When pressed, puss burst out, and the lump disappeared immediately.

Mylabris phalerata (banmao 斑蝥) has a pungent taste and cold yinyang nature. It is very poisonous, and should be handled with caution. It goes into the liver, spleen, kidney meridians. It opens up water passages, breaks down abscesses, removes stagnation and nodules, clears liver wood, dissolves malignant sores and dogged scaly rash. Mylabris phalerata (banmao) paste will leave a mark/scar on the skin, and could take a year to heal.

Another 53-year-old woman had the root of one of her teeth exposed and whenever she ate fruit or anything sweet, in about day or two she would have severe toothache that felt like the bone was broken. To treat the problem, I use 50g of Zanthoxylum bungeanum (huajiao), two tablespoons full of unrefined sea salt, 500ml of water, and boiled them together for 10 minutes. When toothache occurs, warm the Zanthoxylum bungeanum (huajiao), salt water and gargle with the mixture. When the salty Zanthoxylum bungeanum (huajiao) water reaches the aching tooth, the pain can be worse but only for a few seconds. Then the toothache will subside. Keep rinsing the mouth with this solution until the pain is completely gone. The patient was also advised to use unrefined sea salt instead of toothpaste to clean the teeth twice a day to prevent toothache; from then on, her toothache happened much less frequently and with less severity. She was also able to eat fruit without suffering from severe toothaches.

Zanthoxylum bungeanum (huajiao 花椒) has a pungent taste and warm yinyang nature. It goes into the spleen, lung and kidney meridians. It dispels cold, removes dampness, clears liver wood, detoxifies poison, and stops pain.
Unrefined sea salt (haiyan 海盐) has a salty taste and upward moving yinyang nature. It goes into the lung, kidney and liver meridians. It cools blood, clears liver wood, detoxifies poison, and stops pain.

Treating liver wood yin and yang damage with symptoms of acne

An 18-year-old girl came to see me for acne. The girl had acne all over her face. She also suffered from sticky difficult bowel motions, was restless, and had nightmares such as being chased. The patient had been eating biscuits, lollies, and drank soft drinks every day. White sugar breeds dampness in the body and damages liver wood yang. Liver wood yang damage and damp poison congest the blood passages, so there is the symptom of acne. Damp poison congests blood in the large intestine, so her bowel motion was sticky and difficult to release. White sugar also exhaust kidney water heat causing kidney water heat loss, then liver wood loses its moistness and becomes dry. With liver wood dryness, the yin qi of the striving zhi is unable to be exercised, so the striving zhi is firm but not smooth, therefore, the patient was restless and had nightmares of being chased. The treatment is to clear dampness, dissolve mucus, clear liver wood, detoxify poison, and warm kidney water with the Erxian Gongying formula.

124

The patient took 10 packets of the herbs and all symptoms were improved. Her bowel motions were easy but a little loose. However, by 13th day of taking the herbs, all her symptoms came back as before. She continued to take the herbs, and two days later her period came and all the symptoms disappeared. The patient took another month of the same herbs. Two days before her next period she had a few pimples and a little restlessness, and her bowel motions were difficult again. Then when her period came the symptoms would again disappear. She took another month of the herbs and none of the symptoms reoccurred.

Acne often occurs in people who enter puberty. Puberty is a time that the body transits from a growing centred period to a reproductive period. The transition demands kidney water heat to get through. When the kidney water heat reserve is low, liver wood becomes dry, forcing blood to rush in the blood passages. At this time, if consuming refined sugar, it further depletes kidney water heat, damages liver wood yang, and helps to breed dampness in the blood passages, then it is difficult to escape from acne.

The reason that the patient's acne returned just prior to her period was because during this time more blood is in the blood passages, rather than in the root of liver wood, and as a consequence there is blood heat. Blood heat then encourages the remaining dampness to flourish, so the symptoms return.

Erxian Gongying formula:

Epimedium brevicornum (yinyanghuo) 30g
Rhizoma curculiginis orchioides (xianmao) 15g
Radix morindae officinalis (bajitian) 15g
Polygala tenufola (yuanzhi) 10g
Angelica sinensis (danggui) 20g
Rhizome anemarrhenae (zhimu) 10g
Phellodendri chinensis (huangbai) 10g
Gentiana scabra (longdancao) 30g
Polygoni multiflori (yejiaoteng) 30g
Zizyphus jujube (fried) (chao suanzaoren) 15g
Concha margaritifera (zhenzhumu) 30g
Concha haliotidis (shijueming) 30g

Concha ostreae (muli) 30g
Ossa draconis (longgu) 30g
Paeonia lactiflora (chishao) 15g
Taraxacum officinale
(pugongying) 30g

Viola yedoensis (zihuadiding)
30g
Rheum officinale (dahuang) 10g
Coptis chinensis (huanglian) 10g

Erxian Gongying formula in Chinese 二仙公英汤:

淫羊藿30g 仙茅15g 巴戟天15g 远志10g 当归20g 知母10g 黄柏10g 龙胆草30g 夜交藤30g 炒枣仁15g 珍珠母30g 石决明30g 牡蛎30g 龙骨30g 赤芍15g 蒲公英30g 紫花地丁30g 大黄10g 黄连10g.

For the Erxian Gongying formula explanation see the section "Treating kidney water yin and yang damage with symptoms of pain and swollen testicle".

Treating liver wood yang damage with symptoms of patchy hair loss

A 24-year-old female patient came to me for a consultation for hair loss. Before the hair loss she had been taking a weight loss drug for a month, then the hair of her eyebrows fell out and she developed a bald patch on the top of her scalp of about 4 or 5cm in diameter. At the first consultation, she had had the bald patch and lost eyebrows for three months, and her period had stopped for two months. She felt anxious, had restless sleep, and her bowel was dry and hard to open. The cause of her problem was the chemical drugs that she had taken. The drugs had damaged her liver wood yang, and caused blood decay. Hair is the extension of the blood, when blood decays then there is hair loss. The drug had also damaged the kidney water yang, which causes the reproduction cycle congestion and the period delay. When there is kidney water heat damage, the yang qi of the enduring zhi of the spirit was unable to be carried through, so her spirit lost its confidence and was anxious. With kidney water heat loss, the large intestine fails to be moistened, so her bowel motions became dry and difficult. The treatment was to invigorate blood, clear dampness, dissolve mucus in the blood passages, refresh liver wood, and warm kidney water with Erxian Gongying formula.

The patient took two weeks of the herbs, her period came, and her bowel motions became easy and regular. After taking the herbs for two months, her eyebrows grew back, the bald patch disappeared, she slept well and was in good spirits again.

Treating liver wood yin and yang damage with symptoms of wet rashes

Wet rashes are those with sticky fluid seeping out of damaged skin. Such rashes are frequently called in biomedicine as eczema, but not all cases of eczema have the symptom of weeping wounds. The degree of weeping indicates the severity of dampness. For example, if the weeping is with a thin liquid, it means there is liver wood yang damage with fluid and dampness blocking the blood passages. The treatment would then emphasize freeing water flow, draining dampness, and invigorating blood. Rashes that have thick sticky liquid and dry skin flakes means the dampness has thickened to become mucus blocking the blood passages, and the treatment would emphasize scattering stagnation, and dissolving blood mucus.

A six-month-old boy suffering a wet rash was brought to me for a consultation. The boy had recently begun drinking milk formula after originally being breast fed. At the first consultation, the baby showed a lot of restlessness and he had millet sized red rashes all over his body; some parts of the skin were broken with sticky white fluid seeping out. His mother had changed between various brands of milk formulas but the rash did not improve. I had to conclude that the milk formulas/powders had ingredients that were blocking the body's yinyang passages and damaging the liver wood yin and yang. Liver wood yang damage would cause dampness in the blood passages, which causes skin rashes. Liver wood yin damage causes blood heat, therefore the rashes were red. Excessive heat in the blood causes wind, so the patient suffered itchiness. As a result, I urged the mother to stop the milk formulas and she changed to rice congee with a little minced meat, green vegetables and sea salt. The treatment was to clear dampness and clear heat with the Ershi formula taken internally, and a vinegar wash externally.

After taking the herbs and wash with vinegar plus the change of food, the boy's rash disappeared within 3 days.

Ershi formula:

Gypsum (shigao) 20g
Talcum (huashi) 20g
Radix rehmanniae (raw) (shengdi) 10g
Radix rehmanniae (cooked) (shudi) 10g
Ophiopogon japonicas (maimendong) 10g

Asparagus cochinchinensis (tianmendong) 10g
Mesobathus martensii (quanxie) 10g
Scolopendra subspinipes (wugong) $\frac{1}{4}$piece,
Glycyrrhiza radix (gancao) 5g.

Ershi formula in Chinese 二石汤:

石膏20g 滑石20g 生地10g 熟地10g 麦冬10g 天冬10g 全蝎10g 蜈蚣$\frac{1}{4}$甘草5g

Gypsum (shigao 石膏) isolates turbidity.

Talcum (huashi 滑石) isolates turbidity, clears heat, and dissolves mucus.

Raw and cooked radix rehmanniae (shengdi 生地 and shudi 熟地) opens blood passages and removes damp poison in the blood.

Ophiopogon japonicas (maimendong 麦门冬) cultivates water and washes out dampness.

Asparagus cochinchinensis (tianmendong 天门冬) cultivates water and clears damp poison.

Mesobathus martensii (quanxie 全蝎) dissolves mucus, expels wind, and stops itch.

Scolopendra subspinipes (wugong 蜈蚣) opens blood passages, expels damp poison in the blood.

Glycyrrhiza (gancao 甘草) detoxifies poison and harmonizes the wuxing organs.

Preparation method and taking the herbs:

Place the herbs into a pot, add 750 ml of cold water and boil it down to 200 ml of water within an hour. Before every feed, give the child a tablespoon full of the herbal concoction, as often as feeding food.

Vinegar wash:

Mix 100 ml of natural fermented vinegar (for example apple cider vinegar) with 200 ml of warm water. Wash the rash affected area of skin. It can be as often as the itch occurs. The vinegar and water wash can be reused after bringing to boil. Make a new vinegar wash each day.

A 17-year-old girl came for help with wet rashes. The patient had had the rash ever since she was a baby. For most of her 17 years she had been using steroid cream to cope with the itch. Her mother said that she had taken her daughter to see the same skin specialist for the past 17 years and the last time they saw him, the doctor offered them a box of steroid cream. The specialist said that the girl has been using the same cream for many years and would always need it. So she might just as well buy the whole box and get a good discount, plus it would save her the consultation fees. By then the mother suddenly realized that there was no cure for her daughter's rash with biomedicine. She declined the box of steroids and began to search for other treatment options. Subsequently, a friend referred them to me, however, the family had no knowledge about traditional Chinese healing and didn't hide their suspicions about the treatment.

At the first consultation, the patient had rashes on her wrists, elbows, neck, groin, behind the knees and ankles. She suffered waves of severe itch. The rashes were dark brown, the skin was thick, and rough, some parts of the skin had oozing fluid, and some other parts were red and swollen. The mother said, when the daughter first developed the rash they were only on her neck, and after using steroid cream it immediately cleared. But not long after, the rash came back and the cream was helping to cope with the itch but did not clear the rash, instead, the rash gradually spread. The patient had to use the cream more and more frequently and the drug had become less and less effective. In the previous three to four years before they visited my practice, the rashes had progressively worsened and she had applied the steroid cream many times a day but still had to bear the itch. The patient was 17 but still had not commenced her menses. Her breasts were undeveloped but she felt otherwise fine.

This was originally a simple case of liver wood yang damage, with damp poison blocking the blood passages and causing the rashes.

But after long term use of steroid cream, it had created another blockage of the yinyang passages. In a normal situation, a woman at the age of thirteen-fourteen, the body is ready for reproduction and the menstrual cycle begins. Although the patient should have had her menses by then, the kidney yinyang passages were blocked and had prevented this from happening. Kidney water maintains the body yang heat, yang heat is the precondition for reproduction, and therefore, the steroid's effects on the body had been to obstruct the yinyang passage of kidney water. Kidney water is the mother of liver wood in the wuxing cycle, the blockage of the yinyang passage of kidney water means liver wood is unsupported, so the wet rashes become worse at this time.

The treatment was in two steps, first was to clear heat, cool blood, expel dampness, remove mucus, and detoxify poisons to support the liver wood ; the second step was to warm kidney water, expel mucus and dampness to promote regeneration of liver wood. For the first step I used the Tubie Diyu formula. And the second step was to warm kidney water, also dissolve mucus, remove dampness, and clear liver wood for which I used the Erxian Difuzi formula.

Because the patient had been using steroids for many years, the drugs hid the true condition of the illness as well as blocked the body's yinyang passages, so to properly cure her illness, the patient had to stop using the steroids. However, stopping the use of steroids is no easy task. Although her rash was worsening year after year, if she were to suddenly stop using the steroids the body would go through a strong retroaction, which means that the rash would become unbearably bad. Rather than stopping the steroids immediately a more comfortable way is to reduce the steroid use gradually.

In the beginning, as the patient and parents were unfamiliar with herbal treatment, they continued to use the steroid ointment. But after taking one week of the herbs, her rash had obviously improved, so the family decided to drop off the steroid treatment. After stopping the steroids for two weeks, the patient's whole body was covered in rash. The rashes were red, swollen, weeping and extremely itchy. The patient, however, resisted using the steroids and continued with the Tubie Diyu formula and used hot vinegar wash to cope with the itch. A month later, the rashes began to improve.

After six months of taking the herbs the rashes were under control, the colour had become lighter, the itch was more bearable and the areas were less and less. But then suddenly the rash became worse, not as bad as previously but it did shake the patient's confidence in the treatment. Nevertheless, she continued to take the herbs, then a week later, she got her first period, and the rash immediately subsided. This was an indication that her liver wood damage had stabilized, but the kidney water yinyang passage blockage caused by the steroids still remained. From that point I changed her formula to Erxian Difuzi to warm the kidney water, clear liver wood, and continue to cleanse the blood mucus. After taking a year of the Erxian Difuzi formula, gradually the rashes disappeared before her period.

Tubie Diyu formula:

Rehmannia glutinosa (raw) (shengdi) 10g
Rehmannia glutinosa (cooked) (shudi) 10g
Eupolyphaga sinensis (tubiechong) 10g
Scolopendra subspinipes (wugong) $\frac{1}{2}$ piece,
Paeonia lactiflora (chishao) 10g
Paeoniae alba (baishao) 10g
Rheum officinale (dahuang) 10g
Cirsium setosum (xiaoji) 10g
Typha angustifolia (puhuang) 10g
Nelumbo nucifera (oujie) 10g
Sanguisorba officinalis (diyu) 10g
Dianthus superbus (jumai) 10g
Angelica sinensis (danggui) 10g
Zaocys dhumnade (wushaoshe) 30g
Mesobathus martensii (quanxie) 10g
Scutellaria baicalensis (huangqin) 10g
Coptis chinensis (huanglian) 10g
Phellodendri chinensis (huangbai) 10g
Kochia scparia (difuzi) 15g
Cortex dictamni (baixianpi) 15g
Dioscorea septemloba (bixie) 10g
Smilax glabra (tufuling) 30g
Sophorae flavescentis (kushen) 10g
Oldenlandia diffusa (baihuasheshecao) 10g
Taraxacum mongolicum (pugongying) 30g
Viola yedoensis makino (zihuadiding) 30g
Gypsum (shigao) 20g
Talcum (huashi) 20g
Ophiopogon japonicas (maimendong) 10g
Asparagus cochinchinensis (tianmendong) 10g
Glycyrrhiza radix (gancao) 10g

Tubie Diyu formula in Chinese 土鳖地榆汤:

生地10g 熟地10g 土鳖虫10g 蜈蚣½ 赤芍10g 白芍10g 大黄10g 小蓟10g 蒲黄10g 藕节10g 地榆10g 瞿麦10g 当归10g 乌梢蛇30g 全蝎10g 黄芩10g 黄连10g 黄柏10g 地肤子15g 白鲜皮15 萆薢10g 土茯苓30g 苦参10g 白花蛇舌草10g 蒲公英30g 紫花地丁30g 石膏20g 滑石20g 麦门冬10g 天门冬10g 甘草10g

Raw and cooked radix rehmanniae glutinosa (shengdi 生地, shudi 熟地) break down damp poison in the blood.

Eupolyphaga sinensis (tubiechong 土鳖虫) breaks down blood stagnation, dissolves masses, and frees the flow of menses.

Scolopendra subspinipes (wugong 蜈蚣) removes mucus and dampness in the blood, clears liver wood, and detoxifies poison.

Paeonia lactiflora (chishao 赤芍) removes collected nodules, eliminates blood stagnation, dissipates intestinal wind and swelling.

Paeoniae alba (baishao 白芍) frees blood flow, eliminates swelling.

Rheum officinale (dahuang 大黄) cools blood, detoxifies poison, breaks down stagnation, removes dampness, opens bowel motions.

Cirsium setosum (xiaoji 小蓟) cools blood, stops bleeding, detoxifies poison, and dissolves swelling.

Typha angustifolia (puhuang 蒲黄) corrects hot or cold yinyang disorder, frees urine flow, and dissolves blood stagnation.

Nelumbo nucifera (oujie 藕节) drains dampness, dissolves mucus, removes dampness and mucus in the blood.

Sanguisorba officinalis (diyu 地榆) cools blood, eliminates dampness, and expels poison.

Dianthus superbus (jumai 瞿麦) clears heat, frees water flow, and opens blood passages.

Angelica sinensis (danggui 当归) nurtures blood and stops wind.

Zaocys dhumnade (wushaoshe 乌梢蛇) has a sweet taste and mild yinyang nature. It goes into the liver meridian. It eliminates wind, opens meridians, and dissolves nodules.

Mesobathus martensii (quanxie 全蝎) opens orifices, dissolves mucus, and stops wind.

Scutellaria baicalensis (huangqin 黄芩) clears heat, and removes dampness.

Coptis chinensis (huanglian 黄连) clears damp heat, and removes stagnation.

Phellodendri chinensis (huangbai 黄柏) clears dampness, removes heat stagnation in all wuxing organs.

Kochia scoparia (difuzi 地肤子) clears heat, detoxifies poison, moistens the skin, and drains dampness.

Cortex dictamni (baixianpi 白鲜皮) drains dampness, clears heat, detoxifies poison, and stops wind.

Dioscorea septemloba (bixie 萆薢) has a bitter taste, and mild yinyang nature. It goes into the urine bladder and lung meridians. It clears heat, drains dampness, opens meridians, and frees urine flow.

Smilax glabra (tufuling 土茯苓) removes damp poisons, and eliminates malignant sores.

Sophorae flavescentis (kushen 苦参) cools blood, removes dampness, detoxifies poison, kills parasites, and moistens skin.

Oldenlandia diffusa (baihuasheshecao 白花蛇舌草) clears heat, eliminates stagnation, clears liver wood, removes swelling, and detoxifies poison.

Taraxacum mongolicum (pugongying 蒲公英) clears heat and eliminates stagnation.

Viola yedoensis makino (zihuadiding 紫花地丁) clears heat, detoxifies poison, dissolves swelling, and clears liver wood.

Gypsum (shigao 石膏) isolates turbidity.

Talcum (huashi 滑石) isolates turbidity, extinguishes fire, and dissolves mucus.

Ophiopogon japonicas (maimendong 麦门冬) nurtures yin, frees water flow, and removes dampness.

Asparagus cochinchinensis (tianmendong 天门冬) nurtures yin, cultivates water, and clears damp poison.

Glycyrrhiza radix (gancao 甘草) harmonizes the wuxing organs and detoxifies poison.

In the Tubie Diyu formula, raw and cooked Radix rehmanniae (shengdi, shudi), Eupolyphaga sinensis (tubiechong), Scolopendra subspinipes (wugong), Paeonia lactiflora (chishao), Paeoniae alba (bai-shao), Rheum officinale (dahuang), Cirsium setosum (xiaoji), Typha angustifolia (puhuang), Nelumbo nucifera gaertn (oujie), Sanguisorba officinalis (diyu), Dianthus superbus (jumai) are chosen for having the effects of removing blood mucus and dampness. Angelica sinensis (danggui) is used to regenerate blood. Zaocys dhumnade (wushaoshe), and Mesobathus martensii (quanxie) are used to stop wind, dissolve mucus and stop itch. Scutellaria baicalensis (huangqin), Coptis chinensis (huanglian), Phellodendri chinensis (huangbai), Kochia scoparia (difuzi), Cortex dictamni (baixianpi), Dioscorea septemloba (bixie), Smilax glabra (tufuling), Sophorae flavescentis (kushen), Oldenlandia diffusa (baihuasheshecao), Taraxacum mongolicum (pugongying), Viola yedoensis makino (zihuadiding) are used to clear heat, dry dampness, and detoxify poison. Gypsum (shigao), Talcum (huashi) are used to isolate and remove mucus. Ophiopogon japonicas (maimendong), Asparagus cochinchinensis (tianmendong) are used to cultivate fresh water to remove dampness and mucus. Glycyrrhiza (gancao) is used to detoxify poison and harmonize the wuxing organs.

Erxian Difuzi formula:

Epimedium brevicornum (yinyanghuo) 30g
Rhizoma curculiginis orchioides (xianmao) 15g
Radix morindae officinalis (bajitian) 15g
Polygala tenufola (yuanzhi) 10g
Angelica sinensis (danggui) 20g
Rhizome anemarrhenae (zhimu) 10g
Phellodendri chinensis (huangbai) 10g
Gentiana scabra (longdancao) 30g
Polygoni multiflori (yejiaoteng) 30g
Zizyphus jujube (fried) (chao suanzaoren) 15g
Concha margaritifera (zhenzhumu) 30g
Concha haliotidis (shijueming) 30g
Concha ostreae (muli) 30g
Ossa draconis (longgu) 30g
Scolopendra subspinipes (wugong) $\frac{1}{2}$ piece,
Mesobathus martensii (quanxie) 10g
Eupolyphaga (tubiechong) 10g
Paeonia lactiflora (chishao) 30g
Cortex dictamni (baixianpi) 15g
Kochia scoparia (difuzi) 15g
Coptis chinensis (huanglian) 10g

Erxian Difuzi formula in Chinese 二仙地肤子:

淫羊藿30g 克仙茅15g 巴戟天15g 远志10g 当归20g 知母10g 黄柏10g 龙胆草30g 夜交藤30g 炒枣仁15g 珍珠母30g 石决明30g 牡蛎30g 龙骨30g 蜈蚣1/2 全蝎10g 土鳖虫10g 赤芍30g 白鲜皮15g 地

肤子15g 黄连10g

The Erxian Difuzi formula is the Erxian formula with the addition of Scolopendra subspinipes (wugong), Mesobathus martensii (quanxie), Eupolyphaga (tubiechong), Paeonia lactiflora (chishao), Cortex dictamni (baixianpi), Kochia scoparia (difuzi), Coptis chinensis (huanglian).

In the Erxian Difuzi formula, the Erxian formula is to warm kidney water, clear liver wood, ground heart fire. Scolopendra subspinipes (wugong), Mesobathus martensii (quanxie), Eupolyphaga (tubiechong), Paeonia lactiflora (Chishao), Cortex dictamni (baixianpi), Kochia scoparia (difuzi), Coptis chinensis (huanglian) are used to cool blood, expel dampness, remove mucus, and detoxify poison.

Treating liver wood yin and yang damage with symptoms of vaginal itch

A 47-year-old woman came for consultation for vaginal itch. In the late afternoon on the previous day before the consultation, she suddenly felt a vaginal itch and within an hour it had become so unbearable that she was unable to sleep during the night. At the first consultation, the skin of her vaginal area was covered with small red rashes that were mostly broken with water seepage.

This case was diagnosed as liver wood yin and yang damage. The yang damage of liver wood provided the condition for damp poison to flourish in the blood; so there was a symptom of rash. The liver wood yin damage caused blood heat and created wind, so the rashes were red. The strong wind caused the severe itch. Dampness damaged the blood passages, and oozed out, so there was seeping fluid. The treatment was to remove dampness, detoxify poison, cool the blood, and stop wind. I used the Tubie Diyu formula.

After the first cup of the herbs, plus a hot vinegar wash of the vagina, the itch was significantly reduced. An hour later, however, the itch recurred. The patient took another 250 ml of the herbs and the itch subsided again. Four hours later, the itch returned, she took the third cup of the herbs and slept the night. The following day the itch was much more bearable. The patient took the herbs in the morning, midday, and after dinner and had a mild itch all day. She took the herbs for another five days and the itch completely disappeared.

Preparing and administering the herbs:

Place a packet of herbs into a pot, add 2 litres of water and boil down to 750 ml in about 1 hour. Drink 250 ml each time.

Another 60-year-old woman had a vaginal itch for six months before the first consultation. She had been using biomedicines externally to control the itch but the symptoms did not show any improvement, instead, it had become progressively worse. At the first consultation, the woman's vagina was very raw, red, swollen, and some parts of the skin were broken and other parts were thickened. The itch had frequently woken her up during the night so she was very tired. She was treated with the Tubie Diyu formula internally and the Bianxu wash externally.

After taking the herbs internally and externally, the patient's itch improved day by day. After two months, she had completely recovered. This case took longer than usual because she had taken biomedical medicines to block the itch. As a result, not only had the original dampness needed to be cleared but also the blockages that the drugs had created. Biomedical drugs often cause illness to become more complicated and frequently delay or hinder the healing effect of herbal treatments.

Bianxu wash:

Polygonum Aviculare (bianxu 萹蓄) 50g, add 700 ml of water, boil for 30 minutes.

Add 50 ml of vinegar into the liquid. While the decoction is still hot place the liquid into a bowl and squat over the bowl so the steam from the herbs reaches the vagina. When the liquid is cooler use it as a wash. The liquid can be reused after boiling, but a new wash should be made fresh each day.

Polygonum Aviculare (bianxu 萹蓄) kills parasites, removes dampness, and stops itch.

Treating liver wood yin and yang damage with symptoms of blister rashes

A blister rash is skin damage with red rashes and blisters on top. The
rash is often very red with significant fluid discharge when the blisters
are broken, and it is itchy and painful. When there is liver wood yang
damage, dampness blocks the blood passages, so the rashes occur.
When there is liver wood yin damage, blood become hot, so the rash
is deep red. Blood heat creates wind, and extreme heat boils water,
wind pushes hot water out, so there are very painful blisters; wind
travels fast in the blood passages and causes the rashes to itch.

A 56-year-old woman had small red rashes on the left side of her
chest and back for a week, then blisters developed on the top of the
rashes. She was in a lot of pain which disturbed her sleep. At the
first consultation, she had had the blisters for two days. The rashes
were small and dark red in colour. They were slightly itchy but with
excruciating waves of pain. The principle for the treatment was to
clear heat, cool blood, detoxify poison, dissolve mucus, and remove
dampness. The Tubie Diyu formula was used to treat this case.

After taking three packets of the herbs, the pain had become
more bearable. She continued taking the herbs for three weeks, and
within this time, the rashes and pain progressively improved to the
point of having completely disappeared.

Another 56-year-old woman had suffered severe headaches. The
patient had had a blister rash three years before, and since then, she
suffered from severe headaches and permanently lived on painkillers.
At the first consultation, there was a line of redness on her left fore-
head which was painful to touch. Although the rashes and blisters
had disappeared, the pain had remained, which was a sign that the
damaged liver wood yin and yang had not recovered, that blood heat,
and mucus stagnation in the blood were not removed. The treatment
and herbs were the same as the above case.

The patient took one packet of the Tubie Diyu formula and felt
the pain reduced. After taking three packets of the herbs, the interval
between bouts of pain had extended. She took another 10 packets

of the herbs, and only occasionally felt slight pain. She took a total of 30 packets of the herbs and a year later she reported that she no longer had the headaches.

A 52-year-old man suffered a condition in which his eyelids, lips, nostrils, and the prepuce suddenly became red, swollen, and numb. Within two hours, his lips, nostrils, and foreskin began to blister and quickly broke with oozing sticky fluid. The palms and fingertips of his hands were a purplish colour as were the areas around his eyes and lips. This seemed to be a case of chemical poisoning damaging liver wood yin and yang, causing damp poison and abnormal heat to obstruct the blood passages. I prescribed Tubie Diyu formula for his treatment. The patient took three packets of the herbs and the blisters subsided. After taking 10 packets of the herbs, the blisters dried out. Four months later, the patient came back with the same condition. After taking one packet of Tubie Diyu formula, the symptoms got better. He took another two weeks of the same herbs and the skin healed.

Treating liver wood yin & yang damage with symptoms of macular rash

The special feature of a macular rash is that the colour of the rash is dark red and when pressed the colour does not disappear. Macular rashes also produce severe itching. When one rash heals another would immediately take its place. Such a condition is a result of liver wood yin and yang being both damaged. With liver wood yin damage, blood rushes out of the root of liver wood into the blood passages, and causes blood heat. On the other hand, liver wood yang damage allows damp poison to grow in the blood passages. Damp poison together with stagnant heat in the blood cause blood decay, therefore, the rashes were dark in colour, and did not disappear when pressed.

A 55-year-old woman had a macular rash for two years. At the first consultation, she had dark red macular rashes over various parts of her body. The colour was deep red, the colour would not disappear when pressed, and was very itchy. She also suffered pains in her joints. The pain tended to travel around her various joints. She slept lightly and frequently woke during the night.

Liver wood yin damage causes heat and dryness which stimulate heart fire to float, and irritates the spirit's night rest, so there are symptoms of light sleep and frequent waking during the night. Liver wood yin damage fails to store blood in its root, blood crowded in the blood passages causes heat and wind. Liver wood yang damage allows damp poison to develop in the blood passages, which causes the rashes. The damp poison and stagnant heat joined together cause the dark red rash. As the stagnation in the blood is solid, when the rashes are pressed the colour does not disappear. High blood heat causes strong wind, so the itch was severe. The damp poison, wind, and blood heat damages the joints, so she had moving joint pains.

As the liver wood yinyang damage had existed for quite a while, both the yin and yang of liver wood was weak, so the treatment was to warm kidney water, nurture liver wood, and at the same time dissolve mucus, detoxify poison, cease wind, and remove stagnant blood with the Erxian Xiegong formula.

After taking seven packets of the herbs, the patient gained more energy and the colour of her body rashes were lighter. Over the following six months or so, she took on and off 100 packets of the herbs. The symptoms progressively became less and less. She continued for another six months, and the rashes disappeared and she no longer had joint pains.

Erxian Xiegong formula:

Epimedium brevicornum (yinyanghuo) 30g
Rhizoma curculiginis orchioides (xianmao) 15g
Radix morindae officinalis (bajitian) 15g
Polygala tenufola (yuanzhi) 10g
Angelica sinensis (danggui) 20g
Rhizome anemarrhenae (zhimu)10g
Phellodendri chinensis (huangbai) 10g
Gentiana scabra (longdancao) 30g
Polygoni multiflori (yejiaoteng) 30g
Zizyphus jujube (fried) (chao suanzaoren) 15g
Concha margaritifera (zhenzhumu) 30g
Concha haliotidis (shijueming) 30g
Concha ostreae (muli) 30g
Ossa draconis (longgu) 30g
Olibanum (ruxiang) 10g
Myrrh (moyao) 10g

Ampelopsis radix (bailian) 10g

Eupolyphaga sinensis
(tubiechong) 10g

Scolopendra subspinipes
(wugong) $\frac{1}{2}$ piece

Paeoniae lactiflora(chishao) 30g

Zaocys dhumnade (wushaoshe)
30g

Mesobathus martensii (quanxie)
10g

Erxian Xiegong formula in Chinese 二仙蝎蚣汤:

淫羊藿30g 仙茅15g 巴戟天15g 远志10g 当归20g 知母10g 黄柏10g 龙胆草30g 夜交藤30g 炒枣仁15g 珍珠母30g 石决明30g 牡蛎30g 龙骨30g 乳香10g 没药10g 白蔹10g 土鳖虫10g 蜈蚣1/2 赤芍30g 乌梢蛇30g 全蝎10g

The Erxian Xiegong formula is the Erxian formula with the addition of Olibanum (ruxiang), myrrh (moyao), Ampelopsis radix (bailian), Eupolyphaga (tubiechong), Scolopendra subspinipes (wugong), Paeoniae lactiflora (chishao), Zaocys dhumnade (wushaoshe), and Mesobathus martensii (quanxie).

Olibanum (ruxiang 乳香) invigorates blood, dissolves poisonous swelling, and removes damp poison in the blood.

Myrrh (moyao 没药) invigorates blood, breaks down nodules and stagnant blood, dissolves swelling, removes dampness, and detoxifies poison.

Ampelopsis radix (bailian 白蔹) has a bitter taste and mild yinyang nature. It goes into the heart and liver meridians. It breaks down all kind of poisons, swelling, and sores.

Eupolyphaga sinensis (tubiechong 土鳖虫) breaks down stagnant blood, dissolves abdominal masses, regulates menses, and treats prolonged stagnations.

Scolopendra subspinipes (wugong 蜈蚣) removes damp poison in the blood.

Paeoniae lactiflora (chishao 赤芍) removes collected nodules, and scatters stagnant blood.

Zaocys dhumnade (wushaoshe 乌梢蛇) disperses wind, opens meridians, and scatters nodules.

Mesobathus martensii (quanxie 全蝎) opens orifices, dissolves mucus, and stops wind.

Within the formula, Olibanum (ruxiang), myrrh (moyao), Ampelopsis radix (bailian), Eupolyphaga sinensis (tubiechong), Scolopendra subspinipes (wugong), and Paeoniae lactiflora (chishao) are used to remove dampness, mucus, and serious poisoning of the blood. Zaocys dhumnade (wushaoshe) and Mesobathus martensii (quanxie) are used to dissolve mucus, cease wind, and open the meridians. The Erxian formula is used to warm kidney water to regenerate liver wood.

Treating liver wood yin and yang damage with symptoms of scaly rash

The specification of scaly rash is that the damaged skin is dry, has peeling silver flakes of skin, bleeds easily, is very itchy, and the rash is persistent and lasting. Such a condition is caused by liver wood yin and yang being both damaged. Liver wood yang damage allows dampness and mucus to accumulate in the blood passages, which causes skin rashes. Liver wood yin damage causes dry heat in the blood passages, so the rashes becomes dry and flaky. Liver wood yin damage causes blood heat and wind, so there are waves of itch.

A 41-year-old male patient came for a consultation complaining of anxiety. The patient had also had palm sized flaky rashes on both of his shanks. The rash had been there for six years, the skin was thickened, peeling with silver flakes, and every now and then he suffered severe itch, so the damaged skin bled through scratching. As the patient had been seeing many skin specialists and nothing had been helpful, so he had given up the hope of healing it. At the first consultation, the patient was suffering from an anxiety attack, loss of sleep, palpitations, and itchiness from the flaking rash.

Simultaneous liver wood yin and yang damage caused the scaly rash. With kidney water heat loss the yang qi of the enduring zhi of the spirit was unable to be fully exercised, which caused the spirit anxiety. The kidney water heat loss also caused the liver wood to become dry, and the heart fire floats leading to symptoms of palpitations and loss of sleep. The treatment was to warm kidney water, regenerate liver wood, ground heart fire, remove mucus, invigorate blood, and detoxify poison. I used the Erxian Xionghuang formula.

The patient took herbs for three months, the flaky rash was significantly improved and less itchy; he slept better and his moods were more stable, but occasionally he still had loss of sleep, and anxiety attacks. He took another three months of the same prescription, the loss of sleep and anxiety symptoms stopped, however, there were still small patches of the skin rash left. The patient took on and off another 12 months of the herbs, and at the end of the year the rashes had disappeared.

Erxian Xionghuang formula:

Epimedium brevicornum (yinyanghuo) 30g
Rhizoma curculiginis orchioides (xianmao) 15g
Radix morindae officinalis (bajitian) 15g
Polygala tenufola (yuanzhi) 10g
Angelica sinensis (danggui) 20g
Rhizome anemarrhenae (zhimu) 10g
Phellodendri chinensis (huangbai) 10g
Gentiana scabra (longdancao) 30g
Polygoni multiflori (yejiaoteng) 30g
Zizyphus jujube (fried) (chao suanzaoren) 15g
Concha margaritifera (zhenzhumu) 30g
Concha haliotidis (shijueming) 30g

Concha ostreae (muli) 30g
Ossa draconis (longgu) 30g
Olibanum (ruxiang) 10g
Myrrh (moyao) 10g
Eupolyphaga sinensis (tubiechong) 10g
Scolopendra subspinipes (wugong) $\frac{1}{2}$ piece
Paeoniae lactiflora (chishao) 30g
Mesobathus martensii (quanxie) 10g
Arisaematis rhizoma (tiannanxing) 10g
Aconitum carmichaeli (treated) (zhi caowu) 10g
Coptis chinensis (huanglian) 10g
Rheum officinale (dahuang) 10g
Saposhnikovia divaricate (fangfeng) 30g
Asarum sieboldii (xixin) 10g
Realgar (xionghuang) 0.01g

Erxian Xionghuang formula in Chinese 二仙雄黄汤:

淫羊藿30g 仙茅15g 巴戟天15g 远志10g 当归20g 知母10g 黄柏10g 龙胆草30g 夜交藤30g 炒枣仁15g 珍珠母30g 石决明30g 牡蛎30g 龙骨30g 乳香10g 没药10g 土鳖虫10g 蜈蚣半条g 赤芍30g 全蝎10g 天南星10g 制草乌10g 黄连10g 大黄10g 防风30g 细辛10g 雄黄0.01g

The Erxian Xionghuang formula is the Erxian formula with the addition of Olibanum (ruxiang), myrrh (moyao), Eupolyphaga (tubiechong), Scolopendra subspinipes (wugong), Paeoniae lactiflora (chishao), Mesobathus martensii (quanxie), Arisaematis rhizoma (tiannanxing), Aconitum carmichaeli (treated) (zhi caowu), Coptis chinensis (huanglian), Rheum officinale (dahuang), Saposhnikovia divaricate (fangfeng), Asarum sieboldii (xixin), Realgar (xionghuang).

Olibanum (ruxiang 乳香) invigorates blood, dissolves poisonous swelling, and removes damp poison in the blood.

Myrrh (moyao 没药) invigorates blood, breaks down nodules and stagnant blood, dissolves swelling, removes dampness, detoxifies poison.

Eupolyphaga (tubiechong 土鳖虫) breaks down stagnant blood, dissolves lumps, treats prolonged instances of accumulated stagnation.

Scolopendra subspinipes (wugong 蜈蚣) removes damp poison in the blood.

Paeoniae lactiflora (chishao 赤芍) removes collected nodules, and scatters stagnant blood.

Mesobathus martensii (quanxie 全蝎) opens orifices, dissolves mucus, and stops wind.

Arisaematis rhizoma (tiannanxing 天南星) dries dampness, dissolves mucus, disperses wind, and scatters nodules.

Aconitum carmichaeli (treated)(zhi caowu 制草乌) has a pungent and hot taste; a hot dry yinyang nature. It goes into the heart and kidney meridians. It strengthens heart fire yang heat, and ground heart fire heat into kidney. It disperses wind and cold, opens meridians, and treats stubborn mucus and poisonous swelling.

Coptis chinensis (huanglian 黄连) extinguishes fire, detoxifies poison, dries dampness, and cools blood.

Rheum officinale (dahuang 大黄) cools blood, detoxifies poison, breaks stagnation, and removes dampness.

Saposhnikovia divaricate (fangfeng 防风) opens meridians, disperses wind anywhere in the body.

Asarum sieboldii (xixin 细辛) disperses wind and coldness, removes dampness, frees water flow, and clears lung.

Realgar (xionghuang 雄黄) has a pungent taste and cold yinyang nature. It goes into the liver meridian. It is poisonous and the dosage must be precise. It dries dampness, detoxifies poison, kills parasites, disperses wind, and heals malignant sores.

The Erxian Xionghuang formula is similar to the Erxian Xiegong formula which cleanses liver wood, removes stagnated blood, detoxifies poison, ceases wind, and warms kidney water. By adding Arisaematis rhizoma (tiannanxing), Aconitum carmichaeli (treated) (zhi caowu), Coptis chinensis (huanglian), Rheum officinale (dahuang), Saposhnikovia divaricate (fangfeng), Asarum sieboldii (xixin), Realgar (xionghuang), the Erxian Xionghuang formula has more strength to disperse wind, scatter nodules, dry dampness, and detoxify poison.

Note: This formula, because of the treated aconitum carmichaeli, requires at least two hours of boiling before drinking the decoction.

Treating liver wood yin and yang damage with the symptom of an abscess

A 38-year-old man came for help with a walnut size abscess on his thigh. It was red, swollen, hot and painful to touch. It had a pussy tip but had not yet burst. The man had a slight fever; he was thirsty, and had not had a bowel motion for two days. Liver wood yang damage caused damp poison to block the blood passages, which created blood decay, so there was the symptom of an abscess. Liver wood yin damage caused blood heat, so the abscess was red and swollen. Blood heat creates wind, wind strikes on the poison blockages causing pain. Liver wood poisonous heat damages lung metal yin, so there are symptoms of fever, thirst, and constipation. The treatment was to remove dampness, draw out puss, clear heat, cool blood, and clear lung metal heat. Internally I used the Sihuang Rumo formula and externally I used the Jinhuang formula.

After using the internal and external herbs for three days, the patient's abscess broke and the fever dropped; he no longer felt thirsty and his bowel motions had become normal. He stopped taking the herbs internally but continued to apply the Jinhuang formula externally about four times a day. After 10 days, all the puss had cleared and the skin began to heal.

Sihuang Rumo formula:

Gypsum (shigao) 20g
Talcum (huashi) 20g
Rheum officinale (dahuang) 10g
Olibanum (ruxiang) 5g
Myrrh (moyao) 5g
Radix sophorae flavescentis
(kushen) 10g
Scutellaria baicalensis
(huangqin) 10g
Coptis chinensis (huanglian) 10g
Phellodendri chinensis
(huangbai) 10g
Taraxacum mongolicum
(pugongying) 10g
Viola yedoensis makino
(zihuadiding) 10g
Oldenlandia diffusa
(baihuasheshecao) 10g
Smilax glabra (tufuling) 30g
Dioscorea septemloba (bixie) 10g
Dianthus superbus (jumai) 10g
Glycyrrhiza radix (gancao)10g

Sihuang Rumo formula in Chinese 四黄乳没汤:

石膏20g 滑石20g 大黄10g 乳香5g 没药5g 苦参10g 黄芩10g 黄连10g 黄柏10g 蒲公英10g 紫花地丁10g 白花蛇舌草10g 土茯苓30g 萆薢10g 瞿麦10g 甘草10g

Gypsum (shigao 石膏) isolates turbidity, relieves skin blockage, and frees the lung air passages.

Talcum (huashi 滑石) isolates turbidity, clears fire, dissolves mucus.

Rheum officinale (dahuang 大黄) cools blood, detoxifies poison, and breaks down stagnation.

Olibanum (ruxiang 乳香) removes ulcers, and poisonous swelling; disperses damp poison in the blood.

Myrrh (moyao 没药) breaks down stubborn stagnation and old blood, disperses swelling, removes dampness, and detoxifies poison.

Radix sophorae flavescentis (kushen 苦参) cools blood, removes dampness, detoxifies poison, expels parasites, and moistens the skin.

Scutellaria baicalensis (huangqin 黄芩) clears heat and removes dampness.

Coptis chinensis (huanglian 黄连) extinguishes fire; detoxifies poison, and dries dampness.

Phellodendri chinensis (huangbai 黄柏) clears dampness, and removes trapped heat.

Taraxacum mongolicum (pugongying 蒲公英) clears heat, detoxifies poison, and heals carbuncles and ulcers.

Viola yedoensis makino (zihuadiding 紫花地丁) clears heat, detoxifies poison, and dissolves swelling.

Oldenlandia diffusa (baihuasheshecao 白花蛇舌草) clears heat, disperses stagnation, dissolves swelling, and detoxifies poison.

Smilax glabra (tufuling 土茯苓) opens meridians, removes damp poison, and dissolves malignant wounds.

Dioscorea septemloba (bixie 萆薢) clears heat, and drains dampness.

Dianthus superbus (jumai 瞿麦) clears heat, frees water flow, and opens blood passages.

Glycyrrhiza radix (gancao 甘草) harmonizes wuxing organs and detoxifies poison.

Within the formula, Gypsum (shigao), Talcum (huashi) are used to isolate turbidity and eliminate dampness. Rheum officinale (dahuang), Olibanum (ruxiang), Myrrh (moyao), Radix sophorae flavescentis (kushen) are used to cool and detoxify blood poison. Scutellaria baicalensis (huangqin), Coptis chinensis (huanglian), Phellodendri chinensis (huangbai) are used to clear heat, dry dampness, and detoxify poison. Taraxacum mongolicum (pugongying), Viola yedoensis makino (zihuadiding), oldenlandia diffusa (baihuasheshecao) are used to clear heat, eliminate stagnation, and detoxify poison. Smilax glabra (tufuling), Dioscorea septemloba (bixie), Dianthus superbus (jumai) are used to free water flow, and drain dampness; and Glycyrrhiza radix (gancao) is used to harmonize wuxing organs and detoxify poison.

External use of Jinhuang formula:

Trichosanthes kirilowii radix (tianhuafen) 24g
Phellodendri chinensis (huangbai) 24g
Rheum officinale (dahuang) 24g
Curcuma zedoaria (jianghuang) 24g

Radix angelicae (baizhi) 15g
Magnolia officinalis (houpo) 9g
Citrus tangerine (jupi) 9g
Atractylodis lancea (cangzhu) 9g
Arisaematis rhizoma (tiannanxing) 9g
Glycyrrhiza radix (gancao) 9g.

Jinhuang formula in Chinese 金黄散:

天花粉24g 黄柏24g 大黄24g 姜黄24g 白芷15g 厚朴9g 橘皮9g 苍术9g 天南星9g 甘草9

Trichosanthes kirilowii radix (tianhuafen 天花粉) has a bitter taste, cold yinyang nature. It goes into the kidney and urine bladder meridians. It dispels puss, detoxifies poison, & eliminates swelling.

Phellodendri chinensis (huangbai 黄柏) dispels dampness and removes heat stagnation.

Rheum officinale (dahuang 大黄) cools blood, detoxifies poison, and breaks down stagnation.

Curcuma zedoaria (jianghuang 姜黄) has a pungent and bitter tastes, and warm yinyang nature. It goes into liver and spleen meridians. It breaks down blood stagnation, eliminates swelling, and promotes qi flow.

Radix angelica dahurica (baizhi 白芷) dissolves mucus and dispels nodules.

Magnolia officinalis (houpo 厚朴) has a bitter taste and warm yinyang nature. It goes into the spleen and stomach meridians. It warms spleen soil, dispels mucus, and moves qi downward.

Citrus tangerine (jupi 橘皮) has a pungent taste and warm yinyang nature. It goes into the spleen, liver meridians. It promotes qi flow and eliminates mucus.

Atractylodis lancea (cangzhu 苍术) has a sweet taste and warm yinyang nature. It goes into the spleen and stomach meridians. It removes malignant qi, dispels dampness, mucus and stagnant fluid.

Arisaematis rhizoma (tiannanxing 天南星) dries dampness, dissolves mucus, dispels wind, and scatters nodules.

Glycyrrhiza radix (gancao 甘草) harmonizes wuxing organs and detoxifies poison.

The Jinhuang formula is from *The Orthodox Manual of External Illnesses* 外科正宗 by Ming Dynasty yi scholar Chen Shigong 陈实功, and it is an effective external use mixture for removing toxins and drawing pusses. Within the formula, Radix trichosanthis (tianhuafen), Phellodendri chinensis (huangbai), Rheum officinale (dahuang) are used to clear heat and detoxify poisons, eliminate swellings, and dissolve nodules. Curcuma zedoaria (jianghuang),

Radix angelica dahurica (baizhi), Magnolia officinalis (houpo), Citrus tangerine (jupi), Atractylodis lancea (cangzhu) and Arisaematis rhizoma (tiannanxing) are used to promote qi flow, dissolve nodules, disperse wind, and expel toxins. Glycyrrhiza radix (gancao) is used to harmonize the wuxing organs as well as detoxify poison.

Method for using the Jinhuang formula: Grind all the herbs into powder, then mix with 70% alcohol, so that it becomes a paste. Apply the paste on the top of the abscess and cover with a dressing. Change the dressing twice a day.

Another case was a 27-year-old man who had suffered abscesses inside his anus on three occasions within one year. The abscesses seemed to happen after he was overworking and not getting enough sleep, and always came with constipation. The first two times he took antibiotic treatments and the abscesses cleared quickly. On the third occasion he took antibiotics again but the abscess failed to get any better. By the time he came to see me he had had the abscess for two weeks. The abscess was about the size of an apricot kernel and slightly raised on the skin. There was no damage or colour change to the skin, but it was hot and painful to touch and had a soft and hollow inside. It was painful for him to defecate and there was blood in his stool.

Blood in the stool indicated that the abscess had burst within his anus, so it was not advisable to apply drawing herbs such as the Jinhuang formula externally on the skin, in case the skin broke and caused an anal fistula, so only internal herbs were used in treating this case. With liver wood yang damage, damp poison in the blood causes the symptom of abscess as in the previous case, but the difference is that in this case, the abscess happens after exhaustion or late night sleep, which means that after kidney water heat loss the symptom appears. Kidney water heat loss causes liver wood yin and yang deficiency. Liver wood yin deficiency causes blood heat; liver wood yang deficiency leads to the damp poison flourishing in the blood, therefore, the symptoms comes up after exhaustion. The principle of treatment is to warm kidney water, clear liver wood, cool blood, and detoxify poison with the Erxian Gongying formula.

The patient took three packets of the herbs; the swelling, pain, and heat of the abscess all improved. After seven packets of the herbs, the abscess was significantly reduced, and after another seven days of the herbs, all the symptoms had disappeared, but he took another seven packets of the herbs to consolidate the recovery.

Erxian Gongying formula:

Epimedium brevicornum (yinyanghuo) 30g

Rhizoma curculiginis orchioides (xianmao) 15g

Radix morindae officinalis (bajitian) 15g

Polygala tenufola (yuanzhi) 10g

Angelica sinensis (danggui) 20g

Rhizome anemarrhenae (zhimu) 10g

Phellodendri chinensis (huangbai) 10g

Gentiana scabra (longdancao) 30g

Polygoni multiflori (yejiaoteng) 30g

Zizyphus Jujube (fried) (chao suanzaoren) 15g

Concha margaritifera (zhenzhumu) 30g

Concha haliotidis (shijueming) 30g

Concha ostreae (muli) 30g

Ossa draconis (longgu) 30g

Paeonia lactiflora (chishao) 15g

Taraxacum officinale (pugongying) 15g

Viola yedoensis (zihuadiding) 15g

Rheum officinale (dahuang) 10g

Coptis chinensis (huanglian) 10g

The Erxian Gongying formula in Chinese 二仙公英汤:

淫羊藿30g 仙茅15g 巴戟天15g 当归20g 知母10g 黄柏10远志10g 龙胆草30g 夜交藤30g 炒枣仁15g 珍珠母30g 牡蛎30g 石决明30龙骨30g 赤芍30g 蒲公英15g 紫花地丁15g 大黄10g 黄连10g

For the formula explanation, see the section "Treating kidney water yin and yang deficiency with symptoms of pain & swollen testicle".

Treating liver wood yang damage with symptoms of malignant sores

Malignant sores are a symptom of liver wood yang damage, poisonous dampness and mucus blocking blood passages, with long lasting broken and pussy swelling wounds. A 50-year-old woman had an egg size lump on the right side of her groin and after a year the skin broke. At the consultation, the wound was pussy, wet, and the surrounding area was swollen and hard. It was painful to touch. The treatment was to dry dampness, remove mucus, break down nodules, cleanse liver wood, and detoxify poison with the Xiongchan formula.

In the beginning when she applied the herbs, it was very painful, and the pain would last for 1-2 hours and much liquid would ooze out. After three months of applying the herbs, the swelling and hard lump disappeared and left an egg sized hollow. There was a small amount of liquid seeping out after applying the herbs, but the wound was not yet healed. Mylabris (banmao) was removed from the formula to promote coalescence, which made it much less painful when applying the paste. Six months later, the wound was smaller and after a year, the wound had healed.

Xiongchan Formula (external use only):

Realgar (xionghuang) 5g   Mylabris pustulata (banmao) 5g

Bufonis Venenum (chansu) 5g   Olibanum (ruxiang) 5g

Calomelas (qingfen) 5g   Myrrh (moyao) 5g

Cinnabaris (zhusha) 5g

Xiongchan formula in Chinese 雄蟾:

雄黄5g 蟾酥5g 轻粉5g 朱砂5g 斑蝥5g 乳香5g 没药5g。

Realgar (xionghuang 雄黄) has a pungent taste and cold yinyang nature. It goes into the liver meridian. It is a poisonous herb and to be used with caution. It dries dampness, detoxifies poison, kills parasites, eliminates wind, and heals malignant sores.

Bufonis venenum (chansu 蟾酥) breaks down stagnation, cleanses liver wood, removes poison, and treats malignant sores and stubborn scaly tetter.

Calomelas (qingfen 轻粉) has a pungent taste and cold dry yinyang nature. It is a poisonous herb and dosage should be within safe limits, internally it should not be taken long term. It goes into kidney and liver meridians. It breaks down stagnation, scatters nodules, eliminates poison, removes rotten flesh, and regenerates new flesh.

Cinnabaris (zhusha 朱砂) has a sweet taste and cool yinyang nature. It goes into the heart meridian. It is a poisonous herb and the dosage must be within safe limits. It grounds heart fire and calms the spirit; it opens blood passages, removes poisonous qi and all kinds of sores.

Mylabris pustulata (banmao 斑蝥) opens water passages, draws pusses, breaks stagnation, and dissolves lumps, malignant sores, and stubborn scaly tetter.

Olibanum (ruxiang 乳香) invigorates blood, removes mucus and dampness in the blood; it cleanses liver wood, detoxifies poison, and resolves carbuncle and ulcers.

Myrrh (moyao 没药) breaks down nodules and stagnant blood, dissolves swelling, removes dampness, and detoxifies poison.

Among the above herbs, Realgar (xionghuang), Bufonis Venenum (chansu), Calomelas (qingfen), Cinnabaris (zhusha) and Mylabris (banmao) all have strong effects in breaking down stagnation, attacking poison, removing stubborn mucus and pussy swelling. Olibanum (ruxiang) and Myrrh (moyao) invigorate the blood and eliminate swelling.

Preparation:

Grind the herbs into a fine powder, take a tablespoon of the powder and mix with honey then apply on the wound once every 3 days.

Treating liver wood yang damage with symptoms of sticky bowel motions

A 45-year-old woman had sticky and very smelly faeces for over 20 years. Her bowel motions were always loose, and she never felt that she could completely empty her bowels, but she only sought help when she developed a large haemorrhoid. When there is liver wood yang damage, dampness and mucus flourishing causing blood decay in the large intestine area, which leads to the symptoms of sticky and smelly faeces. Prolonged damp poison that block the blood passage causes haemorrhoids. The treatment focuses on removing dampness, dissolving turbidity, cleansing the large intestine, and cooling the

151

blood. The Tujingpi formula was used.

The patient took one cup of the decoction, and three hours later, her stomach was rumbling loudly; she had slight lower stomach pain and needed to open her bowels. She then expelled a large quantity of faeces with a slimy liquid, all of which were quite smelly. Half an hour later she had another bowel movement which was mostly liquid; this time she didn't have any stomach pains, and the faeces was not as smelly. She drank a cup of water, then she had another clean out, and it did not smell. She had a total of eight bowel motions that day with one drink of the decoction. The following day, she took the remainder of the decoction, two hours later she had three very loose bowel motions within an hour. There was no smell nor stomach pains. The haemorrhoid was significantly smaller. By the third day, she made a new batch of the decoction. After taking one cup of the herbs she had one formed clean bowel motion. Later in the day, she took the second cup of the decoction, and she had another bowel motion which was a little loose. She stopped the herbs for two days, and during the two days, each day she had one clean formed bowel motion, something she had not had in the previous twenty years. However, after stopping the herbs for seven days, her bowel motions became a little sluggish again. She took three more packets of the herbs, and was able to take the decoction twice a day which led only to a bowel motion once a day. Sometimes the bowel motion was loose and other times formed. In the following six months or so, she would take a packet or two of the herbs as soon as she felt the symptoms of constipation coming back. A year later, she came for a consultation for a minor lung condition and informed me that the constipation and haemorrhoid symptoms had not appeared again.

Tujingpi formula:

Nepeta cataria (jingjie)15g

Saposhnikovia divaricate (fangfeng) 15g

Periostracum cicadae (chanyi) 15g

Gypsum (shigao) 20g

Paeonia lactiflora (chishao) 30g

Paeonia suffruticosa (mudanpi) 15g

Lium usitatissimum (humaren) 10g

Pseudolarix amailis (tujingpi)10g

Rheum officinale (dahuang) 10g

Tujingpi formula in Chinese 土荆皮汤:

荆芥15g 防风15g 蝉衣15g 石膏20g 赤芍30g 牡丹皮15g 胡麻仁10g 土荆皮10g 大黄10g

Tujingpi formula is a modification of Zijingpi formula which takes out (zijingpi), and adds Pseudolarix amailis (tujingpi) from 5 gram to 10 gram. The purpose of which is to increase the strength of invigorating blood and opening bowel motions.

Nepeta cataria (jingjie 荆芥) opens the breathing passages of the lungs, dissolves qi stagnation, discharges blood stagnation, and removes dampness in the joints.

Saposhnikovia divaricate (fangfeng 防风) opens meridians, stops wind, and removes turbidity.

Periostracum cicadae (chanyi 蝉衣) cools blood, frees the breathing passages of the lung, stops wind, draws out poison.

Gypsum (shigao 石膏) isolates turbidity and removes dampness.

Paeonia lactiflora (chishao 赤芍) cools blood, removes collected nodules, disperses blood stagnation, breaks down wind and swelling in the large intestine.

Paeonia suffruticosa (mudanpi 牡丹皮) cools blood, breaks down accumulated nodules, removes blood stagnation in the stomach and large intestine.

Lium usitatissimum (humaren 胡麻仁) cools the blood, detoxifies poison, clears turbidity, and removes dampness.

Pseudolarix amailis (tujingpi 土荆皮) invigorates blood, expels parasites, and has a strong effect on opening bowel motions and stopping itchiness.

Rheum officinale (dahuang 大黄) cools blood, detoxifies poison, breaks down stagnation, opens bowel motions, and removes dampness.

Each ingredient in the formula has the effect of cooling the blood and removing dampness. Nepeta cataria (jingjie), Saposhnikovia divaricate (fangfeng), Periostracum cicadae (chanyi) also free qi flow and cease wind. Gypsum (shigao) isolates turbidity. Paeonia lactiflora (chishao), Paeonia suffruticosa (mudanpi), Lium usitatissimum (humaren), Pseudolarix amailis (tujingpi), and Rheum officinale (dahuang) break down nodules, detoxify poison, and open bowel motions.

Preparation and taking the herbs:
Place a packet of the formula in a pot and add 1.25 litters (5 cups) of cold water, bring to boil and keep on a rolling boil for approximately one hour until 250ml (1 cup) of liquid is left. Strain the liquid into a jug. Add another 500 ml of cold water into the pot and cook the herbs a second time, bringing it to boil and cooking for 20 minutes to reduce the liquid down to 250 ml again. Strain the liquid out and combine with the first cup. Now discard the dregs of the decoction. Drink 250 ml of the decoction each time.

Treating liver wood yin and yang damage with symptoms of damp feet

Damp feet is a symptom of liver wood yin and yang damage, with blood heat and damp poison blocking the blood passages in between the toes. I had a 21-year-old male patient who suffered from rashes between the toes and smelly feet. His feet were also itchy, and painful because the skin was broken around where it itched. The patient always felt hot and perspired easily, especially his hands and feet. He was always thirsty and drank a lot of soft drinks.

This was a case of white sugar draining the kidney water heat and damaging the liver wood yang qi which caused dampness in the blood passages. White sugar damages liver wood yang and breeds damp poison. Liver wood yang damage enables damp poison to obstruct the blood passages in the toes, so there is the symptom of rashes between the toes. Damp poison causes blood decay, so the feet are smelly. White sugar damages kidney water heat, and kidney water heat loss causes liver wood dry heat, which pushes blood to rush out of liver wood root and results in blood heat, so there is the symptom of the feeling hot and sweaty. Blood heat creates wind, so the rashes are itchy. Kidney water heat loss fails to raise water to the upper body, so there is the symptom of thirstiness. The treatment was to remove dampness, detoxify poison, cool blood, and cleanse the liver wood. As for the kidney water heat loss and dry heat in the liver wood, once the patient stopped drinking soft drinks, the kidney water heat loss would recover, so the precondition of the treatment was to stop the white sugar intake. The formula was Tubie Diyu for internal use and naturally fermented vinegar as an external wash.

Three days later the patient came back for a second consultation, his body was cooler, less sweaty, the itchiness in his feet was improved. After taking another 7 days of herbs and washing his feet with vinegar, his feet no longer had the rash or itchiness, or bad smell, and he no longer had a problem with over perspiration.

If damp feet is localized without other symptoms, using a vinegar wash twice a day the symptoms will stop within one or two days without internal treatment.

Method for vinegar wash:

Any kind of naturally fermented vinegar (for example: apple cider vinegar. Rice vinegar or coconut vinegar) 200 ml, heat to warm, then soak feet for 5-10 minutes, two to three times a day.

Treating liver wood yang damage with symptoms of timidity

When trees are in a moist and airy space they spread and are supple. When a person's liver wood is moist and open the person has courage and is flexible. On the other hand, a yinyang disorder of liver wood makes the liver wood either dry or decaying, and causes the striving zhi of the spirit to be either inflexible or unable to be firm, as a result, there is emotional discomfort.

A seven-year-old boy came for a consultation because, for the previous two months, he could no longer bear the thought of going to school. His parents said, prior to this, the boy had been very active. He enjoyed sports, had good school results, and he had no problems with his schoolmates. It seemed to happen suddenly that one morning he woke up and said he didn't want to go to school, and from that point got progressively worse. He cried every morning with the thought of going to school. He didn't want to see anyone, and didn't have any interest in school work. His skin was itchy here and there but with no obvious rash. Also the boy had been drinking soft drinks every day.

The boy did not have obvious physical discomfort nor apparent external disturbance to his spirit. However, we know that the spirit in liver wood governs the courage of a person, if liver wood yang is damaged, the yang qi of the striving zhi of the spirit is unable to be exercised, so the striving zhi is not solid, and a person feels timid and overcautious.

Because the patient drank soft drinks, the white sugar damaged the liver wood yang, which encouraged the growth of dampness and mucus in the blood. White sugar also drains kidney water heat, and with kidney water heat loss the liver wood yin becomes deficient, which causes blood heat and wind. Finally wind causes the body to itch. Thus this case was diagnosed as liver wood yang damage, causing spirit discomfort and showing symptoms of timidness and over-cautiousness. The treatment was to expel decay, remove turbidity, and invigorate blood with the Sihuang Rumo formula.

The patient stopped taking any form of white sugar during the treatment and after taking seven packets of the herbs, the boy stopped crying over the thought of going to school but still didn't want to see people. He took another seven packets of the same herbs and returned to his normal happy self.

Sihuang Rumo formula:

Gypsum (shigao) 20g

Talcum (huashi) 20g

Rheum officinale (dahuang) 10g

Olibanum (ruxiang) 5g

Myrrh(moyao) 5g

Radix sophorae flavescentis (kushen) 10g

Scutellaria baicalensis (huangqin) 10g

Coptis chinensis (huanglian) 10g

Phellodendri chinensis

(huangbai) 10g

Taraxacum mongolicum (pugongying) 10g

Viola yedoensis makino (zihuadiding) 10g

Oldenlandia diffusa (baihuasheshecao) 10g

Smilax glabra (tufuling) 30g

Dioscorea septemloba (bixie) 10g

Dianthus superbus (jumai) 10g

Glycyrrhiza radix (gancao)10g

Sihuang Rumo formula in Chinese 四黄乳没汤:

石膏20g 滑石20g 大黄10g 乳香5g 没药5g 苦参10g 黄芩10g 黄柏10g 黄连10g 蒲公英10g 紫花地丁10g 白花蛇舌草10g 土茯苓30g 萆薢10g 瞿麦10g 甘草10g

For the formula explanation of Sihuang Rumo formula see the section "Treating liver wood yin & yang damage with symptom of abscess."

Treating liver wood yin deficiency with symptoms of anger

An eight-year-old boy was brought to me by his parents because of his bad temper. From the time of his early infancy the boy suffered from restless sleep. He was continually agitated and easily angered. He was often in trouble in school for fighting with other children. Anger is a sign of liver wood yin deficiency that the yin qi of the striving zhi of the spirit is unable to be exercised. It is similar to the branches of a tree that have insufficient water and have lost flexibility and cannot bend without snapping or breaking. Liver wood dryness and heat causes the striving zhi to be firm but unable to bend, so there are symptoms of agitation and anger. Liver wood yin deficiency makes liver wood dry and hot, which stimulates the heart fire to float and prevents the spirit from resting, so there is the symptom of restless sleep. The treatment is to warm kidney water to soften liver wood, and ground heart fire. I used the Erxian formula.

The boy took seven packets of the Erxian formula and became so calm and good natured that his father felt the boy had become a totally different person.

A 48-year-old patient came for a consultation because his biomedical practitioner told him that he had 5 years to live. Before he came to me, the patient had been taking six kinds of drugs for over 10 years, which began with drugs to calm him, and drugs to enlarge his blood vessels so that he could sleep and keep his blood pressure down. Soon he was given drugs to reduce the water content in the blood, and drugs to kill blood cells were added to make less pressure on his blood vessels. Later a drug to slow the heart rate was also added to reduce blood in the blood vessels. At the first consultation, although he was on drugs to calm him, he found it difficult to hold back his temper. His muscles were tight, he often suffered headaches, and shortness of breath; his face was reddish, the tongue was dry, and deep red, the texture of the tongue was firm and thick, the coating of the tongue was greasy, and his pulse was tight.

157

With liver wood yin deficiency, the yin qi of the striving zhi of the spirit is unable to be exercised; the striving zhi is not supple and, therefore, the patient would easily lose his temper. With liver wood yin deficiency the body becomes rigid, and then there are symptoms of body and pulse tightness. The liver wood yin deficiency fails to store blood in its root, blood rushes in the blood passages creating heat, and the face becomes reddish and the tongue a deep red. In addition the heart fire floats, which disturbs the rest of spirit, so there is the symptom of sleeplessness. When the heart fire floats it indicates that the heart fire yin is weak. In such a condition, the heart fire yang departs from heart fire body yin, so the heart feels tightness.

The texture of the tongue is the reflection of the heart fire organ, when the heart fire organ is tight, the texture of the tongue appears hardened and thick. Liver wood yin deficiency with blood heat also causes wind, and wind rushing in the yinyang passages causes symptoms of headaches. Although the direct cause of the patient's agitated temperament was the liver wood yin damage, it was the kidney water heat loss, which fails to moisten liver wood, that was the root cause of the liver wood yin deficiency. With kidney water heat loss, water is unable to rise to moisten lung metal, then this leads to lung metal yin deficiency, which further leads to the symptom of dry tongue. The yin deficiency of lung metal fails to gather qi, so there is a symptom of shortness of breath. Because the patient had been regularly eating food with a high content of white sugar, this damaged the spleen soil yang and caused fluid not to drain away, and which dampness would grow upon, so the tongue coating was greasy. The treatment was to warm kidney water, soften liver wood, ground heart fire, and cease wind to stop headaches with the formula Erxian Xiongzhi.

After taking the herbs for a month, the patient also changed his diet by avoiding sugar, alcohol, coffee, and dairy products, and the greasy coating on his tongue was cleared. He took the herbs regularly for a year and all the symptoms disappeared. At this point, the patient began to reduce the dosage of the pharmaceutical drugs, but kept taking the herbs. After five years, he was able to give away all his drugs and was in good spirits, without headaches, and breathed freely. His face was no longer reddish, and he slept well.

Erxian Xiongzhi formula:

Epimedium brevicornum (yinyanghuo) 30g

Rhizoma curculiginis orchioides (xianmao) 15g

Radix morindae officinalis (bajitian) 15g

Polygala tenufola (yuanzhi) 10g

Angelica sinensis (danggui) 20g

Rhizome anemarrhenae (zhimu) 10g

Phellodendri chinensis (huangbai) 10g

Gentiana scabra (longdancao) 30g

Polygoni multiflori (yejiaoteng) 30g

Zizyphus jujube (fried)(chao suanzaoren) 15g

Concha margaritifera (zhenzhumu) 30g

Concha haliotidis (shijueming) 30g

Concha ostreae (muli) 30g

Ossa draconis (longgu) 30g

Angelica dahurica (baizhi) 15g

Gastrodia elata (tianma) 15g

Uncaria rhynchophylla (gouteng) 15g

Ligusticum wallichii (chuanxiong) 10g

Erxian Xiongzhi formula in Chinese 二仙芎芷汤:

淫羊藿30g 仙茅15g 巴戟天15g 远志10g 当归20g 知母10g 黄柏10g 龙胆草30g 夜交藤30g 酸枣仁15g 珍珠母30g 石决明30g 牡蛎30g 龙骨30g 白芷15g 天麻15g 钩藤15g 川芎10g

For the formula explanation see the section "Treating liver wood yin deficiency with symptoms of headache".

Heart Fire

The heart is a fire organ, a yang organ, and has a floating nature. Yang likes yin, and heart fire yang attracts kidney water yin, so that its fire heat can be grounded. Heart fire is the house of the spirit, it protects the spirit, and governs the activeness and quietness of the spirit. When the yang qi of heart fire is dominant, the spirit is active and this leads the body to be active. When a person becomes lively, they inevitably consume the body's yinyang qi storage and then the body tires. When the yin of heart fire is dominant, the spirit is quiet, the body is relaxed, a person falls into sleep, and the body is rejuvenated.

The spirit comes from outside the body and remains connected with the outside world. As such, it connects a person to the outside world. Because of the connection with the outside world, the body responds to the yinyang transformations of heaven and earth, and people have emotional feelings with each other and all else within heaven and earth. When the yinyang of heart fire is in harmony, the activeness and the rest of the spirit is in regular order, so that a person is active during the day and sleeps well at night. As the heart fire is an extremely yang organ, it is the impetus for the body's movements, so the spirit relies on the heart fire to exercise its aspiring zhi. When the spirit and heart fire coordinate, a person is ardent but poised.

Overall, the heart fire governs the activeness and quietness of a person, it enables a person to be both active and serene. Heart fire also hosts the spirit, and maintains the intimacy of the spirit and the body.

Yinyang disorders of heart fire disturb a person's activeness and rest. Prolonged or severe heart fire yinyang disorder will then disrupt the intimacy of spirit and body.

Causes of heart fire yinyang disorder

Heart fire has a nature of floating, and is a yang organ. Yinyang disorders of heart fire are frequently related to a deficiency of yin, so that the yang fire loses its grounding and then floats. Exhaustion drains kidney water heat, which causes liver wood dryness and encourages the heart fire yang qi to overpower its yin qi. This is the main reason that heart fire yin becomes deficient. Staying up late will force the yin qi of heaven and earth to travel through the body's yang meridians, which will then exhaust the yang heat of heart fire, and this is one of the most common causes of heart fire yang damage. On the other hand, chemicals in our food congests the yinyang passages of the heart fire, so that the heart fire yinyang cannot be replenished by heaven and earth, which will cause either yin or yang damage, and even simultaneously both yin and yang damage of the heart fire. A yinyang disorder of heart fire causes a spirit and heart fire un-cooperativeness, which in turn results in discomfort to the spirit.

Symptoms

The yang deficiency of heart fire causes a person to be slow, sluggish, inactive, or bodily heavy and have difficulty walking. The yin deficiency of heart fire causes a person to be unable to rest, and have symptoms such as palpitations, and insomnia. Emotionally, the yin deficiency of heart fire prevents the yin of the aspiring zhi of the spirit from being exercised, so the aspiring zhi is ungrounded, and will show symptoms of a panicky spirit. Yang deficiency of the heart fire deprives the yang qi of the aspiring zhi from being exercised, so the aspiring zhi of the spirit is suppressed, and will exhibit symptoms of a despondent spirit.

Tongue

The texture of the tongue is the mirror of the texture of the heart. When the yinyang of the heart fire is bound together, the texture of the tongue is soft and flexible. When the yin qi of the heart fire is weak, the fire floats, which means the yang qi is separating from the body yin, then the heart becomes tight, and the texture of the tongue is solid and thick. The yang deficiency of heart fire means the overwhelming yin qi buries the yang qi, so the heart fire is empty, and the tongue is bloated.

Pulse

A yin deficiency of heart fire means that the yang qi is floating and ungrounded, so the pulse is floating. A floating pulse can be felt on the surface, but pushing down on the pulse, it disappears with no feeling of a middle or deep pulse. A floating pulse occurs first on the left cun pulse, but when it affects the liver wood, the left guan pulse is also floating. When it affects the kidney water, the left chi pulse floats. When the lung metal is affected, the right cun pulse floats. When it affects the spleen soil, the right guan pulse floats, and when it affects the kidney reserve, the right chi pulse will float.

Heart fire yang deficiency means the yang fire is buried by yin, so the pulse is unable to float, therefore, only by pressing down to the deep pulse can one feel the pulse bouncing. It is like a balloon without enough space to bounce. It is called a sinking pulse. It occurs first on the left cun, then the other affected wuxing organs will have the same sinking pulse.

As heart fire is the house of the spirit, when heart fire yin deficiency causes the spirit unease, the pulse is bumpy and unsteady, which means when pressed down to the deep pulse it is like landing on pebbles, jumping sideways, unevenly, with one high, one low. This is called a bumpy pulse. It first occurs on the left cun pulse, but when it affects other wuxing organs, there will be a bumpy pulse accordingly. When the heart fire yang qi begins to diminish, the spirit is about to leave the body, every position of the pulse becomes a very small bead, floating as if the balloon would jump out of the skin. When a pulse is like this, the life is in deep danger, and it is called the death pulse.

Skin

Heart fire is the house of the spirit, the spirit connects with heaven and earth and brings a shine to the life. When the yinyang of heart fire is in regular order, the spirit is settled in the body, and when it is connected with heaven and earth, a person has a bright complexion.

Yang damage of heart fire inhibits the spirit's ability to rise and connect with heaven and earth, so a person has a dull complexion. The yin deficiency of heart fire makes the spirit unable to ground inside heart fire, and a person has a very pale complexion.

Principles for treating heart fire yinyang disorder

The principle for treating heart fire yang deficiency is to strengthen the yang heat of heart fire. However, while strengthening heart fire yang heat, one must also ground the heat into kidney water, so that the heart fire doesn't float, and that the dry and warm herbs don't damage the liver wood yin. The principle for treating heart fire yin deficiency is to ground heart fire heat, raise kidney water, and soften liver wood.

Treating heart fire yang deficiency with symptoms of tightness of chest

A 62-year-old woman consulted me for tightness in the chest. Before the consultation, she was diagnosed in biomedicine as having hydropericardium, which is to say that there was fluid retention in her pericardial cavity. She had been treated twice with an injecting needle to her chest to draw the fluid out but the fluid returned almost immediately. At the first consultation, the patient had severe chest tightness and sometimes with sharp pains. She could not sleep, her complexion was dull, and her face was puffy. She walked slowly and unsteadily. Her pulse was sunken and slippery. The patient also had loss of appetite for many years, and often had reflux. She found food tasteless, and sometimes, she suffered severe stomach ache and at the worst, it caused her to lose conciousness. She had many medical examinations but nothing was found to have caused her condition.

Deficiency of heart fire yang heat makes a person lose vitality, so she had a slow and unsteady walk and sunken pulse. Heart fire yang heat is the source of kidney water heat, when it is exhausted, kidney water heat is also lost. Kidney water heat loss makes water flow sluggish and causes water retention, so her pulse was slippery and the face was puffy. With heart fire yang damage, the spirit is unable to rise and congests the connection of the spirit with heaven and earth, so her face had a dull complexion. Heart fire yang damage will cause loss of control over lung metal, and lung metal loses its softness, and the qi passages become rough and congested, so there is a symptom of tight chest. When the qi passages are uneven, the qi flow is not smooth, then the qi strikes the yinyang passages and causes chest pain. When there is heart fire yang damage, spleen soil is not nurtured, which causes both yin and yang deficiency of the spleen soil. When spleen soil yin deficiency fails to bear food, there is a lack of good appetite. When spleen soil yang deficiency fails to transform food, the congestion of food causes her reflux and the food seems tasteless. When there is spleen soil yang deficiency the spleen soil loses its permeability, and qi cannot pass through the spleen soil, therefore she would have stomach pains. The lengthy suffering of loss of appetite and stomach pain and other symptoms of spleen soil yinyang disorder indicated that her current heart fire yang damage was the result of a spleen soil yinyang disorder, that the heart fire yang qi was unable to store in the kidney water but was dissipated.

The treatment was to strengthen heart fire yang heat, ground fire heat into kidney water, remove dampness, dissolve mucus, and free the water passages. However, spleen soil is the pivot of the wuxing organs, if spleen soil is impermeable, the heart fire yang qi will not store in the kidney water; also, the retention of fluid and stagnant qi will not be able to pass through the spleen soil, and the yinyang transformation of wuxing organs will not get onto the right path. So the treatment began with loosening spleen soil to open the water and qi passages, and was followed by strengthening heart fire yang qi, nurturing spleen soil and warming kidney water. The treatment began with loosening spleen soil with the formula Xianglian Yuling and strengthening heart fire yang with the formula Erxian Wutou Yuxu.

The patient took three packets of the Xianlian Yuling formula, her chest tightness was slightly improved, and she was able to have several hours of sleep. This indicated that there was some permeability of spleen soil. Then I changed to the Erxian Wutou Yuxu formula. She took seven packets of the herbs, all the symptoms improved, but after another three packets of the same herbs, she suddenly had a severe stomach ache. So I changed back to the Xianglian Yuling formula. After one packet of the herbs, the stomach pain was relieved, and she took another seven packets of Xianglian Yuling formula to consolidate the yinyang order of spleen soil, then changed to the Erxian Wutou Yuxu formula. Thereafter, for six months, I would alternate between these two formulas according to her condition. At the end of the six months, she regained her strength and the tightness in her chest was no longer evident.

Xianlian Yuling formula:

Zingiberis rhizoma (ganjiang) 10g

Aucklandia lappa (muxiang) 10g

Cyperus rotundus (xiangfu) 10g

Alpinia officinarum (gaoliangjiang) 10g

Magnolia officinalis (houpo) 10g

Areca catechu (dafupi) 10g

Lindera aggregata (wuyao) 10g

Caryophylli flos (dingxiang) 10g

Evodia rutaecarpa (wuzhuyu) 10g

Aurantii fructus (zhiqiao) 10g

Toosendan fructus (chuanlianzi) 10g

Cinnamomum cassia (guizhi) 10g

Paeoniae lactiflora(baishao) 10g

Glycyrrhiza radix (gancao) 10g

Sepiella maindroni (wuzeigu) 30g

Concha arcae (forged) (duan walengzi) 30g

Typha angustifolia (puhuang) 10

Trogopterpri faeces (wulingzhi) 10g

Poria cocos (fuling) 30g

Polyporus umbellatus (zhuling) 30g

Maydis stigmata (yumixu) 30g

Lygodium japonicum (haijinsha) 10g

Alisma orientalis (zexie) 10g

Xianglian Yuling Formula in Chinese 香楝玉苓汤:

干姜10g 木香10g 香附10g 高良姜10g 厚朴10g 大腹皮10g 乌药10丁香10g 吴茱萸10g 枳壳10g 川楝子10g 桂枝10g 白芍10g 甘草10g 乌贼骨30g 锻瓦楞子30g 蒲黄10g 五灵脂10g 茯苓30g 猪苓30g 玉米须30g 海金沙10g 泽泻10g

Zingiberis rhizoma (ganjiang 干姜) has a pungent taste and warm yinyang nature. It goes into the liver and lung meridians. It expels cold and disperses wind.

Aucklandia lappa (muxiang 木香) has a pungent taste and warm yinyang nature. It goes into the liver, spleen, and lung meridians. It warms spleen soil, resolves damp poison, and removes poisonous qi.

Cyperus rotundus (xiangfu 香附) has a pungent taste and slightly warm yinyang nature. It goes into the liver, spleen, stomach, lung meridians. It opens meridians, removes qi stagnation, warms spleen soil, and frees snarls.

Alpinia officinarum (gaoliangjiang 高良姜) has a pungent taste and warm yinyang nature. It goes into the liver, spleen, and stomach meridians. It warms and loosens spleen soil.

Mangnolia officinalis (houpo 厚朴) has a bitter taste, and warm yinyang nature. It goes into spleen and stomach meridians. It warms spleen soil, dissolves mucus, and moves gas downward and out.

Areca catechu (dafupi 大腹皮) has a pungent taste and slightly warm yinyang nature. It goes into spleen and lung meridians. It moves gas downward and out, drains dampness, expels wind, and relaxes the intestines.

Lindera aggregata (wuyao 乌药) has a pungent taste and warm yinyang nature. It goes into spleen and lung meridians. It frees qi flow, ceases bloating, stops stomach pain, and frees snarls.

Caryophylli Flos (dingxiang 丁香) has a pungent taste and warm yinyang nature. It goes into the stomach, lung, and kidney meridians. It heals cold gassy stomach pain.

Evodia rutaecarpa (wuzhuyu 吴茱萸) has a pungent taste and warm yinyang nature. It goes into liver, spleen, and kidney meridians. It warms spleen soil, moves stomach gas downward, removes dampness, and stops pain.

Aurantii fructus (zhiqiao 枳壳) has a pungent and bitter taste, and slightly cool yinyang nature. It goes into the lung, spleen, stomach, and large intestine meridians. It breaks down gas, dissolves mucus, and improves digestion.

Toosendan fructus (chuanlianzi 川楝子) has a bitter taste and cold yinyang nature. It goes into spleen, stomach meridians. It removes gas, clears liver wood fire, and stops all abdominal pain.

Cinnamomum cassia (guizhi 桂枝) has a pungent and sweet taste, and warm yinyang nature. It goes into lung, urine bladder meridians. It disperses hidden coldness in between skin and muscle, expels irregular qi.

Paeoniae alba (baishao 白芍) has a sour taste and mild yinyang nature. It goes into liver and spleen meridians. It softens liver wood, opens and smooths blood passages, and dissolves swelling.

Glycyrrhiza radix (gancao 甘草) dissolves cold or hot irregular poisonous qi of all wuxing organs.

Sepiella maindroni (wuzeigu 乌贼骨) has a salty taste, and slightly warm yinyang nature. It goes into kidney and spleen meridians. It removes dampness and mucus, opens meridians, dissolves blood stagnation, and stops bleeding.

Concha arcae (walengzi 瓦楞子) has a salty taste, and mild yinyang nature. It goes into the liver and spleen meridians. It breaks down lumps, nodules, and stagnating mucus, blood and gas. Forged concha arcae is dryer and has a stronger effect in dissolving dampness.

Typha Angustifolia (puhuang 蒲黄) has a sweet taste and mild yinyang nature. It goes into the spleen meridian. It clears chest, stomach and urine bladder cold and hot stagnation. It smooths urine flow, and dissolves blood stagnation.

Trogopterpri faeces (wulingzhi 五灵脂) has a sweet taste and mild yinyang nature. It goes into spleen and liver meridians. It smooths blood flow, and disperses cold air in the chest and stomach.

Poria cocos (fuling 茯苓) has a sweet taste and mild yinyang nature. It goes into lung, spleen, and stomach meridians. It strengthens spleen soil yang, drains water, opens the appetite, & calms the spirit.

Polyporus umbellatus (zhuling 猪苓) has a sweet taste and mild yinyang nature. It goes into the spleen, kidney, and urine bladder meridians. It drains dampness, and frees water passages.

Maydis stigmata (yumixu 玉米须) has a sweet taste and slightly warm yinyang nature. It goes into kidney meridian. It frees water passages and soothes water flow, and removes dampness.

Lygodium japonicum (haijinsha 海金沙) has a sweet taste and mild yinyang nature. It goes into spleen and kidney meridians. It removes damp heat and swelling, and tonifies spleen soil yang qi.

Alisma orientalis (zexie 泽泻) has a sweet taste and cold yinyang nature. It goes into the kidney and urine bladder meridians. It removes stale water, and nurtures fresh water, frees urine flow, eliminates water retention, drains dampness, and alleviates thirst.

In the Xianglian Yuling formula, Zingiberis rhizoma (ganjiang), Aucklandia lappa (muxiang), Cyperus rotundus (xiangfu), Alpinia officinarum (gaoliangjiang), Magnolia officinalis (houpo), Areca catechu (dafupi), Lindera aggregata (wuyao), Caryophylli flos (ding-xiang), Evodia rutaecarpa (wuzhuyu) are all fragrant and warm herbs that loosen spleen soil, dissolve dampness, and remove stomach gas. Fructus aurantii (zhiqiao), Toosendan fructus (chuanlianzi) are very effective herbs to remove stomach gas. The sour and sweet herbs of Cinnamomum Cassia (guizhi), Paeoniae alba (baishao) and Gly-cyrrhiza radix (gancao) are used to relax spasms, smooth qi flow, and stop pain. Sepiella maindroni (wuzeigu), Concha Arcae (walengzi), Typha Angustifolia (puhuang), and Faeces Trogopterpri (wulingzhi) these four herbs are used to remove hard mucus in the spleen soil and stop stomach pain. Poria cocos (fuling), Polyporus umbellatus (Zhuling), Maydis stigmata (yumixu), Lygodium japonicum (haijin-sha), and Alisma orientalis (Zexie) are used to drain dampness, free water passages, and eliminate swelling.

Erxian Wutou Yuxu formula:

Aconitum carmichaeli (treated) (zhi caowu) 15g
Radix aconite carmichaeli (treated) (zhi fuzi) 10g
Cortex cinnamomi (rougui) 10g
Olibanum (ruxiang) 10g
Myrrh (moyao) 10g
Arisaematis rhizoma (tiannanxing) 10g
Maydis stigmata (yumixu) 30g
Alisma orientalis (zexie) 15g
Typha angustifolia (puhuang) 10g
Dioscorea septemloba (bixie) 10g
Epimedium brevicornum (yinyanghuo) 30g
Rhizoma curculiginis orchioides (xianmao) 15g
Radix morindae officinalis

(bajitian) 15g
Polygala tenufola (yuanzhi) 10g
Angelica sinensis (danggui) 20g
Rhizome anemarrhenae (zhimu) 10g
Phellodendri chinensis (huangbai) 10g
Gentiana scabra (longdancao) 30g
Polygoni multiflori (yejiaoteng) 30g
Zizyphus Jujube (fried) (chao suanzaoren) 15g
Concha margaritifera (zhenzhumu) 30g
Concha haliotidis (shijueming) 30g
Concha ostreae (muli) 30g
Ossa draconis (longgu) 30g.

Erxian Wutou Yuxu Formula in Chinese 二仙乌头玉须汤:

制草乌10g 制附子10g 肉桂10g 乳香10g 没药10g 天南星10g 玉米须30g 泽泻15g 蒲黄10g 萆薢10g 淫羊藿30g 仙茅15g 巴戟天15g 远志10g 当归20g 知母10g 黄柏10g 龙胆草30g 夜交藤30g 炒枣仁15g 珍珠母30g 石决明30g 牡蛎30g 龙骨30g.

The Erxian Wutou Yuxu formula is the Erxian formula with the addition of Aconitum carmichaeli (treated) (zhi caowu), Radix Aconite carmichaeli (treated) (zhi fuzi), Cortex cinnamomi (rougui), Olibanum (ruxiang), Myrrh (moyao), Arisaematis Rhizoma (tiannanxing), Maydis stigmata (yumixu), Alisma orientalis (Zexie), Typha angustifolia (puhuang) and Dioscorea septemloba (bixie).

Aconitum carmichaeli (treated) (zhi caowu 制草乌) has a pungent taste and hot yinyang nature, it goes into heart, kidney, and spleen meridians. It is one of the most powerful herbs for strengthening heart fire yang heat, and opening meridians. It also dissolves hard mucus, and ceases liver wind. It is poisonous and requires at least two hours of cooking to render it safe.

Radix Aconite carmichaeli (treated) (zhi fuzi 制附子) has a pungent taste and hot yinyang nature. Like Aconitum carmichaeli it is poisonous but by boiling for two hours will also detoxify the poison. It goes into kidney, mingmen, heart, spleen meridians. It strengthens heart fire yang heat, and grounds heart fire heat into kidney. It disperses wind, cold, and damp poisonous qi; it also breaks down collected lumps and nodules, and relieves lower back and knee pain caused by cold and dampness.

Cortex cinnamomi (rougui 肉桂) nourishes heart yang qi, strengthens kidney and mingmen heat, opens blood passages, and strengthens the effects of all other herbs.

Olibanum (ruxiang 乳香) strengthens blood vitality, dissolves abscesses, ulcers and swelling, removes damp poison in the blood.

Myrrh (moyao 没药) invigorates blood, breaks down lumps and blood stagnations; dissolves swelling, removes dampness, and detoxifies poison.

Arisaematis rhizoma (tiannanxing 天南星) dries dampness, dissolves mucus, dispels wind, and disperses nodules.

Maydis stigmata (yumixu 玉米须) opens water passages, and removes dampness.

Alisma orientalis (Zexie 泽泻) removes old water, nurtures fresh water, frees urine flow, dissolves water retention, drains dampness, and quenches thirst.

Typha Angustifolia (puhuang 蒲黄) treats cold or hot damage of heart, stomach, and urine bladder. It frees urine flow, and dissolves blood stagnation.

Dioscorea septemloba (bixie 萆薢) clears heat, dissolves dampness, opens meridians, and frees urine flow.

In the formula, Aconitum carmichaeli (treated) (zhi caowu), Radix aconite carmichaeli (treated) (zhi fuzi), and Cortex cinnamomi (rougui) strengthen heart fire yang and warm kidney water. Olibanum (ruxiang), Myrrh (moyao), Arisaematis rhizoma (tiannanxing) are used to dissolve mucus and remove dampness. Maydis stigmata (yumixu), Alisma orientalis (Zexie), Typha Angustifolia (puhuang) and Dioscorea septemloba (bixie) are used to free water passages and drain the dampness. The Erxian formula warms kidney water, clears liver wood, and grounds heart fire.

Note: This formula, because of the aconitum carmichaeli (treated), zhi caowu and zhi fuzi, requires at least two hours of boiling before drinking the decoction.

Treating heart fire yin deficiency with symptoms of palpitations

A 63-year-old woman had palpitations with a heart rate of 280 per minute. She had been admitted into a hospital emergency department for three days. When all the medication that she had been administered with had no beneficial effect, the patient phoned me for help. As the local legal regulations prevented natural healing from interfering with conventional biomedical procedures, I told her that I would see her after she was out of hospital. The patient then immediately checked herself out of hospital and came for a consultation.

At the first consultation, the patient felt her heart was going to jump out of her body, she could not sleep, was panicky, and had no strength. Heart fire yin deficiency causes floating heat, which leads to the symptom of palpitations. Floating heart fire prevents the spirit to rest in its house, so she could not sleep. Floating fire prevents heat to store inside the kidney water, so there is kidney water heat loss which causes the patient to be weak. The spirit's inability to get into its house causes feelings of panic. The treatment was to warm kidney water, clear liver wood heat, and ground heart fire with the Erxian Doukou formula.

After taking the herbs for seven days, the patient's palpitations were sometimes better, sometimes still severe. After taking the herbs for a month, the palpitations happened mostly in the morning, and after drinking the herbs it would calm her down. She took the herbs without break for a year, all the symptoms disappeared and she felt energetic and calm. Ten years later, the patient had the same palpitations again but not as severe, and after taking the same herbs for a week, the palpitations stopped. She continued taking the herbs for another 6 weeks to consolidate the recovery.

Erxian Doukou formula:

Epimedium brevicornum (yinyanghuo) 30g
Rhizoma curculiginis orchioides (xianmao) 15g
Radix morindae officinalis (bajitian) 15g
Polygala tenufola (yuanzhi) 10g
Angelica sinensis (danggui) 20g
Rhizome anemarrhenae (zhimu) 10g
Phellodendri chinensis (huangbai) 10g
Gentiana scabra (longdancao)
Epimedium brevicornum 30g
Polygoni multiflori (yejiaoteng) 30g
Zizyphus Jujube (fried) (chao suanzaoren) 15g
Concha margaritifera (zhenzhumu) 30g
Concha haliotidis (shijueming) 30g
Concha ostreae (muli) 30g
Ossa draconis (longgu) 30g
Myristica Fragrans (Roudoukou) 10g.

Erxian Doukou Formula in Chinese 二仙豆蔻汤:

淫羊藿30g 克仙茅15g 巴戟天15g 远志10g 当归20g 知母10g 黄柏10g 龙胆草30g 夜交藤30g 炒枣仁15g 珍珠母30g 石决明30g 牡蛎30g 龙骨30g 肉豆蔻 10g

Erxian Doukou formula is the Erxian formula with the addition of Myristica Fragrans (Roudoukou).

Myristica Fragrans (Roudoukou) has a pungent taste, and warm yinyang nature. It goes into the spleen and large intestine meridians. It warms spleen soil, promotes qi flow, and stops diarrhoea.

The patient had cold spleen soil, which caused her easily to suffer from indigestion and diarrhoea. The herb Gentiana scabra (longdancao) in the Erxian formula is cold and may cause the spleen soil to be colder, and affect her digestion, so it was gradually increased from 5 gram to 30 grams. And by adding Myristica Fragrans Houtt (Roudoukou) further protected her spleen soil.

For the Erxian formula explanation see the chapter "Kidney Water."

Treating heart fire yin deficiency with symptoms of loss of sleep

A 30-year-old female patient came for a consultation suffering from loss of sleep. Before the visit, she had been suffering loss of sleep for two years after she had had a child. In every week there were four nights that she could not sleep at all. The patient was constantly fatigued, her body was tight and aching, she felt agitated and easily upset.

Heart fire yin deficiency causes fire heat to float, so that the spirit could not rest in its house, so there is the symptom of sleep loss. Heart fire yang heat that floats instead of storing in the kidney water causes kidney water heat reserves to be low. Yang heat is the body's energy, when there is insufficient yang heat reserves in the kidney water, then there is a symptom of fatigue. Kidney water yang heat deficiency deprives the yang qi of the enduring zhi of the spirit from being exercised, so when there is any task to carry out, the spirit is agitated. When kidney water heat is low it fails to moisten the liver wood, and the liver wood loses its flexibility, so the body is tight, which further restricts the flow of yinyang qi in the meridians, and so the body is also aching. With liver wood dryness and heat, the yin qi of the striving zhi is unable to be fully exercised, so the striving zhi is firm but without suppleness, and there is a symptom of being easily angry. The treatment is to ground heart fire heat, warm kidney water, and moisten liver wood with the Erxian Yanghua formula.

After the first dosage of the herbs, the patient had a good sleep. She took 14 days of the herbs, all the symptoms disappeared, and she stopped the herbs. A month later, she felt difficulty getting into sleep, and took the same herbs for seven days, and slept well again. In the following six months, she occasionally had light sleep, and whenever that happened, she would take a packet of the same herbs and feel good again.

Erxian Yanghua formula:

Epimedium brevicornum (yinyanghuo) 30g
Rhizoma curculiginis orchioides (xianmao) 15g
Radix morindae officinalis (bajitian) 15g
Polygala tenufola (yuanzhi) 10g
Angelica sinensis (danggui) 20g
Rhizome anemarrhenae (zhimu) 10g
Phellodendri chinensis (huangbai) 10g
Gentiana scabra (longdancao) 30g
Polygoni multiflori (yejiaoteng) 30g
Zizyphus jujube (fried) (chao suanzaoren)15g
Concha margaritifera (zhenzhumu) 30g
Concha haliotidis (shijueming) 30g
Concha ostreae (muli) 30g
Ossa draconis (longgu) 30g
Rhododendron molle (naoyanghua) 2 petals.

Erxian Yanghua Formula in Chinese 二仙羊花:

淫羊藿30g 仙茅15g 巴戟天15g 远志10g 当归20g 知母10g 黄柏10g 龙胆草30g 夜交藤30g 炒枣仁15g 珍珠母30g 石决明30g 牡蛎30g 龙骨30g 闹羊花 2个花瓣

The Erxian Yanghua formula is the Erxian formula with the addition of Rhododendron molle (naoyanghua) to soothe liver wood, and calm the spirit.

Rhododendron molle (naoyanghua 闹羊花) has a pungent taste and warm yinyang nature. It is a poisonous herb, the dosage should be within safe limits. It goes into heart and liver meridians. It expels wind, removes dampness, opens meridians, stops pain, and grounds the spirit inside heart fire.

173

Treating heart fire yin and yang deficiency with symptoms of forgetfulness

An 80-year-old female patient sought my help for her forgetfulness and inattentiveness, which had been afflicting her for around six months. The month prior to her consultation, she found it difficult to manage her daily life and the family found her responses very slow. The patient was also unable to fall asleep, and was afraid to be alone at night.

When there is heart fire yin deficiency, the yang heat floats, which prevents the spirit residing in its house, so there is a symptom of insomnia. When heart fire yang heat floats instead of storing into kidney water, the kidney water heat reserve becomes low. With kidney water heat loss, the yang qi of the enduring zhi of the spirit is deprived of being exercised, so the enduring zhi is constrained, which causes the spirit to be in fear. Kidney water heat loss will fail to nurture liver wood, and the heart fire becomes low as fire has no wood to burn upon. The yang deficiency of heart fire causes the spirit to be inactive and uninvolved with the outside world, so the patient is forgetful and slow to respond. Treatment is to strengthen the heart fire yang heat, and ground heart fire yang qi into kidney water with the formula Erxian Fugui.

After taking 10 packets of the herbs, the patient was able to sleep, her memory was better, and the anxiousness at night significantly improved. She stopped the herbs for a month, and the symptoms returned. She took the herbs again for a month, then all symptoms disappeared and she was able to take care of herself again.

Erxian Fugui formula:

Radix aconite carmichaeli (treated) (zhi fuzi) 10g
Cortex cinnamomi (rougui) 10g
Epimedium brevicornum (yinyanghuo) 30g
Rhizoma curculiginis orchioides (xianmao) 15g
Radix morindae officinalis

(bajitian) 15g
Polygala tenufola (yuanzhi) 10g
Angelica sinensis (danggui) 20g
Rhizome anemarrhenae (zhimu) 10g
Phellodendri chinensis (huangbai) 10g
Gentiana scabra (longdancao)

30g
Polygoni multiflori (yejiaoteng)
30g
Zizyphus jujube (fried) (chao
suanzaoren)15g
Concha margaritifera

(zhenzhumu) 30g
Concha haliotidis (shijueming)
30g
Concha ostreae (muli) 30g
Ossa draconis (longgu) 30g

Erxian Fugui formula in Chinese 二仙附桂汤:

制附子10g 肉桂10g 淫羊藿30g 仙茅15g 巴戟天15g 远志10g 当归20g
知母10 g 黄柏10g 龙胆草30g 夜交藤30g 炒枣仁15g 珍珠母30g 石决
明30g 牡蛎30g 龙骨30g.

This formula is the Erxian Fugui Dahuang formula minus Rheum officinale (dahuang). As the patient did not have significant signs of damp heat poison, or bowel motion difficulties, so she did not need the Rheum officinale (dahuang). For the formula explanation see "Treating kidney water heat loss with symptoms of dry mouth" section.

Note: This formula, because of the aconitum carmichaeli (treated), requires at least two hours of boiling before drinking the decoction.

Spleen Soil

The spleen is a soil organ, it has a nature of being adhesive and is a yin organ. Yin needs yang, the adhesive yin nature of spleen soil needs to be loosened. Because of its adhesive yin nature, spleen soil is able to hold and store food, and nourish the body. The yang nature of spleen soil is friable, so it facilitates yinyang transformation and food digestion. Spleen soil stores the body's food. The food is not only from what people eat and drink, it also exists everywhere in the body, so the spleen soil can absorb and transform yin and yang qi from everywhere in the body to meet the yinyang needs of the wuxing organs, which includes the skin.

Spleen soil is the connecting junction of the wuxing organs and also the connecting junction of the body with heaven and earth. Because of the adhesive nature of spleen soil, it is the gathering place of all wuxing organs. It is also because of the adhesive nature of spleen soil, that people can ingest food and water. Drinking and eating is the main path that the body maintains its yinyang order to be coherent with heaven and earth. When the yin of spleen soil is plentiful, it provides the gathering place for the wuxing organs, and enables spleen soil to acknowledge the yinyang needs of the other wuxing organs and transfers such messages into food cravings. For example, when kidney water needs more warmth, people have an appetite for richer food, such as meat, egg and beans. In the same way, when spleen soil needs to be more loosened, people crave for pungent and hot food, such as pepper or ginger; when lung metal needs more moistness, people crave for watery food, such as water melon; when liver wood needs more flexibility, people crave for sour food, such as lemon, vinegar; when heart fire needs more grounding, people crave for bitter tasting food, such as strong tea. When the wuxing organs receive their yinyang needs, food is flavoursome and enjoyable.

Each of the wuxing organs relies on the adhesiveness of spleen soil to provide the nexus for their connectivity and interdependence. However, this connectivity and interdependence could not be establish without spleen soil's friable nature. It is because of the friable nature of spleen soil that each of the wuxing organs can interact. For example, heart fire can store its heat into kidney water by traversing through spleen soil; liver wood can reach kidney water for growth by traversing through spleen soil. Similarly, kidney water can reach lung metal and be replenished by traversing through spleen soil, and lung metal can store clean water in kidney water by traversing through spleen soil.

Spleen soil is not just the provider for the other wuxing organs, it receives heart fire to be replenished; kidney water to be adhesive; liver wood to be stable; and lung metal to be friable.

Because of the adhesive and friable nature of spleen soil, the spirit interacts with spleen soil to exercise its reasoning zhi—that of accepting and sorting out information. The cooperation of spirit and spleen soil provides a person with orderly thoughts.

Overall, spleen soil is capable of bearing and transforming; it allows the wuxing organs to meet, to connect, and to transform. Spleen soil receives, stores, and transforms food, in which it nurtures the entire body. It governs the body's food passages. The harmony of the spleen soil yinyang order makes the body satiated without being heavy, and the spirit in an orderly manner.

Yinyang disorders of spleen soil will cause digestion disorders, and the connectivity disturbance of the wuxing organs. If the spleen soil then fails to respond to the demands of the spirit, a person will suffer emotional disorders such as worry and boredom.

Causes of Spleen Soil Yinyang Disorder

Hunger, overeating, or having food that has chemical and artificial additives are the common causes of spleen soil yinyang disorders. Being hungry for too long means that the yinyang of spleen soil does not get replenished by heaven and earth and is weakened. Following a long period of hunger, then quickly eating too much, which the weakened spleen soil cannot readily transform in time, the food becomes a blockage to the spleen soil, and damages spleen soil yin and yang. Eating synthetic food damages the spleen soil yin and yang because synthetic food doesn't follow the normal regulation of yinyang transformation, and blocks the normal yinyang transformation of the wuxing organs, and causes the yinyang disorders of the wuxing organs. But because spleen soil is the doorway of food getting into the body, so the spleen soil is often the first victim of unhealthy food.

Symptoms

A yang deficiency of spleen soil means the loss of its permeability. In a situation when qi cannot pass through, bloating and stomach pain occur. When fluid cannot get through spleen soil, dampness will grow and cause a greasy coating on the tongue. Fluid and dampness regurgitated causes reflux. When there is spleen soil yang deficiency, food is not transformed, which causes bad breath. Spleen soil yin deficiency means the loss of its bearing ability. In such a situation, as spleen soil cannot respond to the yinyang needs of the other wuxing organs, food then becomes uninteresting and tasteless, so there is the symptom of low appetite, or even no desire for food. When spleen soil fails to adhere, the wuxing organs lose their connections with each other, which then causes disordered yinyang transformations of all the wuxing organs and, as a result, a person becomes over time emaciated.

Spleen soil yang deficiency means the loss of its permeability, which means it holds but does not transform, thus, the yang qi of the reasoning zhi is unable to be exercised, so it holds thoughts but is unable to sort them out, and this makes the spirit to be overly suspicious. On the other hand, when spleen soil yin is deficient, the yin qi of the reasoning zhi is unable to be exercised, so the spirit fails to receive thoughts, and with no thoughts to be sorted out the spirit becomes bored.

Overall, symptoms relating to eating, digestion, and qi and fluid stagnation caused by the disconnection of the wuxing organs are spleen soil yinyang disorders. Emotionally, spleen soil yinyang disorders cause people to be either overly suspicious or to suffer boredom.

The tongue

When the yinyang of spleen soil is in a normal order, each of the wuxing organs interacts without obstruction, so the coating of the tongue is clean and thin. The yin of spleen soil governs its adhesiveness; the yang of spleen soil governs its looseness. When the yin qi of the spleen soil is deficient, it loses its adhesiveness, and the coating of the tongue is bare like a mirror, or has mirror-like patches. When the yang qi of the spleen soil is deficient, it loses its ability of loosening; food and water become stuck and dampness and mucus occur, so the coating of the tongue is greasy and thick.

The pulse

When spleen soil loses its yang qi, soil becomes sticky, the pulse is heavy and it is like a balloon wrapped with mud, being dragged and difficult to bounce. First the right guan pulse of the spleen soil becomes heavy, if it extends to the lung metal, then the right cun pulse becomes heavy. When the sticky spleen soil affects the kidney reserve the right chi pulse is heavy. When the sticky spleen soil affects the heart fire organ, the left cun pulse is heavy. When it affects the liver wood organ, the left guan pulse is heavy. When it affects the kidney water organ, the left chi pulse is heavy.

On the other hand, when spleen soil loses its yin qi, the soil becomes sandy, and metal, wood, water and fire lose their connection. The pulse will feel empty, the balloon is like a shallot leaf, pressed a little harder it will be flat, and all affected wuxing organs will have an empty pulse.

Skin

Spleen soil is the transformation and transportation junction of the wuxing organs. The yin of spleen soil is sticky which closes the skin, so the yinyang qi of the wuxing organs can remain inside the body. The yang of spleen soil is loosening, which opens the skin, so the yinyang qi of the wuxing organs can connect with heaven and earth. Therefore, disorders of the skin opening and closing reflects the disorders of yinyang of spleen soil. For example, when the yang of spleen

179

soil is damaged, a person feels hot but cannot sweat; when the yin of spleen soil is damaged, a person sweats as soon as there's a little movement.

Principles for treating spleen soil yinyang disorder

Spleen soil is a yin organ, the yinyang disorders of the spleen soil are often a lack of yang so that it becomes too damp and gluey. Warming the spleen soil, draining dampness, and opening qi passages are the most common treatments for spleen soil yinyang disorder. Treating spleen soil yin deficiency is to moisten and enrich soil. However, as spleen soil has a tendency of being damp, when moistening and enriching spleen soil one should be cautious of dampness occurring. Treating a simultaneous spleen soil yin and yang deficiency is to enrich the soil, while at the same time loosening the soil.

Treating spleen soil yang damage with cold, damp, and qi stagnant stomach pain

A 30-year-old woman was admitted into a hospital for stomach pain while she was travelling. She then immediately received an appendectomy. But her pain continued. Half a year later she was informed that she had a large intestine adhesion as a result of the appendectomy and she received another operation to repair her large intestine. However, it did not stop her stomach pain. When she made the first visit to me, she had had continuous stomach pain for more than three years. Coldness, and hunger aggravated the pain; a hot water bottle pressed against the abdomen could reduce the pain. She also felt stomach bloating, and passed quite a lot of wind; her sleep was often restless; her tongue had a thick greasy coating, and her pulse was heavy and slippery.

When spleen soil yang deficiency loses its permeability, it leads to air and fluid flow congestions. Where there is blockage, there is pain. The stomach is where the spleen soil root is situated; in this case, the qi congestion of spleen soil caused the stomach pain, bloating, and the passing of wind. Cold and hunger further weakened the spleen soil yang, so the pain became worse. Warmth and pressing strengthened the yang and loosened the spleen soil, so it lessened the pain. When spleen soil loses its permeability, kidney water flow is restricted, so the pulse is slippery. The fluid stagnation allows dampness to grow, which shows on the tongue as a thick coating. With spleen soil yang deficiency, the soil is sticky, so the pulse is heavy. The pain disturbs the spirit, so there was a symptom of restless sleep. The treatment was to warm and loosen spleen soil, drain dampness, and promote qi flow with the Xianglian formula.

The patient took three packets of the herbs and came back to my clinic three years later to say that since the three packets of the herbs she had not had any more stomach pain.

Xianglian formula:

Rhizoma zingiberis (ganjiang) 10g
Aucklandia lappa (muxiang) 10g
Rhizoma cyperi (xiangfu) 10g
Rhizoma galangae (gaoliangjiang) 10g
Magnolia officinalis (houpo) 10g
Areca catechu (dafupi) 10g
Lindera aggregata (wuyao) 10g
Caryophylli flos (dingxiang) 10g
Evodia rutaecarpa (wuzhuyu) 10g
Fructus aurantii (zhiqiao) 10g
Toosendan fructus (chuanlianzi) 10g
Cinnamomum cassia (guizhi) 10g
Paeoniae lactiflora (baishao) 10g
Glycyrrhiza radix (gancao) 10g
Sepiella maindroni (wuzeigu) 30g
Concha arcae (forged) (duan walengzi) 30g
Typha angustifolia (puhuang) 10g
Faeces Trogopterpri (wulingzhi) 10g

Xianglian Formula in Chinese 香楝:

干姜10g 木香10g 香附10g 高良姜10g 厚朴10g 大腹皮10g 乌药10g 丁香10g 吴茱萸10g 枳壳10g 川楝子10g 桂枝10g 白芍10g 甘草10g 乌贼骨30g 锻瓦楞子30g 蒲黄10g 五灵脂10g

Rhizoma zingiberis (ganjiang 干姜) has a pungent taste and warm yinyang nature. It goes into the liver and lung meridians. It expels cold and disperses wind.
Aucklandia lappa (muxiang 木香) has a pungent, fragrant taste and warm yinyang nature. It goes into the liver, spleen, and lung

meridians. It warms spleen soil, resolves damp poison, and removes poisonous qi.

Rhizoma cyperi (xiangfu 香附) has a pungent and fragrant taste and slightly warm yinyang nature. It goes into the liver, spleen, stomach, lung meridians. It opens meridians, removes qi stagnation, warms spleen soil, and frees snarls.

Rhizoma galangae (gaoliangjiang 高良姜) has a pungent and fragrant taste and warm yinyang nature. It goes into liver, spleen and stomach meridians. It warms and loosens spleen soil.

Magnolia officinalis (houpo 厚朴) has a bitter and fragrant taste, and warm yinyang nature. It goes into the spleen and stomach meridians. It warms spleen soil, dissolves mucus, and moves gas downward and out.

Areca catechu (dafupi 大腹皮) has a pungent and fragrant taste and slightly warm yinyang nature. It goes into the spleen and lung meridians. It moves gas downward and out, drains dampness, chases out wind, and relaxes the intestine.

Lindera aggregata (wuyao 乌药) has a pungent and fragrant taste and warm yinyang nature. It goes into the spleen and lung meridians. It frees qi flow, resolves snarls, ceases bloating, stops stomach pain.

Caryophylli flos (dingxiang 丁香) has a pungent and fragrant taste and warm yinyang nature. It goes into the stomach, lung, and kidney meridians. It heals cold gassy stomach pain.

Evodia rutaecarpa (wuzhuyu 吴茱萸) has a pungent and fragrant taste and warm yinyang nature. It goes into the liver, spleen, and kidney meridians. It warms spleen soil, moves stomach gas downward, removes dampness, and stops pain.

Fructus aurantii (zhiqiao 枳壳) has a pungent, bitter, and fragrant taste, and slightly cool yinyang nature. It goes into the lung, spleen, stomach, and large intestine meridians. It breaks down gas, dissolves mucus, and improves digestion.

Toosendan fructus (chuanlianzi 川楝子) has a bitter taste and cold yinyang nature. It goes into the spleen, and stomach meridians. It removes gas, clears liver wood fire, and stops all abdominal pain.

Cinnamomum cassia (guizhi 桂枝) has a pungent and sweet taste, and warm yinyang nature. It goes into the lung and urine bladder meridians. It disperses hidden coldness in between skin and muscles, and expels irregular qi.

Paeoniae Alba (baishao 白芍) has a sour taste and mild yinyang nature. It goes into the liver and spleen meridians. It softens liver wood, opens and smooths blood passages, and dissolves swelling.

Glycyrrhiza radix (gancao 甘草) dissolves cold or hot irregular poisonous qi of all wuxing organs.

Sepiella maindroni (wuzeigu 乌贼骨) has a salty taste, and slightly warm yinyang nature. It goes into the kidney and spleen meridians. It removes dampness and mucus, opens meridians, dissolves blood stagnation, and stops bleeding.

Concha arcae (walengzi 瓦楞子) has a salty taste, and mild yinyang nature. It goes into the liver and spleen meridians. It breaks down lumps, nodules, and stagnating mucus, blood, and gas. Forged concha arcae is dryer and has a stronger effect in removing dampness.

Typha angustifolia (puhuang 蒲黄) has a sweet taste and mild yinyang nature. It goes into the spleen meridian. It clears chest, stomach and urine bladder cold and hot stagnation. It smooths urine flow, and dissolves blood stagnation.

Faeces Trogopterpri (wulingzhi 五灵脂) has a sweet taste and mild yinyang nature. It goes into the spleen and liver meridians. It smooths blood flow, and disperses cold air in the chest and stomach.

In the Xianglian formula, Rhizoma zingiberis (ganjiang), Aucklandia lappa (muxiang), Rhizoma cyperi (xiangfu), Rhizoma galangae (gaoliangjiang), Magnolia officinalis (houpo), Areca catechu (dafupi), Lindera aggregata (wuyao), Caryophylli flos (dingxiang) , Evodia rutaecarpa (wuzhuyu) are all fragrant and warm herbs that loosen spleen soil, dissolve dampness, and remove stomach gas. Fructus aurantii (zhiqiao), Toosendan fructus (chuanlianzi) add more strength to remove stomach gas. The sour and sweet herbs of Cinnamomum cassia (guizhi), Paeoniae alba (baishao) and Glycyrrhiza (gancao) are used to relax spasms, and stop pain. Sepiella maindroni (wuzeigu), Concha arcae (walengzi), Typha angustifolia (puhuang), and Faeces Trogopterpri (wulingzhi) are four herbs used to remove hard mucus in the spleen soil and stop stomach pain.

Another case was a 30-year-old man who had severe stomach pain attacks every two to three weeks that resulted in him going into a hospital emergency department. He was diagnosed as having pancreatitis in biomedicine. At the first consultation, the patient had consistent mild stomach pain which would often become worse after eating. He often had reflux and his bowel motions were always loose and sticky. He was tired all the time. The patient often drank soda water to cope with the reflux.

This was a case of spleen soil yang damage causing the loss of spleen soil permeability. In such a condition, qi could not pass through spleen soil and caused stomach pains. When spleen soil has yang damage it fails to transform and transport food, leading to stagnation, so eating adds to the pain. Spleen soil yang damage congests the water passages and causes dampness to flourish; dampness and water pours out as reflux. With spleen soil yang damage, liver wood yinyang qi cannot pass through, which causes liver wood yang damage, and leads to dampness in the blood. When the blood damp poison stays in the large intestine, the bowel motions become sticky and loose. Spleen soil yang damage also causes kidney water to lose its heat as it is unable to receive yang heat from the heart fire. When kidney water heat reserves are low, then there is a symptom of tiredness.

The treatment and formula are the same as the previous case but the patient had to stop the soda drinks. Drinking soda water had two opposite effects to his condition. One is the cold drink would further damage the spleen soil yang qi; and secondly soda water is a catalyst for breeding dampness and stomach gas. It relieves acid reflux temporarily but helps to build more dampness and causes more reflux in the long run.

The patient took 3 packets of the above herbs and the stomach pain was reduced. He took the herbs each day for 100 days, the pain completely stopped and he regained his energy. A year later he came back for a follow up, by then all the symptoms had disappeared.

Another patient was a 33-year-old man who had been having stomach pain for over 10 years. When he was 18 years of age, he was diagnosed with rheumatic fever and was given antibiotic drugs to take for the rest of his life to prevent his arteries from hardening. He took the drugs for two years but then decided to stop. After taking antibiotics for less than a year, he had begun to lose hair significantly; his palms were cold and sweaty and the skin often peeled. He was often tired, and thirsty. For many months of the year he had constant sneezing and running nose; and was frequently suffering from sore throats and fever. He also slept lightly. But the most inconvenient problem was his everlasting painful stomach.

Antibiotics are foreign to our body system; they block our body's yinyang passages creating stagnant areas in the body conducive for the growth of dampness. After taking one course of antibiotic treatment, a person would have symptoms of dampness building in the body such as bad breath, thick coated tongue, and women with thrush. As for this case, the extended taking of antibiotics had obstructed the yinyang passages of every wuxing organ.

The yinyang passage of spleen soil congestion had caused spleen soil yang damage and the impairment of its friability, which led to the stagnation of qi, and the creation and accumulation of dampness which caused the stomach pain. The palms of the hands and soles of the feet are the satellites of spleen soil, the loss of friability of spleen soil causes water passage congestion, which shows on the hands and feet as sweaty hands and/or feet. The congestion of the liver wood yinyang passages caused liver wood yang damage and led to damp poison blocking the blood passages on the palms, which showed as peeling skin on the palms. Hair is the extension of blood, the liver wood damage caused damp poison in the blood and led to the falling hair. Kidney water yinyang passage congestion caused the kidney water heat loss and the inability of water to rise, which caused the symptom of thirstiness. Kidney water heat provides body strength; weak kidney water heat causes tiredness. With kidney water heat loss, water doesn't rise, lung metal loses its moistness and its yin becomes weak, which makes a person vulnerable to suffering sore throats and fever. Lung metal creates water, but water could not permeate into spleen soil and down to kidney water, so there was a constant runny nose. When there are multiple wuxing organ yinyang disorders, the prioritisation is given to the most urgent condition. Because the stomach pain had been bothering the patient's normal daily life, so the first step was to warm and loosen spleen soil, which not only deals with the stomach pain but also facilitates the connection of each wuxing organ to help each other to recover. The formula I used was Xianglian formula. At the same time I also prescribed the Bianxu Gancao formula for external use to clear liver wood, cool blood, and drain dampness, which is to treat the peeling hands.

The patient took 10 packets of the herbs, the stomach pains were significantly reduced. After stopping the herbs for 10 days, the pain came back. He took another 10 packets of the herbs, the pain stopped again. But 2 months later, the pain came back again. Then he took another 10 packets of the herbs. Intermittently he took the herbs for six months, and didn't have stomach pain again. Also his runny nose had significantly improved, and he didn't suffer from sore throats and fever very often any more. This was because the loosening of spleen soil had allowed the kidney water to rise and moisten the lung metal. Also the spleen soil is the creator of lung metal in the wuxing cycle, and when the yinyang order of spleen soil becomes regulated, it enhances the yinyang harmony of lung metal.

The patient washed his hands for 3 days with 3 packets of the Bianxu Gancao formula, his hands stopped peeling, 10 days later the skin on his hands were repaired.

Bianxu Gancao external wash Formula:

Polygonum aviculare (bianxu)   (kushen) 60g
60g   Talcum 60g
Sophorae flavescentis radix   Glycyrrhiza (gancao) 10g

Bianxu Gancao external wash formula in Chinese 萹蓄甘草汤:

萹蓄60g 苦参60g 滑石60g 甘草10g

Polygonum aviculare (bianxu 萹蓄) has a bitter taste and mild yinyang nature. It goes into stomach and urine bladder meridians. It kills parasites, drains dampness, and stops itch.
Sophorae flavescentis radix (kushen 苦参) removes dampness, detoxifies poison, and kills parasite.
Talcum (huashi 滑石) dissolves dampness.
Glycyrrhiza radix (gancao 甘草) harmonizes the wuxing organs.

The first three herbs in the Bianxu Gancao formula are used to remove dampness; Glycyrrhiza (gancao) is used to promote healing.

186

Preparation and method of use of the Bianxu Gancao wash:

Place the herbs into a saucepan, add 3 cups of cold water, and boil for 30 minutes. Strain the liquid into a bowl, place the hands over the steaming decoction and when cooler then soak the hands in the liquid for 10 minutes.

Treating spleen soil yang deficiency with food stagnant stomach pain

A 70-year-old woman had years of mild stomach pain and belching. For three months, the pain had gotten worse, especially after eating. She was diagnosed in biomedicine as having gall bladder stones. The size of the stone was as large as a chicken egg and it was suggested that she have an operation. She was too afraid to have an operation and thought to try herbs. At the first consultation, the patient was in a lot of stomach pain and had no appetite for food or drink. Whenever she had even a small amount food the pain would become much worse and she had a lot of belching. Her tongue had a greasy yellow coating; her pulse was tight and slippery.

Spleen soil yang deficiency blocked the qi passages, so there were symptoms of belching and stomach pain. The yang deficiency of spleen soil failed to permit the transportation and transformation of food and drink, which became blockages in the yinyang passage, and added to the stagnation. The stagnation caused more pain and belching and suppressed her appetite. Spleen soil impermeability created dampness, so her tongue had a greasy coating. Dampness that ferments causes heat; heat turns the tongue coating to yellow. Losing the permeability of spleen soil caused water passage congestion, so her pulse was slippery. Kidney water flow disorder caused liver wood dryness, so the pulse was also tight. The treatment was to warm spleen soil, smooth qi flow, dissolve dampness, and breakdown food stagnation. When spleen soil regains its friability, kidney water can flow, and liver wood is supple without other treatment. I used the Qianhu formula.

After taking one packet of the herbs, the patient felt hungry and wanted to eat, her stomach pain improved. But after eating oily food, the pain came back. She drank a cup of the herbal concoction immediately, and the pain stopped straight away. She took the herbs each day for three months, and no longer had the pain. Her eating and drinking all became normal again. Five years later, the patient had a stomach ultrasound and found the stone had not changed and her doctor wanted her to have an operation but as she felt normal so she didn't have the operation nor take any more herbs.

Qianhu formula:

Aucklandia lappa (muxiang) 10g
Cyperus rotundus (xiangfu) 10g
Alpinia officinarum (gaoliangjiang) 10g
Magnolia officinalis (houpo) 10g
Areca catechu (dafupi) 10g
Aurantii fructus (zhiqiao) 10g
Fructus toosendan (chuanlianzi) 10g
Glycyrrhiza radix (gancao) 10g
Scutellaria baicalensis (huangqin) 10g
Pinellia ternate (banxia) 10g

Reynoutria japonica (huzhang) 10g
Lysimachia christinae (jinqiancao) 30g
Lygodium japonicum (haijinsha) 10g
Radix stellariae (chaihu) 10g
Curcuma radix (yujin) 10g
Crataegus fructus (charcoaled) (shanzhatan) 30g
Gallus gallus domesticus brisson (jineijin) 15g

Qianhu formula in Chinese 钱虎汤:

木香10g 香附10g 高良姜10g 厚朴10g 大腹皮10g 枳壳10g 川楝子10g 甘草10g 黄芩10g 半夏10g 虎杖10g 金钱草30g 海金沙10g 柴胡10g 郁金10g 山楂炭30g 鸡内金15g

Aucklandia lappa (muxiang 木香) warms spleen soil, detoxifies damp poison, expels turbid qi.

Cyperus rotundus (xiangfu 香附) smooths qi flow, warms spleen soil, and frees snarls.

Alpinia officinarum (gaoliangjiang 高良姜) warms spleen soil.

Magnolia officinalis (houpo 厚朴) warms spleen soil, dissolves mucus, and moves qi downward and out.

Areca catechu (dafupi 大腹皮) moves down the adverse qi, removes dampness, and disperses wind.

Aurantii fructus (zhiqiao 枳壳) breaks down stagnant qi, dissolves mucus, and improves digestion.

Toosendan fructus (chuanlianzi 川楝子) smooths qi flow, and

188

stops stomach pain.

Glycyrrhiza radix (gancao 甘草) detoxifies hot or cold poisonous qi in all wuxing organs.

Scutellaria baicalensis (huangqin 黄芩) expels wind, clears heat, and removes dampness.

Pinellia ternate (banxia 半夏) has a pungent taste and mild yinyang nature. It goes into the spleen, stomach, and gall bladder meridians. It dissolves mucus, opens the appetite, and harmonizes the yinyang order of the spleen soil.

Reynoutria japonica (huzhang 虎杖) has a bitter taste and cool yinyang nature. It goes into spleen, liver, and gall bladder meridians. It dispels wind, removes dampness, detoxifies poison, disperses cold, and opens meridians.

Lysimachia christinae (jinqiancao 金钱草) has a slightly sweet taste and cool yinyang nature. It goes into the liver and spleen meridians. It disperses wind, removes dampness, detoxifies poison, and stops pain.

Lygodium japonicum (haijinsha 海金沙) clears dampness and heat, dissolves swelling and bloating. It harmonizes the yinyang order of spleen soil.

Bupleurum chinense (chaihu 柴胡) has a bitter taste and cool yinyang nature. It goes into the liver, gall bladder, and spleen meridians. It unclutters liver wood, relaxes muscles, lightens the spirit, smooths qi flow, and stops recurring chills and fevers.

Curcuma radix (yujin 郁金) smooths qi flow, and relieves snarls.

Crataegus fructus (charcoaled) (shanzhatan 山楂炭) has a sour and sweet tastes, and slightly warm yinyang nature. It goes into spleen, stomach meridians. It breaks down food stagnation, removes tangled qi, and dissolves stomach gas. The charcoaled Crataetus fructus is dryer and has a stronger effect to break down food stagnation than uncharcoaled Crataegus fructus.

Gallus gallus domesticus (jineijin 鸡内金) has a sweet taste and mild yinyang nature. It goes into spleen and stomach meridians. It relaxes stomach tension, loosens spleen soil, and breaks down food stagnation.

In the Qianhu formula, Aucklandia lappa (muxiang), Cyperus rotundus (xiangfu), Alpinia officinarum (gaoliangjiang), Magnolia of-

189

ficinalis (houpo), Areca catechu (dafupi), Aurantii fructus (zhiqiao), Fructus toosendan (chuanlianzi) have the function of warming spleen soil, dissolving dampness, relieving stagnant qi, and stopping stomach pain. Glycyrrhiza (gancao) is used to detoxify damp poison. Scutellaria baicalensis (huangqin), Pinellia ternate (banxia), Reynoutria Japonica (huzhang), Lysimachia christinae (jinqiancao), Lygodium japonicum (haijinsha) are used to remove dampness, dissolve mucus, and stop pain. Bupleurum chinense (chaihu), Curcuma Radix (yujin) are used to smooth qi flow, and relieve snarls. Charcoaled Crataegus fructus (shanzhatan), Gallus gallus domesticus brisson (jineijin) are used to breakdown food stagnation.

Treating spleen soil yang deficiency with blood stagnating stomach pain

A 60-year-old man had stomach pain and was diagnosed in biomedicine as having stomach cancer. During a stomach laparotomy, the surgeon found the cancer tumour was all over his stomach cavity, and felt that it was not possible to operate on, and sewed him back up without other procedures. His general medical practitioner then told him frankly that he only had time to organize his funeral. After the patient organised his funeral, he came to me for a consultation. At the first consultation, he had continuous sharp pain in his upper stomach, and now and then he would have severe cramping pain lasting for at least two to three hours. The stomach pain disturbed his sleep, his stomach was big, bloated, solid, and he did not like to have it touched. He did not have any appetite and was constipated. He was cold and emaciated, he had a slow tottering walk and shaking hands held up in front of his chest. His complexion was dark; his tongue was dark red with a thick yellow greasy coating. His pulse was sunken, heavy, slippery, and with no clear definition.

Such symptoms suggest qi, fluid, and blood flow being blocked. In the external world, if a water passage is free the water will be clear and we will call it clean water. In the body, the clean water is called fresh fluid of the body. When water passages are blocked, water will become stale and unclear, in such a condition water may be called sewage, the sewage water in the body is called dampness. When filthy sewage water thickens it becomes mould, in the body it is called mucus. When prolonged stagnation of accumulated mucus becomes hardened and swollen, it can be called a tumour.

As for this case, the spleen soil yang deficiency blocked the qi passages so there was stomach pain and bloating. Liver wood yang deficiency caused mucus and dampness to accumulate, blocking the blood passages, so the stomach was hardened, and the complexion was dark. When there is spleen soil yang deficiency, the heart fire yang heat cannot store in the kidney water but is dissipated, so the body is cold. When kidney water heat reserve is low, the body has no strength, and there is a symptom of slow tottering walk. When liver wood lacks kidney water moistening, blood becomes hot and creates wind, so there is a symptom of shaking. When spleen soil loses its friability, food cannot be transformed and transported, so there is no appetite. When spleen soil loses its friability, the yinyang transformation of the wuxing organs become disconnected, so his body was emaciated. The pain alerts the spirit, so he could not sleep. The liver is the blood storage, the colour of the tongue is an indication of whether the blood is fresh. A dark red tongue indicated liver wood yang deficiency, and there was stagnation in the blood. When spleen soil loses its friability the water passages congest and dampness accumulates, so the tongue coating was greasy. Dampness that fermented created heat, so the tongue coating was yellow. Heart fire yang qi dissipation caused the pulse to be inactive, so the pulse was sunken. With spleen soil yang deficiency, soil loses its friability, so the pulse is heavy. When kidney water heat is low, water flow is restricted, so the pulse is slippery. When yang damage to liver wood causes a loss of its erectness, the pulse has no clear definition. Treatment was to warm spleen soil, invigorate blood, dissolve blood stagnation, and free the qi passage with the Maqian formula. In addition to the Maqian formula, each day the patient would take 50 grams of Panax ginseng boiled in water for 2 hours and taken as tea to calm the spirit in all the wuxing organs.

After taking two weeks of the herbs, the patient's stomach pain was reduced. He took the herbs for 18 months and all the pains were gone, then he resumed work.

Maqian formula:

Rheum officinale (dahuang) 10g
Coptis chinensis (huanglian) 10g
Reynoutria japonica (huzhang) 10g
Lysimachia christinae (jinqiancao) 30g
Lygodium japonicum (haijinsha) 10g
Aconitum carmichaeli (treated) (zhi caowu) 10g
Radix aconite carmichaeli (treated) (zhi fuzi) 10g
Arisaematis rhizoma (tiannanxing) 10g
Curcuma zedoaria (ezhu)10g
Trigonobalanus doichangensis (sanleng) 10g
Strychnos nux-vomica (maqianzi) 0.5g
Faeces trogopterpri (wulingzhi) 10g
Typha angustifolia (puhuang) 10g

Eupolyphaga sinensis (tubiechong) 10g
Curcuma longa (jianghuang) 20g
Sepiella maindroni (wuzeigu) 30g
Concha Arcae (forged) (duan walengzi) 30g
Olibanum (ruxiang) 10g
Myrrh (moyao) 10g
Evodia rutaecarpa (wuzhuyu) 10g
Lindera aggregata (wuyao) 10g
Asarum sieboldii (xixin) 10g
Fructus toosendan (chuanlianzi) 10g
Magnolia officinalis (houpo) 10g
Curcuma radix (yujin) 10g
Aurantii fructus (zhiqiao) 10g
Rhizoma cyperi (xiangfu) 10g
Rhizoma galangae (gaoliangjiang) 10g
Cortex cinnamomi (rougui) 10g
Glycyrrhiza radix (gancao) 10g

Maqian formula in Chinese 马钱汤:

大黄10g 黄连10g 虎杖10g 金钱草30g 海金沙10g 制草乌10g 制附子10g 天南星10g 莪术10g 三棱10g 马钱子0.5g 五灵脂10g 蒲黄10g 土鳖虫10g 姜黄20g 乌贼骨30g 煅瓦愣子30g 乳香10g 没药10g 吴茱萸10g 乌药10g 细辛10g 川楝子10厚朴10郁金10g 枳壳10g 香附10g 高良姜10g 肉桂15g 甘草10g

Rheum officinale (dahuang 大黄) cools blood, detoxifies poison, breaks down all stagnations, removes dampness, and opens bowel motions.

Coptis chinensis (huanglian 黄连) detoxifies poison, dries dampness, and cools blood.

Reynoutria japonica (huzhang 虎杖) expels wind pain, removes dampness, detoxifies poison, disperses cold, and opens meridian.

Lysimachia christinae (jinqiancao 金钱草) expels wind pain, removes dampness, and detoxifies poison.

Lygodium japonicum (haijinsha 海金沙) removes damp heat, dissolves swelling, and strengthens the yinyang harmony of spleen soil and stomach.

Aconitum carmichaeli (treated) (caowu 制草乌) strengthens yang qi of all wuxing organs, opens meridian, stops cold pain, dissolves mucus, and stops cramp.

Radix Aconite carmichaeli (treated) (fuzi 制附子) strengthens kidney and mingmen heat, disperses wind, cold, and damp stagnations; it breaks down abdominal masses, and heals damp cold pain in the knees and lower back.

Arisaematis rhizoma (tiannanxing 天南星) dries dampness, dissolves mucus, expels wind, and disperses nodules.

Curcuma zedoaria (ezhu 莪术) has a bitter and pungent taste, and warm yinyang nature. It goes into liver and spleen meridians. It breaks down qi and blood stagnation, disperses nodules, and eases pain.

Trigonobalanus doichangensis (sanleng 三棱) has a slightly bitter taste and mild yinyang nature. It goes into liver and spleen meridians. It softens hard lumps, disperses nodules, and eliminates poisonous blood stagnation.

Strychnos nux-vomica (maqianzi 马钱子) has a bitter taste, and cold yinyang nature. It is a poisonous herb. It goes into the liver and kidney meridians. It opens meridians, dissolves mucus, disperses nodules, eliminates swelling, and eases pain.

Faeces Trogopterpri (wulingzhi 五灵脂) eases blood flow, disperses cold air in the chest and stomach.

Typha angustifolia (puhuang 蒲黄) removes cold or hot stagnation in the chest and stomach, and eliminates blood stagnation.

Eupolyphaga sinensis (tubiechong 土鳖虫) breaks down blood stagnation, eliminates abdominal masses, and heals long lasting stagnations.

Curcuma longa (jianghuang 姜黄) has a sweet taste and cold yinyang nature. It goes into the liver meridian. It breaks down blood stagnation, eliminates swelling, and eases qi flow.

193

Sepiella maindroni (wuzeigu 乌贼骨) removes dampness and mucus, opens meridian, dissolves blood stagnation, and stops bleeding.

Concha arcae (walengzi 瓦楞子) breaks down abdominal masses and nodules; it also dissolves stagnations of mucus, blood and qi.

Olibanum (ruxiang 乳香) invigorates blood; eliminates abscesses, ulcers and poisonous swellings, and removes damp poison in the blood.

Myrrh (moyao 没药) invigorates blood, breaks down nodules and stagnated blood, disperses swellings, and removes damp poison.

Evodia rutaecarpa (wuzhuyu 吴茱萸) warms spleen soil, moves stomach gas downwards and out, removes dampness, and eases pain.

Lindera aggregata (wuyao 乌药) eases qi flow, resolves snarls, eases pain, and disperses bloating.

Asarum sieboldii (xixin 细辛) disperses wind and cold, and opens the meridians.

Toosendan Fructus (chuanlianzi 川楝子) eases qi flow, stops all stomach pain.

Magnolia officinalis (houpo 厚朴) warms spleen soil, dissolves mucus, and moves stomach gas downward and out.

Curcuma radix (yujin 郁金) eases qi flow, and resolves snarls.

Aurantii fructus (zhiqiao 枳壳) breaks down stagnated qi, dissolves mucus, and eliminates food stagnation.

Rhizoma cyperi (xiangfu 香附) opens meridians, eases qi flow, strengthens spleen soil yang qi, and relieves snarls.

Rhizoma galangae (gaoliangjiang 高良姜) warms and loosens spleen soil.

Cortex cinnamomi (rougui 肉桂) warms kidney water, strengthens kidney heat reserve, opens blood passages, and ignites the effectiveness of all herbs.

Glycyrrhiza radix (gancao 甘草) harmonizes wuxing organs.

In the Maqian formula, Rheum officinale (dahuang), Coptis chinensis (huanglian), Reynoutria Japonica (huzhang), Lysimachia christinae (jinqiancao), Lygodium japonicum (haijinsha) are used to remove damp poisons. Aconitum carmichaeli (treated) (zhi caowu), Radix aconite carmichaeli (treated) (zhi fuzi), Arisaematis rhizoma (tiannanxing) are used to dissolve mucus and break down nodules. Curcuma zedoaria (ezhu), Trigonobalanus doichangensis (sanleng),

Strychnos nux-vomica (ma-qianzi), Faeces Trogopterpri (wulingzhi), Typha angustifolia (puhuang), Eupolyphaga sinensis (tubiechong), Curcuma longa (jianghuang), Sepiella maindroni (wuzeigu), Concha arcae (duan walengzi), Olibanum (ruxiang), myrrh (moyao) are used to break down mucus and damp poison in the blood. Evodia rutaecarpa (wuzhuyu), lindera aggregata (wuyao), Asarum sieboldii (xixin), Fructus toosendan (chuanlianzi), Magnolia officinalis (houpo), Curcuma radix (yujin), Aurantii fructus (zhiqiao), Rhizoma cyperi (xiangfu) are used to disperse stagnated qi. Rhizoma galangae (gaoliangjiang) and cortex cinnamomi (rougui) are used to warm spleen soil. Glycyrrhiza radix (gancao) is used to harmonize the wuxing organs.

Note: This formula, because of the aconitum carmichaeli (treated) requires at least two hours of boiling before drinking the decoction.

Treating spleen soil yang deficiency with external heat and dampness residing

A 15-year-old girl came for a consultation on the day when she suddenly felt nauseated, had frequent loose bowel motions, followed by fever. The yang deficiency of spleen soil leads to the loss of permeability, which then permits external heat and dampness residing and blocking its yinyang passages. The heat pushes dampness up so she felt nauseated. Damp heat burning lung metal yin causes fever. The large intestine is the outer extension of lung metal. The yang of lung metal separates turbidity from freshness and excretes turbidity through the large intestine. The damp heat in the spleen soil damages lung metal yang causing the inability to isolate turbidity, so there is diarrhoea. Treatment is to clear heat, dissolve dampness, and loosen spleen soil with the Qingxiang formula.

The patient took 250 ml of the concoction every three hours, and within 10 hours, the fever had dropped and she felt hungry for food. The following day she was completely well.

Qingxiang formula:

Artemisia carvifolia (qinghao) 10g
Anemarrhenae rhizoma (zhimu) 10g
Radix bupleuri (chaihu) 15g
Elsholtzia ciliate (xiangru) 10g
Agastache rugosa (huoxiang) 10g
Zingiber officinale (ganjiang) 10g
Saposhnikoviae radix (fangfeng) 10g
Morus alba (sangye) 10g
Asarum sieboldii (xixin)10g
Lysimachia christinae hance (jinqiancao) 30g
Gypsum (shigao) 20g
Talcum (huashi) 10g
Scutellaria baicalensis (huangqin)10g
Coptis chinensis (huanglian) 10g
Phellodendri chinensis (huangbai) 10g
Glycyrrhiza radix (gancao) 10
Pinelliae rhizoma (banxia) 10g
Eupatorium fortunei (peilan)10g
Paeoniae alba (baishao) 10

The Qingxiang Formula in Chinese 青香汤:

青蒿10g 知母10g 柴胡15g 香薷10藿香10干姜10防风10桑叶10g 细辛10g 金钱草30g 石膏20g 滑石10g 黄芩10g 黄连10g 黄柏10g 甘草10g 半夏10g佩兰10g 白芍10g

Artemisia carvifolia (qinghao 青蒿) has a bitter taste, and very cold yinyang nature. It goes into the heart, liver, and kidney meridians. It expels dampness, clears heat, dissolves mucus, stops periodical fever, and brightens eyesight.
Anemarrhenae rhizoma (zhimu 知母) drains damp turbidity.
Radix bupleuri (chaihu 柴胡) disperses cold, relaxes muscles and skin, and removes mucus.
Elsholtzia ciliate (xiangru 香薷) has a pungent taste and warm yinyang nature. It goes into the lung and stomach meridians. It relaxes muscles and skin; removes irregular qi and dampness, and opens the water passages.
Agastache rugosa (huoxiang 藿香) has a pungent and fragrant tastes and warm yinyang nature. It goes into lung, spleen and stomach meridians. It relaxes muscles and skin, disperses irregular qi, removes wind, and drains dampness.
Zingiber officinale (ganjiang 干姜) warms and loosens spleen soil, disperses wind, and relaxes muscles and skin.

Saposhnikoviae radix (fangfeng 防风) opens meridians.

Morus alba (sangye 桑叶) has a sweet and bitter taste, and a cold yinyang nature. It goes into lung and liver meridians. It disperses wind, relaxes muscles and skin, clears heat, and brightens eyesight.

Asarum sieboldii (xixin 细辛) opens meridians.

Lysimachia christinae hance (jinqiancao 金钱草) disperses wind, removes dampness, detoxifies poison, and stops pain.

Gypsum (shigao 石膏) isolates turbidity.

Talcum (huashi 滑石) isolates turbidity, clears heat, and dissolves mucus.

Scutellaria baicalensis (huangqin 黄芩) disperses wind, clears heat, removes dampness, detoxifies poison, and dissolves swelling.

Coptis chinensis (huanglian 黄连) ceases fire, detoxifies poison, dries dampness, and cools blood.

Phellodendri chinensis (huangbai 黄柏) dries dampness, detoxifies poison, and clears fermenting heat in wuxing organs.

Glycyrrhiza radix (gancao 甘草) resolves hot or cold poisonous qi.

Pinellia rhizoma (banxia 半夏) resolves mucus, opens the appetite, and loosens spleen soil.

Eupatorium fortunei (peilan 佩兰) has a sweet and fragrant tastes and mild yinyang nature. It goes into the lung and stomach meridians. It frees water passages, clears hidden mucus in the chest.

Paeoniae alba (baishao 白芍) smooths blood passages and removes dampness.

All the herbs in this formula remove dampness. Artemisia carvifolia (qinghao), Anemarrhenae Rhizoma (zhimu), Radix Bupleuri (chaihu), Elsholtzia ciliate (xiangru), Agastache rugosa (huoxiang) Zingiber officinale (ganjiang) also warm and loosen spleen soil, as well as clear lung metal heat, relax skin and muscles to expel heat, and stop fever. Saposhnikoviae radix (fangfeng), Morus alba (sangye), Asarum sieboldii (xixin), Lysimachia christinae hance (jinqiancao) also disperse wind, open meridians enhancing the removal of external irregular qi. Gypsum (shigao) and Talcum (huashi) through isolating turbidity facilitate the clearance of dampness and mucus. Scutellaria baicalensis (huangqin), Coptis chinensis (huanglian), Phellodendri chinensis (huangbai) also clear heat and detoxify poison. Glycyrrhiza (gancao) also harmonize wuxing organs, and detoxifies poison. Pinelliae Rhizoma (banxia) and Eupatorium fortunei (peilan) clear stubborn mucus and stop nausea. Paeoniae alba (baishao) frees blood passages to promote recovery.

Method of cooking and drinking the herbs:

Put two packets of the herbs together in a clay pot, add 1500 ml of cold water, bring the water to boil then keep boiling for 50 minutes or so to reduce the liquid down to 500 ml, strain the liquid into a jar, and add another 600 ml of cold water into the pot, bring the liquid to boil then keep boiling for another 10 minutes or so to reduce the liquid down to 500 ml, strain the liquid into the same jar, and take 250 ml of the concoction each time.

Treating spleen soil yang deficiency with symptoms of loose bowels

A 56-year-old man had diarrhoea for three months and came for a consultation. During that three months, he had been taking antibiotics consistently. At the first consultation, he had diarrhoea seven to eight times a day, it was very loose, and had stomach pulling down pain before and during diarrhoea. He had a yellow greasy coating on his tongue, and his pulse was heavy.

This was a case of spleen soil yang deficiency causing diarrhoea. When there is spleen soil yang damage and the soil friability is lost, water passages congest and create dampness and mucus. Therefore the patient's pulse was heavy, and the tongue coating was greasy. Fermenting dampness and mucus creates heat, so the tongue coating was yellow. The large intestine is the outer extension of the lung metal, the lung metal separates turbidity and freshness, and excretes out turbidity through the large intestine. When the damp poison of the spleen soil damages the yang qi of lung metal, it incapacitates lung metal's ability to isolate turbidity from freshness, so the bowel motion was loose and frequent. Damp heat creates wind in the large intestine and causes the symptom of stomach pulling down pain before and during bowel motions. In the "Liver Wood" chapter, I discussed cases of loose bowel motions. The differences between those cases to this case is that in the former cases the liver wood yang damage with blood decay caused loose bowel motions that were sticky, smelly and difficult to excrete. Whereas this case is of frequent bowel motion, stomach pain during the bowel motion, without bad smell. The treatment for this case is to remove dampness, clear heat, loosen spleen soil with the Baitouweng formula.

The patient took 10 packets of the herbs and recovered completely. His bowel motions became formed and regular once more.

Baitouweng formula:

Bupleurum chinense (chaihu) 10g

Pinelliae rhizoma (banxia) 10g

Scutellaria baicalensis (huangqin) 10g

Coptis chinensis (huanglian) 10g

Phellodendri chinensis (huangbai) 10g

Zingiber officinale (ganjiang) 10g

Agastache rugosa (huoxiang) 10g

Eupatorium fortunei (peilan)10g

Pulsatilla chinensis (baitouweng) 15g

Portulaca oleracea (machixian) 30g

Fraxinus rhynchophylla (qinpi) 10g

Glycyrrhiza radix (gancao) 10g

Baitouweng formula in Chinese 白头翁汤:

柴胡10g 半夏10g 黄芩10g 黄连10g 黄柏10g 干姜10g 藿香10g 佩兰10g 白头翁15g 马齿苋30g 秦皮10g 甘草10g

Bupleurum chinense (chaihu 柴胡) disperses cold, relaxes muscles and skin, and removes mucus.

Pinellia rhizoma (banxia 半夏) resolves mucus, opens appetite, and harmonizes yinyang order of spleen soil.

Scutellaria baicalensis (huangqin 黄芩) disperses wind, clears heat, removes dampness, detoxifies poison, and dissolves swelling.

Coptis chinensis (huanglian 黄连) ceases fire, detoxifies poison, dries dampness, and cools blood.

Phellodendri chinensis (huangbai 黄柏) dries dampness, detoxifies poison, clears fermenting heat from the wuxing organs.

Zingiber Officinale (ganjiang 干姜) warms and loosens spleen soil, disperses wind, relaxes muscles and skin.

Agastache rugosa (huoxiang 藿香) relaxes muscles and skin, disperses irregular qi, removes wind, and drains dampness.

Eupatorium fortunei (peilan 佩兰) frees water passages, clears hidden mucus in the chest.

Pulsatilla chinensis (baitouweng 白头翁) has a bitter taste and cold yinyang nature. It goes into large intestine and stomach meridians. It removes dampness, cools blood, detoxifies poison, cleans intestine, and stops diarrhoea.

Portulaca oleracea (machixian马齿苋) has a pungent taste and cold yinyang nature. It goes into the large intestine, and stomach meridians, it removes dampness, clears heat, detoxifies poison, cleanses the intestine, and stops diarrhoea.

Fraxinus rhynchophylla (qinpi 秦皮) has a bitter taste and cold yinyang nature. It goes into large intestine and liver meridians. It clears heat, detoxifies poison, cleans intestine, stops diarrhoea, and brightens eyesight.

Glycyrrhiza radix (gancao 甘草) resolves hot or cold poisonous qi in all wuxing organs.

The intention of the formula with Bupleurum chinense (chaihu), and Pinelliae rhizoma (banxia) is by dissolving mucus to loosen spleen soil. Scutellaria baicalensis (huangqin), Coptis chinensis (huanglian), Phellodendri chinensis (huangbai) are used to dry dampness and clear heat to loosen the spleen soil. The fragrant herbs of Zingiber officinale (ganjiang), Agastache rugosa (huoxiang) Eupatorium fortunei (peilan) are used to resolve dampness, and disperse poisonous qi. Pulsatilla chinensis (baitouweng), Portulaca oleracea (machixian), Fraxinus rhynchophylla (qinpi) are used to guide the healing to the large intestine and stop diarrhoea. Glycyrrhiza (gancao) is used to harmonize the wuxing organs and regenerate their connection.

Treating spleen soil yang deficiency in young children

Spleen soil yang deficiency in young children is mostly caused by inadequate food. A mother brought her 3-year-old child to me for a consultation. The child was very thin and much smaller compared to other children the same age. His tongue had a greasy thick white coating, his complexion was sallow and he suffered constipation a lot. The mother said the child had very little appetite, he only ate some biscuits now and then but never ate a proper meal. Most of the biscuits bought on the market have artificial sweeteners and flavourings, preservatives, puffing agents, and so on. When these chemicals are accumulated in the body, they will block the body's yinyang passages, and lead to illness. In this case, the accumulation of the chemicals damaged the permeability of spleen soil which allowed dampness and mucus to stagnate in the spleen soil, so the patient had no appetite for food. When spleen soil fails to transform food it causes the body to become thin and underdeveloped. Chemical accumulation damaging liver wood yang causes blood passage congestion, so his complexion was sallow. Treatment was to dissolve dampness, eliminate stagnation, and open the appetite with the Jiaomai formula. But the precondition was that the boy had to stop eating biscuits or other food that had too many chemical additives.

The boy took one packet of the formula and ate a little bit of his dinner. The following morning he was hungry. His mother was very pleased. Six months later, the mother brought the boy to my clinic to show her healthy child. The boy had grown taller and stronger, and his complexion was bright.

Jiaomai formula:

Crataegus pinnatifida (scorched) (jiao shanzha) 30g
Fructus hordei germinatus (scorched) (jiao maiya) 30g
Scorched oryza Sativa (jiao guya) 30g
Massa medicata fermentata (liuqu) 30g
Poria cocos (fuling) 10g
Rhizoma atractylodis (baizhu) 10g
Pinellia ternate (banxia) 10g

The Jiaomai formula in Chinese 焦麦汤:

焦山楂30g 焦麦芽30g 焦谷芽30g 六曲30g 茯苓10g 白术10g 半夏10g

Crataegus pinnatifida (jiao shanzha 焦山楂) Scorched hawthorn fruit has a puckery taste, and warm yinyang nature. It goes into the spleen and stomach meridians. It frees qi flow, drains dampness, loosens spleen soil, and breaks down food stagnation.
Fructus hordei germinatus (scorched) (jiao maiya 焦麦芽) has a sweet taste and warm yinyang nature. It goes into the spleen and stomach meridians. It breaks down qi stagnation, drains dampness, loosens spleen soil, and dissolves food stagnation.

Oryza sativa (scorched) (jiao guya 焦谷芽) has a sweet taste and warm yinyang nature. It goes into the spleen, stomach meridians. It drains dampness, frees qi flow, loosens spleen soil, and dissolves food stagnation.

Massa Medicata Fermentata (liuqu 六曲) has a sweet taste and mild yinyang nature. It goes into the spleen and stomach meridians. It frees qi flow, drains dampness, loosens spleen soil, and dissolves food stagnation.

Poria cocos (fuling 茯苓) loosens spleen soil; improves water drainage, whets appetite, and calms the spirit.

Rhizoma Atractylodis (baizhu 白术) disperses head wind, defends external wind attack, drains dampness, and removes mucus.

Pinellia ternate (banxia 半夏) removes mucus, whets appetite, and loosens spleen soil.

In the Jiaomai formula, scorched hawthorn fruit (jiao shanzha), scorched Fructus hordei germinatus (jiao maiya), scorched Oryza sativa (jiao guya), Massa medicata fermentata (liuqu) are used to loosen spleen soil, and break down food stagnation; Poria cocos (fuling) is used to improve water drainage; Rhizoma atractylodis (baizhu) is used to dry dampness; Pinellia ternate (banxia) is used to dissolve mucus.

The formula has a very mild taste, and is suitable for children to take.

Treating spleen soil yang deficiency with prenatal vomiting

A 30-year-old woman who was two months pregnant came for a consultation as she was constantly feeling nauseated, prone to vomiting and was unable to eat. The spleen soil yang deficiency causes foetus fluid congestion and dampness to occur, the regurgitation of dampness causes nausea and vomiting, and loss of appetite. The treatment is to loosen spleen soil, disperse dampness, and arrest vomiting with the Qinchai formula.

After taking two packets of the herbs, the nausea stopped and the patient was able to eat normally. In the next two months, she occasionally had the nausea and vomiting symptoms return, as soon as she took a packet of the same herbs, she returned to normal again.

After 4 months of pregnancy the symptoms disappeared completely. She later had a normal childbirth.

Qinchai formula:

Scutellaria baicalensis (huangqin) 10g
Pinelliae rhizoma (banxia) 10g
Radix stellariae (chaihu) 10g
Atractylodis macrocephalae (baizhu) 15g
Rhizoma zingiberis (ganjiang) 10g
Rhizoma galangae (gaoliangjiang) 10g
Poria cocos (fuling) 10g
Glycyrrhiza radix (gancao) 10g

Qinchai formula in Chinese 芩柴汤:

黄芩10g 半夏10g 柴胡10g 白术15g 干姜10g 高良姜10g 茯苓10g 甘草10g

Scutellaria baicalensis (huangqin 黄芩) clears heat, and dries dampness.
Pinelliae rhizoma (banxia 半夏) dissolves mucus, opens appetite, and loosens spleen soil.
Radix stellariae (chaihu 柴胡) disperses cold, and removes mucus.
Atractylodis macrocephalae (baizhu 白术) removes head wind, consolidates skin protection, removes dampness and mucus.
Rhizoma zingiberis (ganjiang 干姜) warms spleen soil and removes dampness.
Rhizoma galangae (gaoliangjiang 高良姜) warms and loosens spleen soil.
Poria cocos (fuling 茯苓) drains fluid, loosens spleen soil, opens the appetite, and calms the spirit.
Glycyrrhiza radix (gancao 甘草) resolves poisonous qi in all wuxing organs.

Within the formula, Scutellaria baicalensis (huangqin) dries dampness and loosens spleen soil. Pinelliae Rhizoma (banxia), Radix Stellariae (chaihu), and Atractylodis Macrocephalae (baizhu) clear mucus and loosen spleen soil. Rhizoma zingiberis (ganjiang) and Rhizoma galangae (gaoliangjiang) warm and loosen spleen soil. Poria cocos (fuling) drains water and loosens spleen soil. Glycyrrhiza (gancao) harmonizes the wuxing organs to calm the foetus.

Cooking and drinking the herbs:

Place one packet of herbs into a clay pot, add 750 ml of cold water, bring the mixture to boil and keep boiling for another 50 minutes to reduce the liquid down to around 300 ml. Strain the liquid into a jar, discard the dregs of the decoction. Drink a large mouthful of the decoction whenever nausea occurs. According to the degree of the symptoms, the liquid can last up to two days, but no more than one packet a day.

Treating spleen soil yin deficiency with symptoms of dizzy nausea

A 52-year-old woman had dizzy spells on and off for three months. She was taking drugs to manage the dizziness. But two days before she came to me for a consultation, her dizziness was uncontrollable and instead, after taking the western medicine, she felt headaches as well. The patient was unable to walk or stand on her own. She felt nauseated, and sometimes vomited. She had ringing in the ears like ocean waves, and she had no appetite. Her tongue was deep red, with a mirror like coating, and her pulse was big but empty.

The adhesive nature of spleen soil yin facilitates the meeting of the wuxing organs. When there is spleen soil yin damage, soil loses its adhesive nature and bearing capacity, so there is no appetite, and hence the mirror like coating on the tongue, and the empty pulse. Spleen soil controls the water passages of kidney water, the ears are the openings of kidney water. When spleen soil loses its binding ability this causes water passage damage; the kidney water loses control, so water in the kidney water rushes, which causes ringing in the ears. When water goes in waves upward, there are symptoms of nausea and vomiting. With spleen soil yin damage, soil loses its bearing capacity which causes the disconnection of the wuxing organs. When liver wood cannot receive kidney water and becomes dry, it means the blood rushes out of the liver wood root and travels fast in the blood passages and causes heat and wind. The heat and wind in the blood causes the dizziness and a deep red tongue. Treatment is to moisten and enrich spleen soil yin, and smooth water flow, calm the adverse rising energy, soften liver wood, and cease wind with the formula Daizhe.

The patient took one packet of the herbs, the dizziness and ringing ears improved significantly the next day. She took three packets of the herbs all together and all symptoms disappeared.

Daizhe formula:

Codonopsis pilosula (dangshen) 30g
Angelica sinensis (danggui) 24g
Paeoniae alba (baishao) 30g
Nelumbo nucifera (heye)18g

Poria cocos (fuling) 24g
Atractylodis macrocephalae (baizhu) 30g
Pinelliae rhizoma (banxia) 10g
Haematium (daizheshi) 18g

Daizhe formula in Chinese 代赭汤:

党参30g 当归24g 白芍30g 荷叶18g 茯苓24g 白术30g 半夏10g 代赭石18g

Codonopsis pilosula (dangshen 党参) has a sweet taste and mild yinyang nature. It goes into the spleen and lung meridians. It enriches the spleen soil and the qi of lung metal.

Angelica sinensis (danggui 当归) harmonizes yinyang orders of all wuxing organs.

Paeoniae alba (baishao 白芍) softens liver wood, opens and smooths blood passages, and dissolves swelling and mucus.

Nelumbo nucifera (heye 荷叶) has a puckery taste and mild yinyang nature. It goes into the heart, liver, spleen and lung meridians. It raises fresh yang qi, expels turbid qi, and enriches spleen soil yin and yang.

Poria Cocos (fuling 茯苓) loosens spleen soil, improves water drainage, opens appetite, and calms the spirit.

Atractylodis macrocephalae (baizhu 白术) regenerates spleen soil, improves water drainage, expels mucus, expels head wind, and consolidates skin protection.

Pinelliae rhizoma (banxia 半夏) dissolves mucus, opens appetite, and regenerates spleen soil.

Haematium (daizheshi 代赭石) has a slightly sweet taste and mild yinyang nature. It goes into the liver and stomach meridians. It disperses wind, cools blood, loosens spleen soil, and calms down regurgitation.

In the Daizhe formula, the Codonopsis pilosula (dangshen), Angelica sinensis (danggui) are sweet herbs to regenerate spleen soil yin; Paeoniae alba (baishao), Nelumbo nucifera (heye), Poria cocos (fuling), Atractylodis macrocephalae (baizhu) strengthen both the yin and yang of the spleen soil, and removes dampness. Pinelliae rhizoma (banxia) and Haematium (daizheshi) remove mucus, and calm down regurgitation to stop nausea.

Treating spleen soil yin and yang damage with symptoms of fatigue

A 35-year-old woman came for help after she had a mastectomy and was having chemotherapy. At the first consultation, the patient was fatigued; her steps were heavy; she had no appetite for food; she felt nauseated and vomited after eating. Her bowel motions had undigested food and she had patches of mirror-like coating on her tongue.

The chemotherapy had damaged the spleen soil yin and yang. With the spleen soil yin damage, soil losses its adhesiveness and leads to the loss of the wuxing organs' creative and controlling bonds. Thus, kidney water loses its replenishment of heat from food and heart fire, which causes kidney water yang qi reserve to be low, so there is fatigue. As spleen soil could not hold food, so the patient had no appetite for food. Spleen soil yin damage makes it empty, so there are patches of mirror-like coating on the tongue. With spleen soil yang damage, water passages congest, which causes dampness. Water and dampness rise and cause nausea and vomiting. When there is spleen soil yang deficiency, food does not get transformed and transported, so there is undigested food in the stool. Treatment is to restore the spleen soil yin, remove dampness, loosen spleen soil, connect the wuxing organs, and restore energy with the Shenqi formula.

After taking the herbs, the patient gained more strength, the feelings of nausea abated and her appetite improved. Although herbs do help minimize chemotherapy's harsh effects, if the chemotherapy continues its damage to the yinyang passage of wuxing organs would eventually become irreversible.

Shenqi formula:

Panax ginseng (renshen) 30g
Codonopsis pilosula (dangshen) 30g
Astragalus membranaceus (huangqi) 30g
Paeoniae alba (baishao) 30g

Angelica sinensis (danggui) 24g
Poria cocos (fuling) 24g
Pinelliae rhizoma (banxia) 10g
Nelumbo nucifera (heye) 18g
Atractylodis Macrocephalae (baizhu) 30g

Shenqi formula in Chinese 参芪汤:

人参30g 党参30g 黄芪30g 白芍30g 当归24g 茯苓24g 半夏10g 荷叶18g白术30g

Panax ginseng (renshen 人参) warms kidney water and calms the spirit in all wuxing organs.

Codonopsis pilosula (dangshen 党参) enriches the blood, qi, and spleen soil yin.

Astragalus membranaceus (huangqi 黄芪) has a sweet taste and slightly warm yinyang nature. It goes into the lung and spleen meridians. It draws poison out and ejects pusses, nurtures spleen soil yin and yang; enriches muscles and skin, and ceases fire in the lung metal.

Paeoniae alba (baishao 白芍) opens and smooths blood passages, dissolves swelling and mucus.

Angelica sinensis (danggui 当归) harmonizes all wuxing organs.

Poria cocos (fuling 茯苓) drains dampness, loosens spleen soil, and improves appetite.

Pinelliae rhizoma (banxia 半夏) dissolves mucus, opens appetite, and consolidates spleen soil yin and yang.

Nelumbo nucifera (heye 荷叶) raises fresh yang qi, expels turbid qi, and enriches spleen soil yin and yang.

Atractylodis macrocephalae (baizhu 白术) removes dampness and mucus.

In the formula, the sweet Codonopsis pilosula (dangshen) and Astragalus membranaceus (huangqi) are the most favourable herbs to restore spleen soil yin. Panax ginseng, Paeoniae alba (baishao), Angelica sinensis (danggui) nourish both yin and yang of spleen soil. Poria cocos (fuling), Pinelliae rhizoma (banxia), Nelumbo nucifera (heye), and Atractylodis macrocephalae (baizhu) remove mucus to loosen spleen soil and consolidate spleen soil yang.

Lung Metal

The lung is a metal organ, it is naturally solid, but becomes soft when it encounters heat. Lung metal gathers qi and moisture, it fills out the body, and stores the entire body's qi; it is a yin organ. Yin attracts yang, the gathering yin ability of lung metal attracts the separating yang qi of lung metal, which allows the qi to gather but not be trapped, the fluid gathers but does not stagnate. The yin of lung metal upholds its gathering and astringent nature. Because of the gathering and astringent nature of lung metal yin, it absorbs qi from heaven and earth and the internal wuxing organs, which maintains the repletion of the body. Also because of the gathering and astringent nature of lung metal yin, it retains moisture from heaven and earth, and the internal body, so the body is moist. Like metal and stones, separating clear water from sludge, the yang of lung metal sustains its dividing nature, and separates turbid and fresh substances of the body. Thus fresh qi is inhaled into the body and turbid qi is exhaled out of the body. Also because of the dividing yang nature of lung metal, body fluid is separated into fresh water and waste, and located into separate passages. Lung metal sits in the top of the body; the fresh water that lung metal has cleared and condensed drizzles down like fog and dew descending to moisten the entire body, and replenishing kidney water. The large intestine is the outer extension of lung metal, which collects and excretes the wastes that lung metal has been sorting, so that lung metal maintains the freshness of the body. Because of the gathering and separating nature of lung metal, the spirit interacts with lung metal to exercises its lofty zhi. The cooperation of spirit and lung metal makes a person dignified and easy going.

In summary, lung metal aggregates qi and collects moisture, it is the storage of body qi. It also divides the turbid from the fresh, and is responsible for keeping the body fresh. Emotionally, it makes the spirit bright.

Yinyang disorders of lung metal causes qi flow disorders, and affects the body's refreshing and moistening function, and can also cause the spirit sadness or isolation.

Causes of lung metal yinyang disorder

If one does not follow the yinyang changes of heaven and earth to work and rest, to drink and eat, the result will be a yinyang disorder of lung metal. Lung metal is the opening where the body qi connects with heaven and earth. A person will become ill when external cold and wind enters the body and damages the lung metal yang qi and adversely affects the separating function of lung metal yang. On the other hand, prolonged exposure to external heat will exhaust the yin qi of lung metal and also cause illness.

In modern times, air pollution has become one of the most common causes for damaging the yinyang order of lung metal. Chemicals in the air that get into the lung breathing passages will block the yinyang transformation of lung metal and cause both yin and yang damage of lung metal. Moreover, the increased use of antibiotics has become a common cause of lung metal yang damage. Antibiotics may kill bacteria, but as antibiotics do not transform following the normal regulation of yinyang change, it becomes obstructive to the body's yinyang passages. In lung metal, the blockages cause dampness and mucus to grow and damage the yang qi of lung metal.

Symptoms

When the lung metal fails to gather qi because of a yin deficiency, then a person has symptoms of shortness of breath. When the yin deficiency fails to collect fluid, which causes dry heat in the lung metal, then a person will suffer from symptoms such as fever, and sore throats. Yang damage of lung metal will mean that the separation of turbid from fresh is inhibited, which in turn causes an inundation of turbid qi, as well as dampness and mucus blocking the qi passages. A person will then suffer from symptoms such as congested nasal passages, runny nose, tightness of chest, coughing out mucus. When the yang damage of lung metal fails to separate turbidity and freshness, this also causes the body to become sticky, damp, and unfresh, as well as difficult to open bowel motions. When there is a yang deficiency of lung metal, qi and moisture can be gathered but the fresh and turbid cannot be separated, and this deprives the yang qi of the lofty zhi of the spirit to be exercised, and then the spirit is muddy and sad. When there is yin deficiency of lung metal then qi and moisture cannot be gathered, which deprives the yin qi of the lofty zhi from being exercised, and causes the spirit qi to be scattered and isolated.

Overall, fever, breathing passage blockages, body un-freshness are symptoms of lung metal yinyang disorders. Emotionally, sadness or feelings of isolation are indications of lung metal yinyang disorders as well.

Tongue

The yin of lung metal gathers, it gathers qi and moisture. The yang of lung metal separates; it separates fresh water from turbid water, fresh qi and stale qi. When the yinyang of lung metal is in harmony, the body is ample and fresh, the tongue is moist. With yin deficiency, lung metal fails to gather moisture and the tongue is dry—even cracked. With yang deficiency, lung metal fails to isolate turbidity and the tongue is wet with sticky saliva.

Pulse

The yinyang harmony of lung metal means that fresh qi can gather inside the body, and that turbid qi can exit, which makes a body moist and fresh, so that the balloon of the pulse is smooth and is gently paced. When the lung metal yin is deficient, it fails to gather moisture, and becomes dry and hot; the pulse becomes rapid, which comes urgently but leaves slowly. At first, lung metal yin deficiency shows in the right cun pulse. When the dry heat of lung metal extends to the heart fire organ, the left cun pulse becomes rapid. When the dry heat affects the spleen soil organ, the right guan pulse is rapid. When the liver wood organ is affected, the left guan pulse will be rapid. When it affects the kidney heat storage, the right chi pulse is rapid. When it affects the kidney water organ, the left chi

211

pulse becomes rapid. On the other hand, when lung metal yang is deficient, qi and moisture can gather but are unable to be divided from stale and turbid, and are trapped by dampness and mucus; the pulse then becomes hesitating, rising slowly and descending quickly. All affected wuxing organs will have a hesitating pulse.

Skin

The yin of lung metal gathers qi and fluid; the yang of lung metal separates turbidity and freshness. When the yinyang of lung metal is in regular order, the skin is moist and clean. When the yin of lung metal is damaged, it does not gather moisture, so the skin is dry. When the yang of lung metal is damaged, fluid is gathered but the turbidity is not separated nor discharged, so the skin is damp and greasy.

Principles for treating lung metal yinyang disorder

The treatment for lung metal yin deficiency is to clear heat, and increase lubrication. But as lung metal is a yin organ often lacking yang, while nurturing the lung metal yin, one should always protect the yang. Treating yang damage of lung metal is to isolate what is turbid from fresh and dissolve mucus. Lung metal yinyang disorders that cause emotional symptoms will often recover once the yinyang of lung metal is regulated without other treatment.

Treating lung metal yin damage with external wind and cold

A 36-year-old man called me as he was getting off an aeroplane flight. He said he had caught a chill on the plane, and about two hours earlier he had a high fever. His body was cold and shivering; his throat was sore and dry; his nose was blocked; he had headaches, and body aches.

Exhaustion depletes the body fluid and qi and damages the yin of lung metal. Lung metal then fails to gather fluid, which leads to the dryness and heat in lung metal. The dry heat then attracts external abnormal cold and wind to stay in the lung metal and causes illness. The lung metal qi travels between skin and flesh, abnormal cold qi that travels between flesh and skin causes body coldness. Wind travelling between flesh and skin causes shivering. Cold obstructed between flesh and skin causes heat to be trapped inside the body so there is fever. The nose and throat are the doorways of lung metal to heaven and earth; when lung metal fails to congregate fluid it causes dryness in lung metal, so there are symptoms of dry and sore throat. The dry heat in the lung metal collapses the qi passages of lung metal, so there is the symptom of blocked nose. External cold and wind travel up to the head causing headaches; when they travel in between muscle and bones it causes body aches.

The treatment is to disperse wind, expel cold, free skin and flesh passages, and detoxify poison, which is to remove foreign abnormal qi. At the same time, lung metal needs to be moistened to strengthen its yin, and isolate turbid qi to consolidate the yang of lung metal. I used the Cangzhi formula.

The patient cooked two packets of the herbs in a large pot with 2 litres of cold water and boiled down to one litre of liquid in about an hour. Each time he would drink 250 ml of the liquid and often at two hour intervals. By midnight, he had drunk three cups of the herbal decoction and fell asleep. The following morning when he woke, his temperature had dropped down to normal. And he went to work as usual.

Cangzhi formula:

Ephedra sinica (mahuang) 10g
Cinnamomum cassia (guizhi) 10g
Puerariae lobatae (gegen) 10g
Aster tataricus (ziyuan) 15g
Anthium sibiricum (cangerzi) 15g
Angelica dahurica (baizhi) 15g

Magnolia liliflora (xingyihua) 10g
Asarum sieboldii (xixin) 5g
Rhizoma ligustici (gaoben) 5g
Vitex trifolia (manjingzi) 10g
Notopterygium incisum (qianghuo) 5g

---

[6]Sophora Tonkinensis (shandougen) is a very effective herb to stop sore throat, but some people will suffer nausea or severe vomiting after taking it. However, after vomiting once, the feeling of nausea will disappear. To avoid nausea and vomiting, when someone is taking the herb for the first time, use 2-3 grams to see whether

Sophora tonkinensis (shandougen)[6] 5g

Belamcandae rhizoma (shegan) 10g

Sapindus mukorossi (muhuangen)30g

Evodia lepta (sanyaku) 30g

Trichosanthes kirilowii (gualouren) 15g

Stemona japonica (baibu) 15g

Fritillaria cirrhosa (chuanbeimu) 15g

Amygdalus communis (xingren) 10g

Gypsum (shigao) 20g

Anemarrhenae asphodeloides (zhimu)10g

Platycodon grandiflorus (jiegeng) 10g

Allium macrostemon (xiebai) 10g

Spina gleditsiae (zaojiaoci) 10g

Arctii fructus (niubangzi) 15g

Oldenlandia diffusa (baihuasheshecao) 30g

Sauropus rostratus (longliye) 15g

Glycyrrhiza radix (gancao) 10g

Cangzhi Formula in Chinese 苍芷汤:

麻黄10g 桂枝10g 葛根10g 紫苑15g 苍耳子15g 白芷15g 辛夷花10g 细辛5g 藁本5g 蔓荆子10g 羌活5g 山豆根5g 射干10g 木患根30g 三丫苦30g 瓜蒌仁15g 百部15g 川贝母15g 杏仁10g 石膏20g 知母10g 桔梗10g 薤白10g 皂角刺10g 牛蒡子15g 白花蛇舌草30g 龙利叶15g 甘草10g

Ephedra sinica (mahuang 麻黄) opens skin and flesh passages, removes turbid qi from all wuxing organs, and frees blood passages.

Cinnamomum cassia (guizhi 桂枝) disperses external disordered qi, opens skin and flesh passages, and frees meridians.

Puerariae Lobatae (gegen 葛根) has a sweet taste and mild yinyang nature. It goes into the lung and urine bladder meridians. It clears cold and wind headaches, frees flesh passages, and induces sweat.

Aster tataricus (ziyuan 紫苑) has a pungent taste and slightly warm yinyang nature. It goes into lung meridian. It opens the lung meridian, dissolves cold or hot stagnant qi in the chest.

Anthium sibiricum (cangerzi 苍耳子) has a pungent taste and warm yinyang nature. It goes into the lung meridian. It disperses wind, expels cold, stops pain, and opens nasal passages.

---

they can cope with it. Also many herb shops in China and around the world, substitute Menispermi Rhizoma (beidougen) for Sophora tonkinensis (shandougen). The two have similar effect, but Menispermi Rhizoma (beidougen) is much weaker in effectiveness.

Angelica dahurica (baizhi 白芷) has a strong pungent taste, and warm yinyang nature. It goes into lung, large intestine, and stomach meridians. It expels wind, disperses cold, dissolves mucus, eliminates nodules, primes other herbs to go to the upper body, opens nasal passages, and stops headaches.

Magnolia liliflora (xinyihua 辛夷花) has a pungent taste and warm yinyang nature. It goes into the lung meridian. It disperses wind, and opens nasal passages.

Asarum sieboldii (xixin 细辛) disperses wind; expels coldness, and opens meridians and nasal passages.

Rhizoma Ligustici (gaoben 篙本) has a pungent taste, and warm yinyang nature. It goes into urine bladder meridian. It removes mucus, expels puss, and stops headache.

Vitex trifolia (manjingzi 蔓荆子) has a pungent and bitter taste, and slightly cold yinyang nature. It goes into the urine bladder meridian. It cools blood, and stops headache.

Notopterygium incisum (qianghuo 羌活) has a pungent and bitter taste, and warm yinyang nature. It goes into the urine bladder meridian. It stops headaches that occur at the back of the head, and stops all joint pains.

Sophora tonkinensis (shandougen 山豆根) has a bitter taste and cold yinyang nature. It goes into the lung meridian. It clears heat, detoxifies poisons, expels swelling, soothes throat, and stops pains.

Belamcandae rhizoma (shegan 射干) has a bitter taste and slightly cold yinyang nature. It goes into the lung, liver, and spleen meridians. It clears heat, detoxifies poison, draws pusses, dissolves swelling, and stops sore throat.

Sapindus mukorossi (muhuangen 木患根) has a bitter taste and cool yinyang nature. It goes into lung and liver meridians. It clears heat, detoxifies poison, dissolves mucus, and removes dampness.

Evodia Lepta (sanyaku 三丫苦) has a bitter taste and cold yinyang nature. It goes into the lung, stomach, liver and gall bladder meridians. It clears heat, detoxifies poison, cools blood, removes mucus, and opens meridians.

Trichosanthes kirilowii (gualouren 瓜蒌仁) has a sweet taste and cold yinyang nature. It goes into lung and large intestine meridians. It moistens lung metal, dissolves mucus, relieves oppression, and opens bowel motions.

215

Stemona Japonica (baibu 百部) has a sweet taste, and slightly warm yinyang nature. It goes into lung and stomach meridians. It moistens lung metal, and stops coughing.

Fritillaria cirrhosa (chuanbeimu 川贝母) has a sweet and bitter taste, and mild yinyang nature. It goes into lung meridian. It moistens lung metal, dissolves mucus, stops coughing, and disperses qi stagnation in the chest.

Amygdalus Communis (xingren 杏仁) has a bitter taste and warm yinyang nature. It goes into lung and large intestine meridians. It moistens lung metal, dissolves mucus, and stops coughing.

Gypsum (shigao 石膏) separates turbid and freshness, and opens the lung breathing passage.

Anemarrhenae asphodeloides (zhimu 知母) cools lung heat, and clears dampness and turbidity.

Platycodon grandiflorus (jiegeng 桔梗) has a bitter and pungent taste, and mild yinyang nature. It goes into the lung meridian. It loosens tight chest, removes pusses in the lung, stops sore throat, and opens nasal passages.

Allium macrostemon (xiebai 薤白) has a pungent taste, and warm yinyang nature. It goes into lung and heart meridians. It warms stomach, disperses nodules and detoxifies poison.

Spina gleditsiae (zaojiaoci 皂角刺) has a pungent taste and warm yinyang nature. It primes other herbs to go to the upper body, disperses wind, dissolves mucus, and counteracts toxic poison.

Arctii fructus (niubangzi 牛蒡子) has a pungent taste and mild yinyang nature. It goes into the lung meridian. It dissolves swelling, and detoxifies poison.

Oldenlandia diffusa (baihuasheshecao 白花蛇舌草) has a sweet and slightly sour taste, and cold yinyang nature. It clears heat, disperses stagnations, dissolves puss, and detoxifies poisons. It is especially effective in clearing pusses in the lung.

Sauropus rostratus (longliye 龙脷叶) has a mild yinyang nature. It goes into and opens the lung meridian, and dissolves mucus.

Glycyrrhiza radix (gancao 甘草) detoxifies poison.

Within the Cangzhi formula, Ephedra sinica (mahuang), Cinnamomum Cassia (guizhi), Puerariae Lobatae (gegen), and Aster tataricus (ziyuan) are used to relieve skin blockage, and free flesh and skin passages, so the external abnormal cold and wind can be expelled. Anthium sibiricum (cangerzi), Angelica dahurica (baizhi), Magnolia liliflora (xingyihua), and Asarum sieboldii (xixin) are used to expel wind, disperse cold, and open nasal passages. Rhizoma ligustici (gaoben), Vitex trifolia (manjingzi), Notopterygium incisum (qianghuo) are used to prime herbs upward, and stop headaches. Sophora tonkinensis (shandougen), Belamcandae rhizoma (shegan), Sapindus mukorossi (muhuangen), and Evodia lepta (sanyaku) are used to cool lung metal, detoxify poison which would bring down the fever and stop the sore throat. Trichosanthes kirilowii (gualouren), Stemona japonica (baibu), Fritillaria cirrhosa (chuanbeimu), and Amygdalus communis (xingren) are used to nurture the yin and moisten lung metal, and dissolve mucus. Gypsum (shigao), and Anemarrhenae asphodeloides (zhimu) are used to cleanse lung metal and dissolve turbidity which protect the yang qi of lung metal; Platycodon grandiflorus (jiegeng), Allium macrostemon (xiebai), Spina gleditsiae (zaojiaoci), Arctii Fructus (niubangzi), Oldenlandia diffusa (baihuasheshecao), Sauropus rostratus (longliye), Glycyrrhiza (gancao) are used to detoxify poison, dissolve mucus, which further enhance the protection of cleanliness of lung metal yang.

Another 35-year-old man came for a consultation as he suffered from symptoms of headache, severe sore throat and fever for four days. Before the symptoms began, he had been physically working in the hot summer sun consistently for six hours; he had perspired heavily and then had a cold shower. After the cold shower, he begun to have a headache, a sore throat and then a fever began.

Exhaustion and sweating damaged his lung metal yin and caused the lung metal to be dry and hot. The cold shower led the cold qi into the yinyang passages of lung metal, and caused him to fall ill. Cold qi dwelled between the flesh and skin preventing body heat from evaporating and to be trapped inside, so there was fever. The dry heat in lung metal caused the sore throat. The counteracting of cold and heat causes wind. Wind and cold travelling up to the head causes headaches. The treatment is to disperse external cold and wind, clear heat inside the body, strengthen the yin, and moisten the lung metal with the Doushen formula.

After taking first packet of the herbs, the fever dropped a little, after three packets of the herbs there was no longer any fever but he had a slight cough, so he kept taking the herbs for another two days, then all symptoms disappeared.

Doushen formula:

Gypsum (shigao) 20g

Aster tataricus (ziyuan) 15g

Sauropus rostratus (longliye) 15g

Platycodon grandiflorus (jiegeng) 10g

Allium macrostemon (xiebai) 10g

Morus alba (sangye) 10g

Spina gleditsiae (zaojiaoci) 10g

Sophora tonkinensis (shandougen) 3-10g[7]

Belamcandae rhizoma (shegan) 10g

Isatis indigotica (banlangen) 30g

Paris polyphylla (zaoxiu) 10g

Sapindus mukorossi (muhuangen) 30g

Evodia lepta (sanyaku) 30g

Lonicera japonica (jinyinhua) 15g

Forsythia suspensa (lianqiao) 15g

Oldenlandia diffusa (baihuasheshecao) 30g

Anemarrhenae asphodel ides (zhimu)10g

Arctii fructus (niubangzi) 15g

Glycyrrhiza radix (gancao) 10g

Scrophularia ningpoensis (xuanshen) 10g

Stemona japonica (baibu) 15g

Amygdalus communis (xingren) 10g

Doushen Formula in Chinese 豆参汤:

石膏20g 紫苑15g 龙利叶15g 桔梗10g 薤白10g 桑叶10g 皂角刺10g 山豆根3-10g 射干10g 板蓝根30g 蚤休10g 木患根30g 三丫苦30g 金银花15g 连翘15g 白花蛇舌草30g 知母10g 牛蒡子15g 甘草10g 玄参10g 百部15g 杏仁10g

Gypsum (shigao 石膏) isolates turbidity, and opens the lung breathing passages.

Aster tataricus (ziyuan 紫苑) opens the lung meridian, relieves hot or cold stagnated qi in the chest.

Sauropus rostratus (longliye 龙脷叶) opens the lung meridian, and dissolves mucus.

---

[7]See footnote 6.

Platycodon grandiflorus (jiegeng 桔梗) free tightness in the chest, clears abscesses in the lung metal, stops sore throat, and unblocks nasal passages.

Allium macrostemon (xiebai 薤白) opens the lung breathing passage, dissolves nodules, and detoxifies poison.

Morus alba (sangye 桑叶) disperses wind, clears heat, brightens eyesight, and induces sweat.

Spina gleditsiae (zaojiaoci 皂角刺) disperses wind, dissolves mucus, and removes poison.

Sophora tonkinensis (shandougen 山豆根) clears heat, removes dampness, detoxifies poison, eliminates swelling, stops pains, and clears sore throat.

Belamcandae rhizoma (shegan 射干) clears heat, detoxifies and draws out poison, dissolves swelling, and stops sore throat.

Isatis indigotica (banlangen 板蓝根) has a bitter taste and cool yinyang nature. It goes into liver and lung meridians. It dissolves all poisonous sores, and purges intense heat.[8]

Paris polyphylla (zaoxiu 蚤休) has a bitter taste and cold yinyang nature. It goes into the liver meridian. It disperses all kinds of poisons.

Sapindus mukorossi (muhuangen 木患根) clears heat, detoxifies poisons, dissolves mucus and dampness.

Evodia lepta (sanyaku 三丫苦) clears heat, detoxifies poison, cools blood, removes dampness, and opens meridians.

Lonicera Japonica (jinyinhua 金银花) has a sweet taste and cold yinyang nature. It goes into lung meridian. It clears heat, drains dampness, and cools blood.

Forsythia suspensa (lianqiao 连翘) has a bitter taste and cool yinyang nature. It goes into liver and gall bladder meridians. It clears heat, expels pusses, disperses nodules, and dissolves swelling.

Oldenlandia diffusa (baihuasheshecao 白花蛇舌草) clears heat, disperses stagnation, dissolves swelling, and detoxifies poison.

Anemarrhenae asphodeloides (zhimu 知母) clears lung heat, and drains dampness and turbidity.

Arctii fructus (niubangzi 牛蒡子) eliminates swelling, and detoxifies poison.

---

[8]Only wild grown Isatis indigotica has obvious such effects, farmed Isatis indigotica shows very weak effect.

Glycyrrhiza radix (gancao 甘草) detoxifies poison.

Scrophularia ningpoensis (xuanshen 玄参) has a slightly bitter taste and cool yinyang nature. It goes into the lung and kidney meridians. It clears heat, nurtures yin, calms the spirit, and repairs heat caused yin damage.

Stemona japonica (baibu 百部) moistens lung metal, and stops coughing.

Amygdalus communis (xingren 杏仁) moistens lung metal, dissolves mucus, and stops coughing.

In the formula, Gypsum (shigao), Aster tataricus (ziyuan), Sauropus rostratus (longliye), Platycodon grandiflorus (jiegeng), Allium macrostemon (xiebai) open the yinyang passages of lung metal to disperse cold. Morus alba (sangye), Spina gleditsiae (zaojiaoci) expel wind. Sophora tonkinensis (shandougen), Belamcandae rhizoma (shegan), Isatis indigotica (banlangen), Paris polyphylla (zaoxiu), Sapindus mukorossi (muhuangen), Evodia lepta (sanyaku), Lonicera japonica (jinyinhua), Forsythia suspensa (lianqiao), oldenlandia diffusa (baihuasheshecao), Anemarrhenae asphodeloides (zhimu), Arctii fructus (niubangzi), Glycyrrhiza radix (gancao) clear heat and or detoxify poisons; and are used to cease the fever and stop sore throat. Scrophularia ningpoensis (xuanshen), Stemona japonica (baibu), Amygdalus communis (xingren) are used to nurture the yin and moisten lung metal. This case and the previous case are all lung metal yin damage with external cold and wind residing in the lung metal yinyang passages. But in this case, the patient had been having fever and severe sore throat for four days, and didn't feel cold, which indicated that the trapped heat was more of the problem. So the formula used many herbs that clear body heat.

Cooking and taking the herbs:

Place a packet of the herbs in a pot, add 1250 ml of cold water, bring the herbs to boil, continue boiling for 45 minutes to reduce the liquid down to 500 ml. Pour the liquid into a big jar, discard the dregs of the decoction. Drink 250ml of the liquid each time, 4 to 6 times a day, preparing up to 3 packets of the herbs a day until the body heat drops to normal.

Treating lung metal yin deficiency with symptoms of running nose

A 39-year-old male patient came for a consultation for an itchy nose and throat. For about 10 years, every spring and autumn, the patient had suffered itchy throat and nose, constant sneezing, and runny nose. He had been on anti-histamine drugs to cope with the symptoms, but the condition has been gradually getting worse.

When there is lung metal yin damage, fluid cannot be gathered in the lung metal but pours out through the nose which causes the runny nose. Lung metal yin damage causes dry heat, and dry heat creates wind, which causes itch. Although the symptoms only occur in spring and autumn, the yin damage of lung metal has persisted. Because spring and autumn are the seasons that cold and heat are changing positions, dry and hot lung metal attracts cold and wind into the lung passages, so the symptoms become obvious.

Treatment is to expel wind, disperse cold, open nasal passages, clear heat, and moisten lung metal to nurture its yin. But as lung metal is a yin organ, while nurturing its yin, there is often a lack of yang, so the treatment is also to detoxify poison, dissolve mucus to consolidate its yang. The formula I used was Guizhi Canger.

The patient took three packets of the herbs, the blocked and running nose became better and he stopped the herbs. But two weeks later the symptoms returned. He then took another three packets of the same herbs, and the symptoms improved again. The patient took the herbs intermittently to relieve the symptoms for three years, and the frequency of the symptoms occurring were reduced and less severe. His family also said that he had stopped snoring at night.

Guizhi Canger formula:

Cinnamomum cassia (guizhi)10g
Rhizoma zingiberis (ganjiang) 10g
Nepeta cataria (jingjie)10g
Saposhnikovia divaricate (fangfeng)10g
Aster tataricus (ziyuan) 15g

Spina gleditsiae (zaojiaoci) 10g
Atractylodis macrocephalae (baizhu) 10g
Angelica dahurica (baizhi) 15g
Anthium sibiricum (cangerzi) 10g
Asarum sieboldii (xixin) 5g

Magnolia liliflora (xingyihua) 10g

Vitex trifolia (manjingzi) 15g

Paeoniae alba (baishao) 10g

Glycyrrhiza radix (gancao) 10g

Arctii fructus (niubangzi) 15g

Polistes mandarinus (lufengfang) 10g

Oldenlandia diffusa (baihuasheshecao) 30g

Stemona japonica (baibu) 15g

Astragalus membranaceus (huangqi) 10g

Schisandra chinensis (wuweizi) 10g

Guizhi Canger Formula in Chinese 桂枝苍耳汤:

桂枝10g 干姜10g 荆芥10g 防风10g 紫苑15g 皂角刺10g 白术10g 白芷15g 苍耳子10g 细辛5g 辛夷花10g 蔓荆子15g 白芍10g 甘草10g 牛蒡子15g 露蜂房10g 白花蛇舌草30g 百部15g 黄芪10g 五味子10g

Cinnamomum cassia (guizhi 桂枝) disperses cold and wind between skin and flesh, and relieves chills.

Rhizoma zingiberis (ganjiang 干姜) disperses cold, expels wind, warms the stomach, and removes dampness.

Nepeta cataria . (jingjie 荆芥) expels wind, disperses cold, relieves chills, induces sweat, and clears head wind.

Saposhnikovia divaricate (fangfeng 防风) opens meridians, disperses wind in all parts of the body.

Aster tataricus (ziyuan 紫苑) disperses cold or hot stagnated qi in the chest.

Spina gleditsiae (zaojiaoci 皂角刺) disperses wind, dissolves mucus, detoxifies poison, and primes herbs to the upper body.

Atractylodis macrocephalae (baizhu 白术) removes head wind, protects body exterior, and removes dampness and mucus.

Anthium sibiricum (cangerzi 苍耳子) expels wind, disperses cold, stops headache, and opens nasal passages.

Asarum sieboldii (xixin 细辛) expels wind, disperses cold, opens nasal passages and meridians.

Magnolia liliflora (xingyihua 辛夷花) expels wind, disperses cold, and opens nasal passages.

Vitex trifolia (manjingzi 蔓荆子) cools blood, and primes herbs to the head.

Paeoniae alba (baishao 白芍) opens blood passages, and dissolves swelling.

Glycyrrhiza (gancao 甘草) dissolves hot or cold poison.

Arctii fructus (niubangzi 牛蒡子) eliminates swelling, and detoxifies poison.

Polistes mandarinus (lufengfang 露蜂房) disperses cold or hot disordered qi, dissolves swelling, and detoxifies poison.

Oldenlandia diffusa (baihuasheshecao 白花蛇舌草) clears lung metal heat, disperses stagnation, dissolves swelling, and detoxifies poison.

Stemona japonica (baibu 百部) moistens lung metal, stops cough.

Astragalus membranaceus (huangqi 黄芪) has a sweet taste and slightly warm yinyang nature. It goes into lung, and spleen meridians. It harmonizes the yinyang order of all wuxing organs, improves body energy, protects body exterior, and excretes heat from the lung metal.

Schisandra chinensis (wuweizi 五味子) has a sour taste and warm yinyang nature. It goes into the lung meridian. It harmonizes the yinyang order of all wuxing organs, creates moistness, removes heat, and ceases wind.

Within the formula, Cinnamomum cassia (guizhi), Rhizoma zingiberis (ganjiang), Nepeta cataria (jingjie), Saposhnikovia divaricate (fangfeng), and Aster tataricus (ziyuan) free chest tightness, and relax skin to disperse cold. Spina gleditsiae (zaojiaoci), Atractylodis macrocephalae (baizhu), Angelica dahurica (baizhi), Anthium sibiricum (cangerzi), Asarum sieboldii (xixin), Magnolia liliflora (xingyihua), Vitex trifolia (manjingzi) expel wind, and open nasal passages. Paeoniae alba (baishao), Glycyrrhiza radix (gancao), Arctii fructus (niubangzi), Polistes mandarinus (lufengfang) detoxify poison, and eliminate swelling. Oldenlandia diffusa (baihuasheshecao), Stemona japonica (baibu), Astragalus membranaceus (huangqi), Schisandra chinensis (wuweizi) clear lung metal heat, and moisten lung metal.

Treating lung metal yin damage with symptoms of damp poison

A 36-year-old man was travelling in the hot summer and felt pain in his eye. The next day he arrived home with a burning hot body, severe persistent headache, and nausea. He went for biomedical help first and was given antibiotics and steroid drip treatments in a hospital. After 7 days, he had no sign of improvement; so he discharged himself out of the hospital, and sought herbal treatment. At the first consultation, the patient was suffering a high fever. His pulse was rapid. He had a severe headache, his throat was painful, he felt nauseated, was unable to eat, and had difficulty to stand straight.

Yin damage of lung metal attracts external damp poison residing in its yinyang passage. The damp poison ferments and creates heat which further damages the yin of lung metal and causes extreme heat in the lung metal, so there are symptoms such as persistent burning hot body, sore throat, and rapid pulse. The poison heat creates wind, poison heat is pushed by wind up to the head, so there are severe headaches. Poison heat above prevents fresh body qi from rising, so the patient had difficulty in standing. Damp poison travelling upwards causes dry retch.

The treatment was focused on clearing heat, detoxifying poison, dissolving dampness, and expelling wind. I used the Qinghao Dougen formula.

After drinking one packet of the herbal decoction, the patient's fever reduced slightly, and his headache was less severe. After two days of taking the herbs, all the symptoms were further improved. After three days his body temperature had dropped to normal; the headaches and sore throat were gone, and his appetite and strength gradually returning to normal.

Qinghao Dougen formula:

Sophora tonkinensis (shandougen) 30g[9]

Paris polyphylla (zaoxiu) 30g

Belamcandae rhizoma (shegan) 30g

Isatis indigotica (banlangen) 90g

Glycyrrhiza radix (gancao) 30g

Rhizoma ligustici (gaoben) 30g

Puerariae lobatae (gegen) 45g

Notopterygium incisum (qianghuo) 15g

Uncaria rhynchophylla (gouteng) 45g

Ephedra sinica (mahuang) 30g

Gypsum (shigao) 60g

Anemarrhenae asphodeloides (zhimu) 30g

Artemisia apiacea (qinghao) 30g

Elsholtzia ciliate (xiangru) 30g

---

[9]In the first instance, reduce the dosage to 3g if the patient has had no prior use of this herb. See footnote 4.

Qinghuo Dougen Formula in Chinese 青蒿豆根汤:

山豆根30g 蚤休30g 射干30g 板蓝根90g 甘草30g 藁本30g 葛根45g 羌活15g 钩藤45g 麻黄30g 石膏60g 知母30g 青蒿30g 香薷30g

Sophora tonkinensis (shandougen 山豆根) clears heat, removes dampness, detoxifies poison, dissolves swelling, stops pain, and soothes sore throat.

Paris polyphylla (zaoxiu 蚤休) clears heat, disperses all poisons.

Belamcandae Rhizoma (shegan 射干) clears heat, draws out poison, eliminates swelling, and stops sore throat.

Isatis indigotica (banlangen 板蓝根) purges intense heat, and detoxifies poison.

Glycyrrhiza (gancao 甘草) detoxifies poisons.

Rhizoma Ligustici (gaoben 藁本) expels pussy mucus, and stops headache.

Puerariae Lobatae (gegen 葛根) disperses wind and dampness between flesh and skin to relax muscle tension, induces sweat, and stops headache.

Notopterygium incisum (qianghuo 羌活) Expels wind, opens meridians, stops joint pains and headache.

Uncaria rhynchophylla (gouteng 钩藤) expels wind, opens meridians, and stops headache.

Ephedra sinica (mahuang 麻黄) expels colds or heat stagnation between skin and flesh to relax muscle, and induces sweat.

Gypsum (shigao 石膏) opens lung meridian, clears heat, isolates and removes dampness and turbid.

Anemarrhenae asphodeloides (zhimu 知母) clears lung metal heat, and removes dampness and turbid.

Artemisia apiacea (qinghao 青蒿) clears heat, removes dampness, and dissolves mucus.

Elsholtzia ciliate (xiangru 香薷) relaxes skin; removes dampness and disordered qi, and clears fresh water passages.

In the formula, Sophora tonkinensis (shandougen), Paris polyphylla (zaoxiu), Belamcandae rhizoma (shegan), Isatis indigotica (banlangen), and Glycyrrhiza (gancao) are used to clear heat, detoxify poison, and stop sore throat. Rhizoma ligustici (gaoben), Puerariae lobatae (gegen), Notopterygium incisum (qianghuo), Uncaria rhynchophylla (gouteng) are used to prime all herbs upward, to expel wind, and stop headache. Ephedra sinica (mahuang) relaxes skin and flesh, open the meridians to chase out external poison. Gypsum (shigao), Anemarrhenae asphodelides (zhimu) Artemisia apiacea (qinghao), and Elsholtzia ciliate (xiangru) are used to clear heat, and dissolve dampness.

Cooking and drinking:

Place one packet of the herbs into a pot (preferably a clay pot), add 2 litres of cold water, and bring to boil; keep boiling for 40 minutes to reduce liquid down to 1.5 litres. Drink 250ml of the liquid every 4 hours.

Treating lung metal yin and yang damage with symptoms of night coughing

A 37-year-old woman came for a consultation with a cough of two months without signs of improvement. The patient had an itchy throat which gave her coughing fits. She felt there was mucus in her throat but could not bring it out. She coughed more at night, which badly disturbed her sleep.

Lung metal yin damage causes the failure to gather moisture, so the lung metal became dry and hot. Dry heat creates wind, and wind irritating the throat causes coughing fits. During the night, yin qi rises, but the lung metal is dry and hot, the cold yin qi from heaven and earth travels fast into the lung metal breathing passages creating even stronger wind, so at night the cough becomes worse. The yang damage of lung metal causes turbidity to retain in the lung metal and creates mucus. But the dry heat causes the mucus to harden so the mucus could not be expectorated. Treatment is to clear heat, dissolve mucus, cease wind, and moisten lung metal with the Qingdai Haige formula.

After taking three packets of the herbs, the patient's itchy throat was improved and the frequency of coughing had reduced. She coughed up more mucus and they were pussy. The patient was worried that her condition had become worse. The fact is that because of moistening the lung metal, the dry heat had reduced; and by cleansing lung metal, the mucus was isolated, so there was a lot of expectorating.

Therefore, there was no need to change the formula but to continue with the same formula for another three days. After taking six packets of the herbs in total, she had no more itchy throat. Occasionally she would cough just to get the mucus out, and the colour of the mucus had become clear. She took three more packets of the herbs and by the end all the symptoms had disappeared.

Qingdai Haige formula:

Angelica dahurica (baizhi) 15g

Anthium sibiricum (cangerzi) 15g

Magnolia liliflora (xingyihua) 10g

Asarum sieboldii (xixin) 5g

Spina gleditsiae (zaojiaoci) 10g

Trichosanthes kirilowii (gualouren) 15g

Stemona japonica (baibu) 15g

Fritillaria cirrhosa (chuanbeimu) 15g

Amygdalus communis (xingren) 10g

Indigo naturalis (qingdai) 10g

Mactra veneriformis (haigefen) 10g

Platycodon grandiflorus (jiegeng) 10g

Allium macrostemon (xiebai) 10g

Arctii fructus (niubangzi) 15g

Aster tataricus (ziyuan) 15g

Oldenlandia diffusa (baihuasheshecao) 30g

Sauropus rostratus (longliye) 15g

Glycyrrhiza radix (gancao) 10g

Qingdai Haige formula in Chinese:青黛海蛤汤:

白芷15g 苍耳子15g 辛夷花10g 细辛5g 皂角刺10g 瓜蒌仁15g 百部15g 川贝母15g 杏仁10g 青黛10g 海蛤粉10g 桔梗10g 薤白10g 牛蒡子15g 紫苑15g 白花蛇舌草30g 龙利叶15g 甘草10g

Angelica dahurica (baizhi 白芷) disperses wind, dissolves mucus, disperses nodules, and opens the nasal passages.
Anthium sibiricum (cangerzi 苍耳子) disperses wind, dissolves mucus, and opens the nasal passages.
Magnolia liliflora (xingyihua 辛夷花) disperses wind, dissolves mucus, and opens the nasal passages.
Asarum sieboldii (xixin 细辛) disperses wind, dissolves mucus, and opens the meridians and nasal passages.
Spina gleditsiae (zaojiaoci 皂角刺) disperses wind, and dissolves

227

mucus.

Trichosanthes kirilowii (gualouren 瓜蒌仁) moistens lung metal, dissolves mucus, and relieves oppression.

Stemona japonica (baibu 百部) moistens lung metal, and stops coughing.

Fritillaria cirrhosa (chuanbeimu 川贝母) moistens lung metal; dissolves mucus, stops coughing, and disperses qi stagnation in the chest.

Amygdalus communis (xingren 杏仁) moistens lung metal, dissolves mucus, and stops coughing.

Indigo naturalis (qingdai 青黛) has a salty taste and cold yinyang nature. It goes into lung and liver meridians. It nurtures yin, removes heat, detoxifies poison, and dissolves mucus.

Mactra veneriformis (haigefen 海蛤粉) has a salty taste and mild yinyang nature. It goes into lung meridian. It nurtures yin, moistens lung metal, dissolves mucus, and eliminates dampness.

Platycodon grandiflorus (jiegeng 桔梗) dissolves pussy mucus in the lung metal, stops sore throat, opens nasal passages, and frees chest congestion.

Allium macrostemon (xiebai 薤白) dissolves mucus, disperses nodules, and detoxifies poison.

Arctii fructus (niubangzi 牛蒡子) dissolves mucus, eliminates swelling, and detoxifies poison.

Aster tataricus (ziyuan 紫苑) dissolves mucus, opens lung meridian, and disperses hot or cold qi stagnation in the chest.

Oldenlandia diffusa (baihuasheshecao 白花蛇舌草) clears heat, disperses stagnations, dissolves pussy mucus, and detoxifies poison.

Sauropus rostratus (longliye 龙脷叶) opens the lung meridian, and dissolves hard mucus.

Glycyrrhiza radix (gancao 甘草) detoxifies poisons in all wuxing organs.

In the formula, all herbs have the function of clearing mucus and dampness in lung metal; whereas Angelica dahurica (baizhi), Anthium sibiricum (cangerzi), Magnolia liliflora (xingyihua), Asarum sieboldii (xixin), Spina gleditsiae (zaojiaoci) are used to also disperse wind, and open qi passages. Trichosanthes kirilowii (gualouren), Stemona japonica (baibu), Fritillaria cirrhosa (chuanbeimu), Amygdalus communis (xingren), Indigo naturalis (Qingdai), Mactra veneriformis (haigefeng) are used to nurture the yin and moisten lung metal. Platycodon grandiflorus (jiegeng), Allium macrostemon (xiebai), Arctii Fructus (niubangzi), Aster tataricus (ziyuan), oldenlandia diffusa (baihuasheshecao), Sauropus rostratus (longliye), Glycyrrhiza (gancao) are used to detoxify poison and cleanse lung metal.

Treating lung metal yin and yang deficiency with symptoms of chronic cough

A 37-year-old female patient had had a cough for six months. Her throat was dry and itchy. Cold air often triggered the itch and cough. Once the cough started, it could last up to 10 minutes without stop. She was short of breath, and had tightness of chest, but not much mucus came out.

Yin damage of lung metal fails to gather moisture which makes it dry and hot, so her throat was dry. Dry heat creates wind, so there is an itchy throat. External cold air adds to internal wind, triggering the itchy throat and cough. The yin deficiency of lung metal fails to gather qi, so there is shortness of breath. On the other hand, the yang damage of lung metal causes turbid and fresh qi to mix, so mucus is created and blocks the lung metal breathing passage, and there is tightness of chest. Dry heat makes the mucus harden so it is difficult to spit out. Prolonged coughing exhausted both the yin and yang qi of lung metal, so the coughing fits were difficult to stop.

The treatment was to clear heat, dissolve mucus, cease wind, and moisten the dryness. As the cough had been persistent, the yin and yang qi of lung metal was depleted and needed replenishing, so the treatment also included methods for strengthening the spleen soil to build up lung metal with the formula Shenling Qingge.

The patient took three packets of the herbs and the itchy throat was improved, and the frequency of coughing fits became less. She took another seven days of the herbs and the cough stopped.

Shenling Qingge formula:

Angelica dahurica (baizhi) 15g

Anthium sibiricum (cangerzi) 15g

Magnolia liliflora (xingyihua) 10g

Asarum sieboldii (xixin) 5g

Spina gleditsiae (zaojiaoci) 10g
Trichosanthes kirilowii (gualouren) 15g
Stemona japonica (baibu) 15g
Fritillaria cirrhosa (chuanbeimu) 15g
Amygdalus communis (xingren) 10g
Indigo naturalis (qingdai) 10g
Mactra veneriformis (haigefen) 10g
Platycodon grandiflorus (jiegeng) 10g

Allium macrostemon (xiebai) 10g
Arctii fructus (niubangzi) 15g
Aster tataricus (ziyuan) 15g
Oldenlandia diffusa (baihuasheshecao) 30g
Sauropus rostratus (longliye) 15g
Glycyrrhiza (gancao) 10g
Glehnia littoralis (beishashen) 10g
Poria cocos (fuling) 10g
Atractylodis macrocephalae (baizhu) 10g

Shenling Qingge Formula in Chinese 参苓青蛤汤:

白芷15g 苍耳子15g 辛夷花10g 细辛5g 皂角刺10g 瓜蒌仁15g 百部15g 川贝母15g 杏仁10g 青黛10g 海蛤粉10g 桔梗10g 薤白10g 牛蒡子15g 紫苑15g 白花蛇舌草30g 龙利叶15g 甘草10g 北沙参10g 茯苓10g 白术10g

The Shenling Qingge formula is the Qingdai Haige formula with the addition of Glehnia littoralis (beishashen), Poria cocos (fuling), and Atractylodis macrocephalae (baizhu).

Glehnia littoralis (beishashen 北沙参) has a mild taste, and cold yinyang nature. It goes into spleen and lung meridians. It moistens lung metal, strengthens the yinyang order of spleen soil, and stops coughing.
Poria Cocos (fuling 茯苓) frees water passages, and strengthens the yinyang order of spleen soil.
Atractylodis Macrocephalae (baizhu 白术) strengthens the yinyang order of spleen soil, and removes dampness and mucus.

The Shenling Qingge formula incorporates the Qingdai Haige formula to cease wind, moisten dryness, remove mucus, and clear heat. According to the wuxing theory of soil creates metal, I added Glehnia littoralis (beishashen), Poria cocos (fuling) and Atractylodis macrocephalae (baizhu), three spleen soil strengthening herbs to enhance the regeneration of the damaged lung metal.

Treating lung metal yin and yang deficiency with symptoms of tight chest and shortness of breath

A 41-year-old female patient had severe sinus problems since she was 5 years old. For more than 10 years, she had pussy mucus constantly running in her nose and spat thick mucus. When she was around 15 or 16 years old, the pussy mucus gradually disappeared and her nose was clear, but she always felt there was mucus in her throat but nothing would come out. At the first consultation, she was suffering from a tight chest and had been affected by shortness of breath for about six months and the condition was getting worse.

When there is lung metal yang damage, turbidity and freshness fail to be separated, mucus and dampness block the lung metal qi passages, so the patient had pussy mucus running in her nose. Lung metal fails to gather fluid because of yin damage, so the mucus became dry and hardened, which made room to breathe, so the nose was seemingly cleared, but the mucus could be felt in the throat. The persistent yang damage of lung metal allows mucus to build up, and qi can be gathered but is not able to move, so there is tightness of the chest and difficulty breathing. Treatment is to cleanse lung metal, dissolve mucus, and moisten the dry lung with the Ludai formula.

The patient took 7 packets of the herbs and felt easier to breathe, although she still felt mucus stuck in the throat, but as it did not affect her life too much so she didn't go further with the treatment. 5 years later, she came back for shortness of breath again. This time, her chest was so tight that she could not walk up a small hill; running a short distance would make her chest painful, and to lie down in bed at night would cut off her breath. Apart from taking the Ludai formula I also asked the patient to perform a regular daily nasal rinse.

She took 7 packets of the herbs and washed her nasal passages as instructed, she felt the chest tightness was getting less and stopped taking herbs but continued to wash the nose. In the beginning, washing her nose was very painful like a knife stabbing through her head, but after the wash she felt relief from the tight chest, so she persisted. Three months later, her tight chest was almost gone, but her nose was blocked with a lot of pussy mucus running down like her childhood condition. Sometimes, her face was swollen and painful, which is the result of the congealed and hardened mucus breaking down. So the treatment did not change. She took another 7 packets of the herbs and the symptoms got better again. She then stopped the herbs but continued the nasal rinse. Sometimes, when the discharge from the nose became pussy, she would take a few packets of the herbs again. As such, she repeated the process for a year; her chest tightness was completely gone but she still often suffered from thick discharge from the nose. Another five years later, the patient informed me that she still washed her nose regularly, and that the nose had become clear, her breathing normal, and she hardly ever got colds again.

Ludai formula:

Gypsum (shigao) 20g
Angelica dahurica (baizhi) 15g
Anthium sibiricum (cangerzi) 15g
Magnolia liliflora (xingyihua) 10g
Asarum sieboldii (xixin) 10g
Rhizoma ligustici (gaoben) 5g
Vitex trifolia (manjingzi) 10g
Platycodon grandiflorus (jiegeng) 10g
Allium macrostemon (xiebai) 10g
Spina gleditsiae (zaojiaoci) 15g
Arctii fructus (niubangzi) 15g
Aster tataricus (ziyuan) 15g
Oldenlandia diffusa (baihuasheshecao) 30g
Duchesnea indica (shemei) 30g

Trichosanthes kirilowii (seeds of) (gualouren) 15g
Trichosanthes kirilowii (skin of) (gualoupi) 15g
Sauropus rostratus (longliye) 15g
Stemona japonica (baibu) 15g
Fritillaria cirrhosa (chuanbeimu) 15g
Fritillaria thunbergii (zhebeimu) 10g
Glycyrrhiza radix (gancao) 10g
Amygdalus communis (xingren) 10g
Indigo naturalis qingdai) 10g
Mactra veneriformis (haigefen) 10g
Polistes mandarinus (lufengfang) 10g

Ludai formula in Chinese: 露黛汤:

石膏20g 白芷15g 苍耳子15g 辛夷花10g 细辛10g 藁本5g 蔓荆子10桔梗10薤白10g 皂角刺15g 牛蒡子15g 紫苑15g 白花蛇舌草30g 蛇莓30g

瓜蒌仁15g 瓜蒌皮15g 龙脷叶15g 百部15川贝母15g 浙贝母10g 甘草10g 杏仁10g 青黛10g 海蛤粉10g 露蜂房10g

The Ludai formula is the Qingdai Haige formula with the addition of Gypsum (shigao), Rhizoma ligustici (gaoben), Vitex trifolia (manjingzi), Duchesnea indica (shemei), (skin of) Trichosanthes kirilowii (gualoupi), Fritillaria thunbergii (zhebeimu), and Polistes mandarinus (lufengfang).

Gypsum (shigao 石膏) isolates turbidity, removes dampness, and clears the lung breathing passages.

Rhizoma ligustici (gaoben 篙本) removes mucus, expels puss, and stops headache.

Vitex trifolia (manjingzi 蔓荆子) cools blood, primes herbs to the head, and stops headache.

Duchesnea indica (shemei 蛇莓) has a bitter taste and cold yinyang nature. It goes into the lung and liver meridians. It clears heat, dissolves mucus, and removes dampness and mucus in the blood.

Trichosanthes kirilowii (skin) (gualoupi 瓜蒌皮) has a sweet taste and cold yinyang nature. It goes into the lung and stomach meridians. It clears heat, dissolves mucus, and expels stagnated qi in the chest.

Fritillaria thunbergii (zhebeimu 浙贝母) has a bitter taste and cold yinyang nature. It goes into the liver, lung, and kidney meridians. It detoxifies poison, clears mucus, and frees qi flow in lung metal.

Polistes mandarinus (lufengfang 露蜂房) has a sweet taste and mild yinyang nature. It goes into the lung meridian. It disperses cold or hot qi stagnation, dissolves swelling, and detoxifies poison.

The Qingdai Haige formula cleanses and moistens lung metal, dissolves mucus, and opens nasal passages. Adding Gypsum (shigao), Duchesnea indica (shemei), (husk of) Trichosanthes kirilowii (gualoupi), Fritillaria thunbergii (zhebeimu), and Polistes mandarinus (lufengfang) strengthen the removing of dampness, and dissolving mucus effects, as well as clearing heat in the lung metal. Adding Rhizoma ligustici (gaoben), Vitex trifolia (manjingzi) into the Qingdai Haige formula is to enhance the dissolving mucus, expelling puss effect, and also to prime herbs to the head.

Method for nasal rinse:

Use a nasal wash pot or nasal rinse bottle. Alternatively, use a small tea pot without the lid. Place 100 ml of filtered boiled warm water into the pot, add 10 ml of fully saturated Alum water. Tilt the head forward and sideways; pour the Alum solution and water slowly into one nostril and the liquid will come out of the other nostril, then repeat the procedure with the other nostril. After both sides have been washed, blow the nose gently and allow the water and mucus to come out and avoid pushing water back inside the nose. The wash should be done at least once a day or as often as needed.

Potassium Alum (mingfan 明矾) has a sour taste and cold yinyang nature. It goes into lung and liver meridians. It isolates turbidity, dries dampness, dissolves mucus, removes nasal swellings, and stops toothache.

Treating lung metal yang damage with symptoms of loud snoring

A 56-year-old male patient came for a consultation as he had severe snoring that disturbed the sleep of his family members. He was tired, had restless sleep, and often woke up during the night. The patient also often suffered from palpitations. For every 5 or 6 beats of the pulse he had one missing beat.

The yang damage of lung metal becomes unable to isolate turbidity, and allows mucus and dampness to grow and accumulate, then blocks the nasal passages. At night, mucus in the throat is unable to be coughed out, air and mucus struggle for space, which causes the loud snoring. When the mucus stops the breathing, the spirit is disturbed and causes waking and restless sleep. At night when the spirit is awake, the yang meridians are open and let the yin qi of the heaven and earth get through the yang meridians and wreak havoc on the yang qi, so he was tired. Mucus blocking the qi passages causes the spirit to be unsettled in the body, so the pulse was missing. Treatment is to cleanse lung metal, dissolve mucus with the

234

Cangzhi formula, and perform a regular nasal rinse.

The patient took 7 packets of the herbs and did the nasal rinse. He soon lost the palpitations, slept well and his pulse became regular. He stopped taking the herbs internally but kept washing the nose for another month then came back for a consultation. He was no longer feeling palpitated, he slept well, and felt energetic, and his family reported that he now only snored lightly and occasionally.

For Cangzhi formula and explanation see the section "Treating lung metal yin damage with external wind and cold."

Treating lung metal yang deficiency with symptoms of pussy discharge from the ear

A 9-year-old female patient came for a consultation because of a blocked nose and pussy discharge which had been coming out of her left ear and nostrils for a month.

When there is yang damage the lung metal fails to isolate turbidity, which allows the creation and accumulation of dampness and mucus in the lung metal yinyang passage, so there is nasal congestion and pussy discharge. The ear is an opening of the kidney water. Damp poison of the lung metal extends to the kidney water gateways, so there is a pussy discharge out of her ear. The treatment is to cleanse lung metal, detoxify poison, dissolve mucus with the Ludai formula (see above) and also apply eucalyptus oil on the damaged ear, as well as nasal washing.

The patient came back for another consultation three days later, and said after one drop of the Eucalyptus oil into the ear, her ear discharge stopped and she didn't need to use the Eucalyptus oil further. With the nose wash and the herbs, her nose was clearer and the discharges were thinner and less. She took three more days of the herbs plus the nose wash, and all symptoms disappeared.

Eucalyptus oil (anshuyou 桉树油) has a pungent taste and dry yinyang nature. It goes into lung and liver meridians. It clears heat, dissolves mucus, opens meridian, and detoxifies poison.

Method of applying eucalyptus oil:

Place a drop of organic pure eucalyptus oil into the affected ear once a day until recovery. Nasal rinse in the same way as the above case.

Treating lung metal yang deficiency with symptoms of ringing ears

A 44-year-old female patient came because of ringing in her ears. The sound was like ocean waves, day and night, never ending, and her hearing had declined significantly. When she was younger she had once worked in a noisy factory. She thought it might have been the result of the damage from her early noisy working environment, but it was almost 20 years since she left the job and she had never had any hearing problems until recently. Although the patient wasn't aware of any sinus problem, her nasal passages were obviously red and swollen, and the openings were paper thin.

The nose is the gateway of lung metal to heaven and earth, the yang damage of lung metal allows mucus to grow and to block the yinyang passages of lung metal and to congest the nasal chamber. Mucus fights against blood and qi for space making loud sounds next to the ear passage, so there is ringing in the ears. The sounds of internal blood and qi disturb her hearing of external sounds, so the hearing ability was diminished.

Washing the nasal passages was the simplest and most effective way of treating this condition.

The patient performed a nasal rinse twice a day, and after one month the ear ringing had become brief and only occasional. After two months of performing the nasal rinse she came back for a consultation and reported that the ringing ears had stopped, the swollen and red nostrils had reduced and the passage had become freer. Finally, her hearing had significantly improved as well.

Spirit & Body

The spirit is the motive power of human life. A person's activities are directed by the spirit. The spirit is yang, its existence is presented through various zhi, which may be described as the qualities of the spirit. The body is the carrier of the spirit, it is the material base of life, so it is yin. Without the domination of the spirit, the body is unanimated. Without the carrier of the body, the spirit has no material means of manifesting its zhi or will. It is the joining of the body and the spirit that life comes into existence and is sustained. As the body needs to breathe, so too in a sense does the spirit need to breathe. Because the spirit breathes with heaven and earth, it connects the body with heaven and earth and so enables the body's yinyang transformation to respond to heaven and earth. Also because the spirit breathes with heaven and earth, it connects with other spirits, so people have feelings for other people and everything surrounding them.

The zhi (wills) of the spirit are immaterial, so they are yang. Within yang there is yin, so the zhi of the spirit have their yin and yang aspects. The interaction of the yin and yang of the spirit's zhi also inevitably fall into a wood, fire, soil, metal, and water wuxing cycle which forms a wuxing zhi of the spirit. The wood zhi of the spirit is the striving zhi, the fire zhi of the spirit is the aspiring zhi, the soil zhi of the spirit is the reasoning zhi, the metal zhi of the spirit is the lofty zhi. The spirit interacts with the wuxing organs to exercise these zhi, and enables a person to have and express emotions.

In each of the wood, fire, soil, metal, and water wuxing elements, there is yin and yang; in each of the liver, heart, spleen, lung, and kidney wuxing organs there exists yin and yang natures. Each of the striving, aspiring, reasoning, lofty, and enduring zhi of the spirit also have their yin and yang characteristics.

The striving zhi 斗志 dòuzhì

The striving zhi of the spirit is its readiness to struggle—to be a competitive, resilient, and fighting spirit. Whereas the yang of wood is erect, and the yin of wood is supple, which makes wood straight and flexible, similarly the yang of the striving zhi is firm, while the yin of the striving zhi is flexible, which makes the striving zhi to be firm but not brittle. So the striving zhi is classified in wuxing as wood. In the human body, the liver wood yang is upright, the yin is supple, so the body is sturdy and adaptable. Things of one kind come together. As the striving zhi of the spirit has the same yinyang nature of liver wood, so spirit interacts with liver wood to exercise its striving zhi, and makes a person firm but gentle.

The aspiring zhi 立志 lìzhì

The aspiring zhi of the spirit is its desire—to achieve, and be realistic. The yang of fire rises, the yin of fire is grounding, so fire rises but does not float. The yang of the aspiring zhi is ardent, and the yin of the aspiring zhi is poised, so the aspiring zhi of the spirit is enthusiastic but careful, which classifies the aspiring zhi of the spirit in wuxing as fire. In the human body, the heart fire yang qi is active, the yin qi is descending, so a person can be active and quiet. As the heart fire and the aspiring zhi share the same yinyang nature, which allow the spirit to interact with heart fire to exercise its aspiring zhi, so a person has desire but also reserve.

The reasoning zhi 理志 lǐzhì

The reasoning zhi of the spirit is its thinking—to be inquisitive, and logical. The yin of soil is adhesive, the yang of soil is loose, so soil bears and permits the transit of other things. The yin of the reasoning zhi of the spirit is lingering, the yang of the reasoning zhi is sorting, so the reasoning zhi of the spirit receives information and sorts the information into order. This yinyang nature of the reasoning zhi is then classified in wuxing as soil. In the human body, the yin of the spleen soil is sticky, and the yang of the spleen soil is loose, so people can receive food and transform food. As the reasoning zhi of the spirit and spleen soil organ share the same yinyang nature, so the spirit is able to exercise its reasoning zhi through spleen soil, and a person can think before acting.

The lofty zhi 壮志 zhuàngzhì

The lofty zhi of the spirit is its loyalty—to be close, and respected. The yin of metal gathers, the yang of metal cleanses, so the metal is solid and pure. The yin of the lofty zhi of the spirit gathers spirits together, the yang of the lofty zhi filters the gathered spirits and keeps ones alike together, so the lofty zhi of the spirit is inclusive and differentiating. This nature of the lofty zhi is then classified as metal in wuxing. In the human body, the yin of lung metal gathers qi and moisture, the yang of lung metal separates turbidity from freshness, so the body is brimming and fresh. As the lung metal and lofty zhi of the spirit share the same yinyang nature, so the spirit interacts with lung metal to exercise its lofty zhi, which makes a person friendly but dignified.

The enduring zhi 励志 lìzhì

The enduring zhi of the spirit is its faithfulness—to commit, be reliable, and to last. The yin of water is cold and coagulating, the yang of water is moving, so water moves without surging. The yin of the enduring zhi is calm, the yang is excited, so the enduring zhi is prompt and persistent, which gives the enduring zhi the character of water in wuxing. In the human body, the yin of kidney water is cold and stagnant, the yang of kidney water is arousing, so the kidney water provides serenity and strength for bodily action. As the kidney water shares the same yinyang nature as the enduring zhi, the two interact together to realize the enduring zhi of the spirit, which makes a person confident, decisive and calm.

The creative wuxing cycle of the spirit zhi

As wood, fire, soil, metal, and water have a creative cycle, the striving, aspiring, reasoning, lofty, and enduring zhi also have a creative cycle. The striving zhi of the spirit, like wood, has an emulative nature, and is a yang dominant zhi, when the yang of the striving zhi reaches its highest, it raises its desires and becomes the aspiring zhi. The aspiring zhi, like fire, is eager, so it is a yang dominated zhi, when the yang is exhausted, the thoughts are received and the aspiring zhi becomes the reasoning zhi. The reasoning zhi, like soil, bears all thoughts, so it is a yin dominant zhi, it consolidates thoughts and becomes the lofty zhi. The lofty zhi, like metal, is loyal and firm, so it is a yin dominant zhi, when firmness reaches its furtherest extent, it is calm, and turns into the enduring zhi. The enduring zhi, like water, has a nature of continuing, it is an extreme yin zhi, the extreme yin of the enduring zhi attracts yang qi, and when the yang qi of the enduring zhi becomes high, it creates the striving zhi.

The control cycle of the spirit zhi

As wood, fire, soil, metal, and water have a controlling wuxing cycle, the striving, aspiring, reasoning, lofty, and enduring zhi also have a controlling cycle. The striving zhi of the spirit controls the reasoning zhi, so the spirit concentrates. The reasoning zhi of the spirit controls the enduring zhi, so the spirit is not conceited. The enduring zhi controls the aspiring zhi so the spirit is serene. The aspiring zhi controls the lofty zhi, so the spirit is not isolated. The lofty zhi controls the striving zhi so the spirit is unyielding. Thus the zhi of the spirit forms a never ending wuxing cycle.

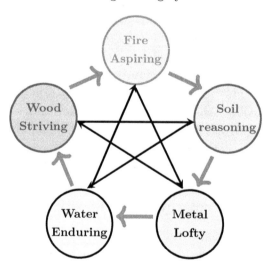

Wuxing Spirit diagram

Causes of spirit damage

In everyday life, an individual may encounter all kinds of problems and things that go against a person's spirit and subsequently threaten the overall well-being of the individual. However, a person's spirit has its resilience, especially when it derives support from other individuals. Nevertheless, if the challenge to a person's spirit exceeds the capacity of the spirit during that time, an individual's spirit is more likely to be hurt.

In the previous chapters, the spirit damaging cases were caused by the body's yinyang disorders that fail to carry through the various zhi of the spirit. In this chapter I discuss spirit damage that causes bodily and spirit zhi disorders.

The symptoms

When the spirit is damaged it will show emotionally, as well as through physical symptoms. When the spirit is damaged, it will lose its intimacy with the body and will then fail to lead the yinyang qi of heaven and earth through the body and cause a yinyang disorder of the body. When the body has a yinyang disorder, it will also show on the pulse, the tongue, and skin.

Striving zhi symptoms

The yang qi of the striving zhi of the spirit makes a person brave, and the yin qi makes a person supple. When the yang qi of the striving zhi is damaged, the courage of the spirit is unable to expand; emotionally it causes a person to suffer symptoms such as timidity. When the spirit qi is inextensible, the yang qi of heaven and earth will not get through to liver wood, and this will cause liver wood yang damage. In such a case, blood flow will be congested, and a person suffers bodily symptoms such as boils, ulcers, or poisonous swellings. When the yin qi of the striving zhi is damaged, the spirit qi loses its suppleness, and the individual suffers an emotional symptom such as anger. Anger will damage liver wood yin qi and cause a person to suffer from symptoms such as body tightness and aches.

Aspiring zhi symptoms

The yang qi of the aspiring zhi makes a person enthusiastic, and the yin qi makes a person grounded and cautious. But when the yang qi of the aspiring zhi is damaged, the spirit hesitates to connect with the outside world and makes a person lose interest in life, and emotionally there will be a symptom such as disheartenment. When the spirit is disconnected with the outside, the yang qi of the heart fire fails to be replenished by the yang qi of heaven and earth, then the heart fire yang qi will be damaged, which will have physical symptoms such as heaviness and indolence. When the yin qi of the aspiring zhi of the spirit is damaged, the spirit will lose its grounding, which will show emotional symptoms such as panic. When the spirit is panicky, it will not settle in the heart fire, so a person will have physical symptoms such as restlessness day and night.

Reasoning zhi symptoms

The yang qi of the reasoning zhi makes a person accessible to reason, and the yin qi enables a person to receive thoughts. When the yang qi of the reasoning zhi of the spirit is damaged, the spirit fails to arrange thoughts, emotionally it causes people to suffer from symptoms such as being overly suspicious. When the spirit is trapped in thoughts, it fails to lead the yang qi of heaven and earth into the spleen soil, which causes spleen soil yang deficiency and loss of its permeability. This congests the body's qi passages, which leads to bodily sufferings such as bloated stomach, and digestion disorders. When the yin qi of the reasoning zhi of the spirit is damaged, emotionally a person becomes bored. For example, if a person spends long hours each day doing a simple repetitive task his or her reasoning zhi yin qi will be damaged through lack of exercise, and the spirit will exhibit listlessness. When the yin qi of the reasoning zhi is damaged, it fails to lead the yin qi of heaven and earth though spleen soil, and bodily a person may suffer a wide range of symptoms depending on which other wuxing organs are affected.

Lofty zhi symptoms

The yang qi of the lofty zhi of a spirit makes a person dignified, and the yin qi makes a person affable. When the yang qi of the lofty zhi is damaged, the spirit qi becomes unclear; emotionally it causes people to suffer from symptoms such as sadness. When the yang qi of the lofty zhi is damaged it fails to lead the yang qi of heaven and earth to the lung metal, then the yang qi of lung metal will be deficient, and turbidity and freshness won't be separated, which causes a person physically to suffer from symptoms such as tight chest, and mucus in the breathing passages. When the yin qi of the lofty zhi is damaged, the spirit qi becomes scattered, emotionally a person suffers symptoms such as loneliness. When the spirit qi is scattered, lung metal qi is also scattered, which causes a person physically to suffer from symptoms such as shortness of breath, and an appearance of being downcast.

Enduring zhi symptoms

The yang qi of the enduring zhi makes a person excited, and the yin qi makes a person calm. When the yang qi of the enduring zhi of the spirit is damaged, the spirit qi stagnates, and causes a person to suffer from fear related symptoms. When the spirit qi stagnates, it fails to lead the yang qi of heaven and earth into kidney water, then the kidney water heat is lost, and a person suffers physical symptoms such as weakness. When the yin qi of the enduring zhi is damaged, the spirit qi loses its calmness and causes a person emotional irritability. When the spirit qi is restless, it exhausts kidney water yin qi, and causes a person to suffer symptoms such as frequent urine, heat in the urine, and dry mouth.

Principles for treating spirit disorders

Spirit disorders that cause emotional and physical symptoms generally recover after the cause of the spirit damage has been removed. Nevertheless, in some cases, after the cause of the spirit damage has been removed, the spirit continues its estrangement from the body and prolongs emotional and bodily suffering. In such situations, strengthening the body's yinyang cooperation will provide a stable material foundation for the spirit to exercise its zhi, which will encourage the recovery of the damaged spirit and promote the restoration of the intimacy of the spirit and body. This is the major concern of this chapter.

After removing the external causes of spirit damage, the principles for treating spirit and body disharmony is the same as treating wuxing organ yinyang disorders.

The principle for treating yang damage of the striving zhi is to invigorate blood, detoxify poison, remove dampness, and restore the yang qi of liver wood. The principle for treating yin damage of the striving zhi is to clear liver wood heat, and soften liver wood.

The principle for treating the yang damage of the aspiring zhi is to strengthen the yang heat of heart fire, and warm kidney water. The principle for treating yin damage of the aspiring zhi is to warm kidney water and raise water to the heart fire, and ground heart fire yang heat into kidney water.

The principle for treating yang damage of the reasoning zhi of the spirit is to loosen spleen soil. Treating the yin damage of the reasoning zhi is to enhance the adhesiveness of spleen soil.

The principle for treating yang damage of the lofty zhi is to relax the chest, and dissolve mucus. The principle for treating the yin damage of the lofty zhi is to nourish and lubricate lung metal, and clear heat.

The principle for treating the yang damage of the enduring zhi of the spirit is to warm kidney water. The principle for treating the yin damage of the enduring zhi is to nurture water yin.

Treating the spirit wandering from the body

When the aspiring zhi of a spirit is excited by an appetence, the spirit is restless in the body and tends to wander off, which will cause the spirit and body discomfort.

Once, a 30-year-old man came to me to have treatment for tightness in his lower jaw and wanted to have acupuncture. Before giving him the treatment, I took his pulse. It was tight like a wire about to break. I asked him: "Are you all right?" He replied calmly: "I am fine. Only my lower jaw is a bit tight, I think it is because I grind my teeth at night." He did not wait for my reply and quickly said: "I just want to have acupuncture." Since he seemed unwilling to discuss his problem further, I therefore chose several acupuncture points according to his pulse.

Tightness of the jaw and the pulse are signs of liver wood inflexibility, but the tight pulse to the extent of almost breaking is a sign that the liver wood yin is almost depleted, and the spirit is in desperation. The treatment is to ground heart fire, calm the spirit, strengthen kidney water, and soften liver wood. I chose Shàohǎi (*少海*), Dàdūn (*大敦*), Xíngjiān (*行间*), Fùliū (*复溜*) and a few A-shì (*阿是穴*) points which are the pain points on his shoulder, neck and lower jaw.

Shàohǎi is a Hé point (*合穴*) of the heart meridian. The Hé point is where the yinyang qi goes deep into the meridian, and is the water of the heart meridian in wuxing. The use of this point is to ground heart fire into kidney water, so the yang heat of heart fire is calm and able to calm the spirit. Dàdūn is a Jǐng point (*井穴*) of the liver meridian. The Jǐng point is where yinyang qi begins to move into the meridian. Xíngjiān is a Yíng point (*荥穴*) of the liver meridian. The Yíng point is where yinyang qi moves through the meridian. The use of Dàdūn and Xíngjiān points is to slow the dry heat from rushing deeper into the liver meridian. Fùliū is a Jīng point (*经穴*) of the kidney meridian. The Jīng point is where yinyang qi moves rapidly in the meridian. Use of the Fùliū point is to promote the kidney water growth, which will nurture the liver wood. A-shì points open meridians locally to relieve the symptom of tightness of the jaw.

The following week the patient returned and said the acupuncture had given him some help so he wanted another treatment. I took his pulse again, and had forgotten what his pulse was like and I was startled when I felt it: "Are you okay?" I said. He replied: "I am fine." I then remembered that he didn't like to be asked too many questions, so I proceeded with the same acupuncture treatment.

On the fifth visit I again asked: "Are you okay?" He stared at me but didn't immediately reply. After a moment he then said, "This is the fifth time you've asked the same question!"

"Did I?" I said. "But your pulse is so tight. It feels like it will break, and it makes me worry."

He hesitated for a moment then told me the following story. Two years before, during a flight from London to Sydney, he felt that he had jumped into the sea, he was pushed by dark waves and large animals came to attack him. He fought with all his strength and felt very afraid. After a long struggle, he came back to the flight and found himself drenched in perspiration.

Since then, he felt very nervous; his jaw was so tight that sometimes he could not open his mouth. So he went to see a doctor and was referred to a psychiatrist. He was then diagnosed as having schizophrenia. The man was a trained designer, he was young and handsome, but with a medical label of schizophrenia, his future was very gloomy. Therefore, he decided never to tell anyone about this again.

I told him that he didn't need to tell me the diagnosis, but I needed to know how he really felt. He then became very frank and told me that he actually felt very nervous and unhappy, sometimes he felt very afraid.

This was a case that the spirit failed to guard the body and went wandering outside; it forced the yang heat of the body to escape with it. So kidney water heat was lost, and liver wood became dry and hot, so the pulse was tight. Kidney water heat loss results in no strength to carry out the enduring zhi of the spirit, so there is the symptom of a fearful spirit. With liver wood dryness, the striving zhi of spirit is firm but inflexible, so he was nervous. An inflexible liver wood also causes the muscle and jaw tightness.

I told him that I thought his kidney water was cold and needed to be warmed, but that a weekly acupuncture treatment was not enough to solve the problem, so he needed to take herbs, since taking herbs twice a day was like having acupuncture twice a day. He happily accepted my suggestion. The principle for the herbal treatment was the same as acupuncture but with the Erxian formula (see chapter: "Kidney Water" for the Erxian formula explanation).

After taking a week of the Erxian formula he felt much lighter, and his pulse had loosened. After taking another two weeks of herbs he felt completely normal and stopped the herbs. I had his Christmas greetings for quite a few years saying that he was completely well and thanked me for the help.

Erxian Formula:

Epimedium brevicornum (yingyanghuo) 30g
Rhizoma curculiginis orchioides (xianmao) 15g
Radix morindae officinalis (bajitian) 15g
Polygala tenufola (yuanzhi) 10g
Angelica sinensis (danggui) 20g
Rhizome anemarrhenae (zhimu) 10g

Phellodendri chinensis (huangbai) 10g

Gentiana scabra (longdancao) 30g

Polygoni multiflori (yejiaoteng) 30g

Zizyphus jujube (fried) (chao suanzaoren) 15g

Concha margaritifera (zhenzhumu) 30g

Concha haliotidis (shijueming) 30g

Concha ostreae (muli) 30g

Ossa draconis (longgu) 30g

Erxian Formula in Chinese 二仙汤:

淫羊藿30g 仙茅15g 巴戟天15g 远志10g 当归20g 知母10g 黄柏10g 龙胆草30g 夜交藤30g 炒枣仁15g 珍珠母30g 石决明30g 牡蛎30g 龙骨30g

Treating yang damage of the aspiring zhi and heart fire yinyang disorder

A 30-year-old woman came for a consultation for feeling heavy and with no desire to do anything. Her marriage had recently ended and since then she had been blaming herself for the breakup, and had lost her self-confidence and interest in life. At the first consultation, she felt her body was heavy, she felt lazy, and had no motivation for doing things. She felt sleepy during the day even though she slept well at night. She was suffering from lower back pain, and she felt hungry all the time and her body weight was rapidly increasing.

The shock of a marriage breakup had damaged the yang qi of the aspiring zhi and caused the spirit to lose interest in life and motivation for doing things. The yang qi damage of the aspiring zhi had caused the spirit to lose the desire to associate with other people, and had suppressed the heart fire yang qi to respond with heaven and earth, which causes heart fire yang heat loss. The yang heat of heart fire is the impetus of the body force; a heart fire yang deficiency causes a loss of liveliness, and feelings of heaviness, lassitude, and difficulty in staying awake. Heart fire yang damage also causes kidney water heat loss as there is no yang heat from the heart fire to ground into kidney water. The lower back is where the root kidney water organ resides, the kidney water heat loss causes its yinyang passages to be obstructed, and so there is lower back pain. Kidney water heat loss fails to nurture the liver wood. In the wuxing cycle, liver wood

247

controls spleen soil so when liver wood is weak, and unable to control spleen soil, then spleen soil becomes excessively loose, which prevents food from being transformed, and the wuxing organs do not get the yinyang qi that they need, so food does not satisfy hunger. As food is not transformed and transported, so the body becomes heavy.

Treatment was to strengthen the yang heat of heart fire and ground the heat into kidney water to establish a harmonized yinyang order of heart fire which would promote the spirit to connect with heaven and earth. The formula used was Erxian Fugui.

The patient took 7 packets of the herbs and all symptoms improved, and after she stopped the herbs for a month all symptoms gradually came back. She took another 7 packets of the same herbs, but drank them only on every second day. Her symptoms were sometimes better and sometimes less so. Then she took a packet of the herbs every day for 8 days, and all the symptoms were stabilised again. She then took the herbs every second day again, most of the time she felt fine, but every now and then she would have thoughts about her ex-husband, which would give her a "sting". She then consistently took one packet of the herbs every day for 30 days, all the symptoms disappeared, and when she thought about her ex-husband, she didn't quite get the sting that she used to. Thereafter, she took a packet of the herbs each day for three months and no longer suffered any symptoms.

Erxian Fugui formula:

Radix aconite carmichaeli (treated) (zhi fuzi) 10g	10g
Cortex cinnamomi (rougui) 10g	Phellodendri chinensis (huangbai) 10g
Epimedium brevicornum (yingyanghuo) 30g	Gentiana scabra (longdancao) 30g
Rhizoma curculiginis orchioides (xianmao) 15g	Polygoni multiflori (yejiaoteng) 30g
Radix morindae officinalis (bajitian) 15g	Zizyphus Jujube (fried) (suanzaoren) 15g
Polygala tenufola (yuanzhi) 10g	Concha margaritifera (zhenzhumu) 30g
Angelica sinensis (danggui) 20g	Concha haliotidis (shijueming)
Rhizome anemarrhenae (zhimu)	

30g   Ossa draconis (longgu) 30g
Concha ostreae (muli) 30g

Erxian Fugui Formula in Chinese 二仙附桂汤:

制附子10g 肉桂10g 淫羊藿30g 仙茅15g 巴戟天15g 远志10g 当归20g 知母10g 黄柏10g 龙胆草30g 夜交藤30g 炒枣仁15g 珍珠母30g 石决明30g 牡蛎30g 龙骨30g

The Erxian Fugui formula is the Erxian formula with the addition of Radix aconite carmichaeli (treated) (zhi fuzi) and Cortex Cinnamomi (rougui) which both are herbs that strengthen the yang heat of heart fire. The Erxian formula meanwhile is to ground the heart fire heat into kidney water, and to nurture the liver wood.
Note: This formula, because of the aconitum carmichaeli (treated) (zhi fuzi), requires at least two hours of boiling before drinking the decoction.

Treating yin and yang damage of the aspiring zhi and heart fire yinyang disorder

I had a young male patient whose girlfriend had left him and he felt so despressed that he didn't wish to live on. He was panicky and for a week he could not sleep, then he made a visit to my practice. Being rejected had damaged the yang qi of the aspiring zhi of the spirit, so his spirit wanted to abandon his body, and he wished to die. The yin qi damage of the aspiring zhi of the spirit caused the patient to lose his steadiness, so he felt panicky. The yin qi damage of aspiring zhi also caused the spirit not to be able to rest in its chamber, so he could not sleep. The treatment was to warm kidney water, soften liver wood, and ground heart fire to invite the spirit to settle back to its home with the Erxian formula. The patient took three packets of the herbs and came back for a follow up visit. He reported that after taking the first packet of herbs, he fell asleep very quickly that night. The next day he went to work, his boss asked him where had he been the previous day and he said he had come to work, it was then that he realized that he had slept two consecutive nights and a day and had missed a day of work. From that point he recovered completely.

Treating yang damage of the reasoning zhi and spleen soil yinyang disorder

An 18-year-old girl came for a consultation for having no appetite. Four years earlier she tried to lose weight by eating very little and exercising hard. At first, it was difficult to control the feelings of hunger, but seeing the size of her waist getting smaller she was happy to keep going.

After three months, although she lost the feelings of hunger, she constantly felt full and bloated in the stomach. If she ate something, it would aggravate the bloated feelings and even cause feelings of nausea. She felt the need to defecate, but it was dry and hard, and not much could come out. She was upset most of the time, but she did not have a clear reason why, and her thoughts were tangled in meaningless things. Every now and then she would even feel afraid. Her periods had begun when she was around thirteen, but two months after her strict dieting her periods stopped.

Over worrying about body shape had tangled the reasoning zhi of the spirit, and damaged the yang qi of the reasoning zhi, which caused the patient not to reason clearly and so the spirit took action against the spleen soil to achieve the goal of losing weight.

The yang qi damage of the reasoning zhi had prevented the spleen soil gaining its yang qi from heaven and earth and caused the spleen soil yang damage. With the yang damage, the spleen soil lost its permeability, the qi passage became congested, and so there was the symptom of bloated stomach. When the water passages are unable to pass through spleen soil, the intestine loses its moistness, so the bowel motion is dry and difficult to open. The loss of permeability of the spleen soil inhibits the transformation and transport of food, so the patient had a lost of appetite. The spleen soil's loss of permeability prevented the heart fire yang heat descending to kidney water, so the kidney water heat reserve became low. Warmth of kidney water ensures regular menses and fertility for women. When kidney water loses its heat, periods become irregular or disappear and fertility becomes problematic. When there is kidney water heat loss, the yang qi of the enduring zhi of the spirit is unable to be exercised, and the spirit is hesitating and fearful. Spleen soil yang damage in turn further damages the yang qi of the reasoning zhi, so her thoughts were tangled like a ball of thread with no beginning nor end.

By the time of the first consultation, the patient's problems were not just that the reasoning zhi of the spirit had been damaged, but also that there was spirit and spleen soil disharmony, spleen soil yinyang disorder, kidney water yinyang disorder, and the spirit and kidney water disharmony. To treat this case, we needed to resolve the conflict between the spirit and spleen soil; at the same time, harmonize the yinyang order of spleen soil, as well as harmonize the yinyang order of the kidney water. As the spirit and kidney water disharmony was caused by the yinyang disorder of kidney water, so once the kidney water yinyang order was regular, then the problem of spirit and kidney water relation would be resolved without further treatment.

To harmonize the relation between spirit and spleen soil is to stop the antagonism of the spirit towards the spleen soil, however, by this time, it was almost impossible to turn around the patient's aversion towards obesity, even though by then she was very thin. The patient had been hospitalized several times for her eating disorder, and she had developed strong emotional resistance towards force feeding. She asked me to help her constipation, bloating stomach and anxiety, but not to force her to eat. I also asked for a precondition before treating her; which was to eat rich for breakfast, full for lunch and little or nothing for dinner. I had given her some examples of people using this method for weight loss and explained the reasons.

The logic behind eating rich for breakfast and full for lunch to lose weight is that during the day, people are active and exhaust a lot of yang qi, and all the food eaten has been transformed into yang qi which is exhausted through the day of working and nothing can be saved. At night, yin qi is rising, people's activities are slowing down, and food gained will be transformed into yin qi presenting as fat accumulating in the body. This is especially the case when not eating enough for breakfast and lunch, the body is more likely to accumulate weight for the need of transforming yang qi the following day. If there is always enough food for yang qi transformation during the day, the body will not have a sense of needing to store excessive yin qi. If one occasionally eats too much food at night, the body will be more likely to dump it than to transform it into yin qi and store it; because yin qi needs the support of yang qi to avoid decay, so excessive yin qi will exhaust yang qi.

The patient happily accepted the explanation and the diet plan. The no evening meal suggestion especially made her relaxed. Having gained the patient's spirit cooperation meant that we achieved the first step of stopping the antagonism of the spirit against the spleen soil, which eliminated some of the barriers for regulating the yinyang order of spleen soil and kidney water.

Although this case had both yin and yang damage of spleen soil, the treatment priority was given to strengthening the spleen soil yang because when spleen soil yang is strong again, food can be transformed and transported then the patient's appetite for food can be improved. The Xianglian Dahuang formula was used for regulating the yinyang disorder of spleen soil. The Xianglian Dahuang formula is the Xianglian formula with the addition of scorched hawthorn fruit (shanzhatan), Rheum officinale (dahuang) and Folium sennae (fanxieye). The Xianglian formula is formulated with herbs to loosen spleen soil, smooth qi flow, and eliminate dampness in the spleen soil. Adding charcoaled hawthorn fruit (shanzhatan), Rheum officinale (dahuang) and Folium sennae (fanxieye) is to promote appetite and move the bowel motions. For detailed explanation of the Xianglian formula see the "Spleen Soil" chapter.

To regulate kidney water yinyang disorder, the Erxian Dahuang formula was used. The Erxian Dahuang formula is the Erxian formula with the addition of Rheum officinale (dahuang) and Folium Sennae (fanxieye). The Erxian formula is formulated with herbs to warm kidney water, nurture liver wood, and ground heart fire. Adding Rheum officinale (dahuang) and Folium sennae (fanxieye) promotes bowel motions. See also the "Kidney Water" chapter.

In the beginning, the patient took one cup of Xianglian Dahuang formula in the morning, and one cup of Erxian Dahuang formula in the afternoon. Sometimes, after taking the Erxian dahuang kidney warming formula, she felt nauseated. She would then have a break from the Erxian dahuang formula for a couple of days. Sometimes after taking the kidney warming herbs, she felt calmer and had better bowel motions, and then she would only take the kidney herbs twice a day. But a few days later, she would feel nauseated with the kidney herbs again; she would again stop the kidney herbs and go back to spleen soil herbs for a few days. Sometimes, her constipation was very bad and she would take one capsule of ground dried Aloe vera that always gave her a little relief. The treated Aloe vera has a bitter and very cold yinyang nature. It goes into the lung and liver meridians; it has a powerful ability to relieve constipation, and clears excessive heat and expels dampness. But Aloe vera cools kidney heat, so it cannot be used often.

After a year of treatment, the patient's menses returned; after three years, the patient's emotions stabilized, her appetite returned, her constipation was much improved and she seldom felt bloated.

Xianglian Dahuang formula:

Rhizoma cyperi (xiangfu) 10g
Toosendan fructus (chuanlianzi) 10g
Lindera aggregata (wuyao) 10g
Cinnamomum cassia (guizhi) 10g
Paeoniae alba (baishao) 10g
Glycyrrhiza radix (gancao) 10g
Rhizoma zingiberis (ganjiang) 10g
Aucklandia lappa decne

(muxiang) 10g
Rhizoma galangae (gaoliangjiang) 10g
Magnolia officinalis (houpo) 10g
Areca catechu (dafupi) 10g
Fructus aurantii (zhiqiao) 10g
Fructus crataegi (shanzhatan) 30g
Rheum officinale (dahuang) 10g
Folium sennae (fanxieye) 1g

Xianglian dahuang formula in Chinese 香楝大黄汤:

香附10g 川楝子10g 乌药10g 桂枝10g 白芍10g 甘草10g 干姜10g 木香10g 高良姜10g 厚朴10g 大腹皮10g 枳壳10g 山楂炭30g 大黄10g 番泻叶1g

Fructus Crataegi (shanzha 山楂) has a sour and sweet taste, and slightly warm yinyang nature. It goes into the spleen and stomach meridians. It breaks down stagnated food, moving the blocked qi, and disposes stomach lumps. Charcoaled Fructus crataegi (shanzhatan 山楂炭) is dryer and is used to add extra strength to eliminate the dampness, loosening the spleen soil, and helping digestion.

Rheum officinale (dahuang 大黄) has a bitter taste, and a cold yinyang nature. It goes into the spleen, stomach, and large intestine meridians. It cools blood, detoxifies poison, breaks down blood stagnation, removes dampness, and moves bowel motions.

Folium Sennae (fanxieye 番泻叶) has a bitter taste, and cold yinyang nature. It goes into the large intestine meridian. It clears the intestines, opens bowel motions, smooths qi flow, dissolves bloating.

Erxian Dahuang formula:

Epimedium brevicornum (yinyanghuo) 30g

Rhizoma curculiginis orchioides (xianmao) 15g

Radix morindae officinalis (bajitian) 15g

Polygala tenufola (yuanzhi) 10g

Angelica sinensis (danggui) 20g

Rhizoma anemarrhenae (zhimu) 10g

Cortex phellodendri chinensis (huangbai) 10g

Gentiana scabra (longdancao) 30g

Polygoni multiflori (yejiaoteng) 30g

Zizyphus Jujube (fried) (chao suanzaoren) 15g

Concha margaritifera (zhenzhumu) 30g

Concha haliotidis (shijueming) 30g

Concha ostreae (muli) 30g

Ossa draconis (longgu) 30g

Rheum officinale (dahuang) 10g

Folium sennae (fanxieye) 0.5g

Erxian dahuang formula in Chinese: 二仙大黄汤:

淫羊藿30g 仙茅15g 巴戟天15g 远志10g 当归20g 知母10g 黄柏10g 龙胆草30g 夜交藤30g 炒酸枣仁15g 珍珠母30g 石决明30g 牡蛎30g 龙骨30g 大黄10g 番泻叶0.5g

Treating the reasoning zhi working against spleen soil

When I was studying at Beijing Chinese Medicine College, one of the compulsory courses was the pathology of biomedicine. During the study of hepatitis, it reminded me of what I went through when I had hepatitis at the age of 14. I now read what was written in the textbook and I began to feel those symptoms described in the text. I felt nausea and a bloating stomach after eating. Sometimes my stomach was even painful. I convinced myself that I had hepatitis again. The more I thought about it, the more symptoms I had. Within two weeks, my complexion had become darker and yellowish.

However, after I had a blood test, the results showed that I didn't have hepatitis, then all the symptoms disappeared overnight.

Nausea, stomach bloating and pain are some of the typical symptoms of hepatitis, but from the traditional Chinese healing point of view, they are symptoms of spleen soil yang damage. The yang damage of spleen soil causes food not to be transformed and transported, so there is nausea after eating. The loss of spleen soil permeability causes qi passage congestion, so there is bloating and pain in the stomach. Loss of spleen soil permeability also causes the inability of liver wood to extend and damages its yang, which causes blood congestion, so the complexion is dark and yellow. Therefore the illness was caused by entangling my thoughts on the hepatitis symptoms. The yang qi of the reasoning zhi was inhibited from being exercised and damaged. Thus the spirit failed to lead the yang qi of heaven and earth through spleen soil, and caused the symptoms of the spleen soil yang deficiency. When the worry of having hepatitis was resolved, the yang qi of the reasoning zhi of the spirit was able to loosen up, and the yinyang order of spleen soil and liver wood quickly caught up with the yinyang order of heaven and earth, so the symptoms disappeared overnight. If the thoughts of having hepatitis didn't stop, the sickness would probably have continued to develop.

Treating yang damage of the lofty zhi and lung metal yinyang disorder

A 68-year-old woman had lost her husband, and she was overwhelmed by sadness. She cried day and night for three months before she came for a consultation. At the first consultation, she couldn't stop crying, her chest was tight, she breathed heavily with the sound of mucus rubbing her qi passages, and she had no strength to walk without help.

The yang qi of the lofty zhi sustains the clarity and dignity of its spirit. The loss of a loved one caused damage to the yang qi of the lofty zhi, so the spirit qi was trapped in sadness and became opaque. As a result of the yang damage, the lofty zhi then failed to bring the yang qi of heaven and earth through to the lung metal and then there was yang deficiency of lung metal. The yang qi of lung metal governs the separation of freshness and turbidity, when the yang qi is damaged, dampness and mucus occurs, so the patient had mucus in the qi passages. Mucus obstructs the qi passages of lung metal and causes tightness in the chest. Kidney water is the storage of body yang qi which gives people strength. In the wuxing cycle, lung metal creates kidney water; with the yinyang disharmony of lung metal it meant that the kidney water wasn't nurtured, and the patient then had insufficient kidney water heat and therefore little strength.

For treatment, the first requirement was to rebuild the intimacy of the spirit with lung metal. While the initial damage to the spirit was over, nevertheless the damage caused a yinyang disorder of lung metal and obstructed the reunion of the spirit with lung metal, which in turn created the feelings of illness. The way to rebuild the intimacy of the spirit and lung metal was to clear lung metal, dissolve mucus, and smooth qi flow to regain the yinyang harmony of lung metal. The yinyang harmony of lung metal provides the resource for the generation of kidney water. In addition, kidney water heat promotes water to rise and moisten the lung metal to dissolve hardened mucus. Also the warmth of kidney water improves the body's strength. Therefore the treatment alternated between clearing lung metal and warming the kidney water. To clear lung metal the Cangzhi formula was used; to warm kidney water the Erxian formula was used.

The treatment procedure:

At first, the patient was given three packets of the Erxian formula to soften the accumulated mucus. After taking the herbs, she felt stronger and breathed more easily, but began to cough up a lot of thick yellow mucus. Then I prescribed the Cangzhi formula to clear the mucus. After taking 7 packets of the Cangzhi formula, the mucus became clearer, and the patient stopped crying. But then she felt weak, and also felt fearful and had restless sleep. So I changed to the Erxian formula again. After taking 10 packets of Erxian formula, she no longer felt fearful and she slept better, but more mucus came out. So I changed her formula to Cangzhi again. For two months I kept changing her formula from Erxian formula to Cangzhi formula, then to the Erxian formula. Eventually the patient recovered from the emotional disorders and the physical tightness of the chest and the lack of strength were resolved.

Cangzhi formula:

Ephedra sinica (mahuang) 10g
Cinnamomum cassia (guizhi) 10g
Puerariae lobatae (gegen) 10g
Aster tataricus (ziyuan) 15g
Anthium sibiricum (cangerzi) 15g
Angelica dahurica (baizhi) 15g
Magnolia liliflora (xingyihua) 10g
Asarum sieboldii (xixin) 5g
Rhizoma ligustici (gaoben) 5g
Vitex trifolia (manjingzi) 10g
Notopterygium incisum (qianghuo) 5g
Sophora tonkinensis (shandougen) 5g
Belamcandae rhizoma (shegan) 10g
Sapindus mukorossi (muhuangen)30g
Evodia lepta (sanyaku) 30g
Trichosanthes kirilowii (gualouren) 15g
Stemona japonica (baibu) 15g
Fritillaria cirrhosa (chuanbeimu) 15g
Amygdalus communis (xingren) 10g
Gypsum (shigao) 20g
Anemarrhenae asphodel ides (zhimu)10g
Platycodon grandiflorus (jiegeng) 10g
Allium macrostemon (xiebai) 10g
Spina gleditsiae (zaojiaoci) 10g
Arctii fructus (niubangzi) 15g
Oldenlandia diffusa (baihuasheshecao) 30g
Sauropus rostratus (longliye) 15g
Glycyrrhiza radix (gancao) 10g

Cangzhi Formula in Chinese 苍芷汤:

麻黄10g 桂枝10g 葛根10g 紫苑15g 苍耳子15g 白芷15g 辛夷花10g
细辛5g 藁本5g 蔓荆子10g 羌活5g 山豆根5g 射干10g 木患根30g 三
丫苦30g 瓜蒌仁15g 百部15g 川贝母15杏仁10g 石膏20g 知母10g 桔
梗10g 薤白10g 皂角刺10g 牛蒡子15g 白花蛇舌草30g 龙利叶15g 甘
草10g

For explanation of Cangzhi formula see the "Lung Metal" chapter.

Erxian formula:

Epimedium brevicornum (yinyanghuo) 30g
Rhizoma curculiginis orchioides
(xianmao) 15g
Radix morindae officinalis (bajitian) 15g

257

Polygala tenufola (yuanzhi) 10g
Angelica sinensis (danggui) 20g
Rhizoma anemarrhenae (zhimu) 10g
Cortex phellodendri chinensis (huangbai) 10g
Gentiana scabra (longdancao) 30g
Polygoni multiflori (yejiaoteng)
30g
Zizyphus jujube (fried) (chao suanzaoren) 15g
Concha margaritifera (zhenzhumu) 30g
Concha haliotidis (shijueming) 30g
Concha ostreae (muli) 30g
Ossa draconis (longgu) 30g

Erxian formula in Chinese: 二仙汤:

淫羊藿30g 仙茅15g 巴戟天15g 远志10g 当归20g 知母10g 黄柏10g 龙胆草30g 夜交藤30g 炒酸枣仁15g 珍珠母30g 石决明30g 牡蛎30g 龙骨30g

For explanation of the Erxian formula see the "Kidney Water" chapter.

Treating yang damage of the enduring zhi with kidney water yinyang disorder

A 44-year-old man came for a consultation as he wanted to stop taking anti-depressant drugs. The patient had a very demanding job, and after a long time working under pressure he gradually became very nervous and sometimes felt uncontrollable fear. At the first consultation, he had been taking the anti-depressant drugs for more than 10 years and the dosage had been progressively increasing. He attempted to stop taking the drugs several times, but each time he stopped, a week or two would pass and then he would become more depressed and fearful than before, and inevitably took more drugs to calm down. He also suffered from loss of sleep and had long lasting headaches and relied on sleeping pills and painkillers to cope with these symptoms.

When the enduring zhi of the spirit over exercises its yang qi, it exhausts kidney water heat reserves and causes kidney water heat loss. Insufficient kidney water heat would then fail to meet up with the spirit expectations and damage the yang qi of the enduring zhi, so the spirit feels fearful. When there is kidney water heat loss there is a failure to nurture liver wood, and liver wood becomes dry. The dry liver wood causes heart fire to over burn and prevents the spirit from resting in its home, so there is loss of sleep. When the liver wood is dry and inflexible, qi flow is uneven and creates wind that causes headache.

The treatment is to warm kidney water, nurture liver wood, and ground heart fire so the body is able to undertake the tasks that the spirit wishes the body to perform. The formula used is Erxian. (See previous case for the formula and details.)

After taking two weeks of the herbs, the patient felt emotionally more stable and slept better, and he didn't have headaches. After he took the herbs for three months he then stopped all his Western pharmaceutical drugs. He continued to take another three months of herbs and he felt well and completed his treatment.

During the period of the patient's treatment I often noticed that he was always on his computer as soon as he sat in the waiting area. Once I said to him "Sorry to make you wait."

"Not at all," he said, "I didn't waste any time, I've been working."

"Maybe you should learn not to be afraid of wasting time," I said.

In fact, when you don't do anything, you don't waste time. Your body and mind have been allowed to have a rest and catch up with the yinyang transformation of heaven and earth. Thereafter, he didn't bring his computer to his consultation and deliberately "wasted" some time.

Another 48-year-old woman came for a consultation for having patches of baldness on her head for six months. At the first consultation, she had an area of around four centimetres in diameter which lacked any hair, and another slightly smaller sized bare area on the side of her head. The patient had a high demanding job and always worked overtime. She also did much of the housekeeping tasks after she got home from work. She felt tired, anxious, had restless sleep, and often felt sharp pains on the side of her scalp.

As in the previous case, when the yang qi of the enduring zhi of the spirit over exercises its will upon the body, it exhausts kidney water yang heat. When kidney water heat is low, and unable to carry out the spirit's will, the yang qi of the enduring zhi will be hurt, so a person feels anxious and afraid. The insufficient kidney water heat delays the body's activities, so she was tired. Kidney water heat loss fails to nurture liver wood, so the liver wood is dry and hot. Hair is the extension of blood, the liver wood is blood storage. The dry and hot liver wood causes hair loss like a dry tree loses its leaves. Dry and hot liver wood stimulates the burning of heart fire which disturbs the peace of spirit in its home, so she had restless sleep. Dry and hot liver wood creates blood heat and wind. Wind striking the blood passages caused sharp pain on the side of her scalp.

The treatment was to warm kidney water, nurture liver wood, and ground heart fire, so that the body becomes capable of undertaking the demands of the spirit and to promote the intimacy of spirit and kidney water. I used the Erxian Xiongzhi formula.

The patient took 10 packets of the herbs, after which new hair began to appear; she felt more confident, and no more sharp pains on her scalp. After taking 40 packets of the herbs, the bald patches disappeared; she slept well and had more energy.

Erxian Xiongzhi formula:

Epimedium brevicornum (yinyanghuo) 30g

Rhizoma curculiginis orchioides (xianmao) 15g

Radix morindae officinalis (bajitian) 15g

Polygala tenufola (yuanzhi) 10g

Angelica sinensis (danggui) 20g

Rhizome anemarrhenae (zhimu) 10g

Phellodendri chinensis (huangbai) 10g

Gentiana scabra (longdancao) 30g

Polygoni multiflori (yejiaoteng) 30g

Zizyphus jujube (fried) (chao suanzaoren) 15g

Concha margaritifera (zhenzhumu) 30g

Concha haliotidis (shijueming) 30g

Concha ostreae (muli) 30g

Ossa draconis (longgu) 30g

Angelica dahurica (baizhi) 15g

Gastrodia elata (tianma) 15g

Uncaria rhynchophylla (gouteng) 15g

Ligusticum wallichii (chuanxiong) 10g

Erxian Xiongzhi formula in Chinese二仙芎芷汤:

淫羊藿30g 克仙茅15g 巴戟天15g 远志10g 当归20g 知母10g 黄柏10g 龙胆草30g 夜交藤30g 炒枣仁15g 珍珠母30g 石决明30g 牡蛎30g 龙骨30g 白芷15g 天麻15g 钩藤15g 川芎10g

For the formula explanation see the section "Treating liver wood yin deficiency with symptom of headache."

Treating yin damage of the striving zhi with liver wood yinyang disorder

A 26-year-old man came for a consultation to control his anger, which frequently arose for insignificant reasons. The man had an unpleasant childhood, being bullied by his father, a veteran of the Vietnam War, who became alcoholic after returning to Australia. The young patient had been feeling angry on the day he came for the consultation. Two days earlier someone had taken a parking spot that he was attempting to get into. He felt so incensed that he felt like killing the other driver. After two days, he still could not calm his anger. He had been breaking bowls, plates and loss his temper with his girlfriend and his mind was running around with all the things that made him feel angry. He felt hot, had body tightness, and was looking for any excuse to lose his temper.

The yang qi of the striving zhi sustains the erectness of the spirit, and the yin qi of the striving zhi sustains the flexibility of the spirit. Being constantly bullied exhausted the patient's yin qi of the striving zhi and caused the striving zhi to be stiff, so the spirit was easily angry. When the yin qi of the striving zhi is damaged, it is firm but not flexible, so when in a situation of conflict, the striving zhi has no flexibility to bend, so the anger became uncontrollably intense. When the yang qi of the striving zhi over exercises upon liver wood yin, it exhausts liver wood yin and prevents the liver wood from storing blood in its root organ. Blood then rushes out of its root storage and into the blood passages and causes body heat. The liver wood becomes inflexible, so the patient's body is tight. Although he was no longer living with his father, the damaged spirit caused the liver wood yinyang disorders, and on the other hand, the liver wood yinyang disorder also further damaged the striving spirit, which then prolonged his mental and physical sufferings.

Treatment was to cool blood, clear heat, and regenerate liver wood. Hot blood running outside of its storage causes liver wood to be dryer; and cooling blood softens the liver wood which brings flexibility to the striving zhi and calms the anger. The formula I used was Erxian Zijingpi.

After taking the first packet of the herbs, the patient had watery bowel motions six times in a day but felt calmer. The next day his bowel motion was still loose but reduced to three times a day. The third day was two times. After taking four days of the herbs, he felt completely calm.

Erxian Zijingpi Formula:

Epimedium brevicornum (yinyanghuo) 30g

Rhizoma curculiginis orchioides (xianmao) 15g

Radix morindae officinalis (bajitian) 15g

Polygala tenufola (yuanzhi) 10g

Angelica sinensis (danggui) 20g

Rhizoma anemarrhenae (zhimu) 10g

Cortex phellodendri chinensis (huangbai) 10g

Gentiana scabra (longdancao) 30g

Polygoni multiflori (yejiaoteng) 30g

Zizyphus jujube (fried) (suanzaoren) 15g

Concha margaritifera (zhenzhumu) 30g

Concha haliotidis (shijueming) 30g

Concha ostreae (muli) 30g

Ossa draconis (longgu) 30g

Nepeta cataria L. (jingjie) 15g

Saposhnikovia divaricate (fangfeng) 15g

Cryptotympana pustulata (chanyi) 15g

Gypsum (shigao) 20g

Paeoniae lactiflora (chishao) 30g

Paeonia suffruticosa (mudanpi) 15g

Lium usitatissimum (humaren) 10g

Cercis chinensis bunge (zijingpi) 15g

Pseudolarix amailis (tujingpi) 5g

Rheum officinale (dahuang) 10g

Erxian Zijingpi formula in Chinese 二仙紫荆皮汤:

淫羊藿30g 仙茅15g 巴戟天15g 远志10g 当归20g 知母10g 黄柏10g 龙胆草30g 夜交藤30g 炒枣仁15g 珍珠母30g 石决明30g 牡蛎30g 龙

骨30g 荆芥15g 防风15g 蝉衣15g 石膏20g 赤芍30g 牡丹皮15g 胡麻仁10g 紫荆皮15g 土荆皮5g 大黄10g

The Erxian Zijingpi formula is the Erxian formula plus the Zijingpi formula. The Zijingpi formula is used to cool blood, the detailed explanation can be found in the section "Treating liver wood yang damage with symptoms of wind rash". The Erxian formula is used to warm kidney water, nurture the liver wood. The detailed formula explanation can be found in the "Kidney Water" chapter.

Difficult & Complicated Yinyang Disorders

So called difficult and complicated cases are no more than the yinyang disorders of wuxing organs. They are difficult because the yinyang disorder has extended to more than one wuxing organ. Like a ball of tangled thread, when pulling one side it tightens the other side. When treating difficult and complicated cases, regulating the yinyang disorder of one wuxing organ can cause other disorders of wuxing organs to have pronounced symptoms. Sorting out a tangled ball of thread first requires finding a place that is relatively loose, then little by little loosening further the tangled ball apart. Treating difficult and complicated yinyang disorders first requires finding a symptom that can be resolved relatively easily, and then step by step further resolving the other complications.

Cases Number One:

A 32-year-old man was suffering from constant body heat, he perspired all four seasons of the year without any physical exertion. He felt his skin was constantly wet and sticky, and after showering he felt even stickier and more uncomfortable. Also he had a lot of mucus going down to his throat, he snored loudly, and sometimes the mucus choked him awake. His fingertips and scalp had burning pains; the fingernails were thickened and rough, there were a dozen or so spots of rash on his skin, which were thick, scaly, and slightly itchy. He became bald when he was 18. His appetite was normal, but he always had loose bowel motions that were sticky and incomplete. He urinated often, but with little quantity and the colour was dark yellow. His sex drive was low with poor erection, premature ejaculation, and lower back pain. He often suffered nervousness. The patient had grown up frequently taking antibiotics as he had often suffered flu symptoms.

His problem was caused by the long term use of pharmaceutical medicines. Chemicals had accumulated and blocked his yinyang passages, disrupting the order of the wuxing organs and made his body constantly uncomfortable.

With lung metal yang damage, turbid and fresh qi are unable to be separated, so the body feels unclean. Turbidity blocks the qi passages, so there is mucus in the throat and snoring while sleeping.

The yang damage of spleen soil causes a loss of permeability, water passage congestion, and the retention of water. Yin damage on the other hand affects the adhering capabilities of spleen soil, the skin opens but is unable to close, so the retained water pours out through the skin, and there is constant perspiration.

In the instance of liver wood yin damage, blood doesn't rest in the root of liver wood but rushes in the blood passages and creates heat, so his body is hot. Heat in the blood creates wind, and wind strikes the blood passages causing burning sensations in his fingertips and scalp. Liver wood yang damage creates mucus in the blood, so he had skin rashes. Old mucus becomes dry, so the rashes were thick and the scalp peeling. Hair is the extension of blood, with liver wood yin and yang both damaged, this restricts the storage of liver for blood, so he had hair loss. Liver wood yang damage causes blood damage in the large intestine, so his bowel motions were sticky and incomplete.

Kidney water yang heat secures the ability of reproduction, so kidney water yang damage causes symptoms of low desire for sex, and weak erection. Kidney water yang deficiency fails to control seminal fluid, so he had premature ejaculation; kidney water yang deficiency fails to move water freely, so he felt lower back heaviness and aching. Kidney water yin deficiency slows the flow of water, and encourages dampness and heat accumulation in the water passages, which also causes dark yellow urine and frequent but small quantities of urine. When there is kidney water heat loss, the yang qi of the enduring zhi, which makes a person high spirited, cannot be exercised, so there is the symptom of a low and nervous spirit.

This was a case that each of the wuxing organs had its yinyang passage congested and had disordered yinyang transformation with heaven and earth. In treatment, the priority was first to clear liver wood, cool blood, remove dampness and mucus in the blood, so the burning pain in his fingertips and scalp, the skin rashes, and the sticky and incomplete bowel motions could be relieved. Second, to loosen spleen soil so that the wuxing organs could be connected and his uncontrollable perspiration could be stopped. Third, to clear mucus in lung metal, isolate turbidity, so the sticky unclean skin and mucus in the throat could be removed. Fourth, to warm kidney water and ground heart fire, so the lower back aches, low sexual desire, premature ejaculation and nervousness could be improved. Fifth, to nurture kidney water yin, drain dampness, free the water passages, so the frequent and dark yellow urine condition could be cleared. Although the plan was in five steps in reality the treatments were intertwined and there was always adjustments according to the patient's response and progress with the treatments.

To clear liver wood, cool blood, remove dampness, and detoxify poisons with the Ershi formula.

Ershi formula:

Gypsum (shigao) 20g
Talcum (huashi) 20g
Radix rehmanniae (raw) (shengdi) 10g
Radix rehmanniae (cooked) (shudi) 10g
Ophiopogon japonicas (maimendong) 10g
Radix trichosanthis (tianhuafen) 10g
Mesobuthus martensii (quanxie) 10g
Scolopendra subspinipes (wugong) $\frac{1}{4}$ piece
Glycyrrhiza radix (gancao) 5g

Ershi Formula in Chinese 二石汤:

石膏20g 滑石20g 生地10g 熟地10g 麦冬10g 天冬10g 全蝎10g 小蜈蚣$\frac{1}{4}$甘草5g

For the formula explanation see section "Treating liver wood yin and yang damage with symptoms of wet rashes".

266

The patient took one mouthful of the herbal decoction and felt as though he were stung by wasps. He immediately felt strong burning pains at his fingertips and scalp. He thought he might be allergic to some herbs in his prescription, so he stopped taking the herbs. Half a day later, the pains subsided.

The burning sensations were already being suffered by the patient, but after taking the herbs the symptoms became more pronounced, which was an effect of the blockages of damp poisons being attacked. It is like an abscess, without touching it, the pain is bearable, but when pressed, the pain becomes unbearable. However, the treatment gave him no relief so an alternative was needed. I changed to a loosen spleen soil method to promote the interaction of the wuxing organs.

Loosening spleen soil

Considering his reaction to the first small formula, the next formula I began with an extremely simple and low dosage prescription. If the herbs could get through, then the dosage could be increased later.

Loosening spleen soil formula:

Cinnamomum cassia (guizhi) 1g   Glycyrrhiza radix (gancao) 1g
Paeoniae alba (baishao) 1g   Rhizoma zingiberis (ganjiang) 1g

Loosening spleen soil formula in Chinese 松脾土方:

桂枝1g白芍1g甘草1g干姜1g

Cinnamomum cassia (guizhi 桂枝) warms and loosens spleen soil, frees the skin to breathe, harmonizes skin and muscles.
Paeoniae Alba (baishao 白芍) frees blood passages.
Glycyrrhiza (gancao 甘草) detoxifies poisons in all the wuxing organs.
Rhizoma zingiberis (ganjiang 干姜) warms and loosens spleen soil, and removes dampness.

After taking one packet of the herbs, he felt less sweaty, and had no uncomfortable feelings. So he took another packet of the herbs, then he felt that his body was hotter, the burning pains in his fingertips and scalp were also more pronounced. He stopped the herbs for two days, then took the third packet of the herbs. He felt the skin was dryer and more comfortable. Then he took another packet of the same formula, but he felt very uncomfortable with sticky heat all over his skin. So I changed the formula to clear lung metal, and remove mucus and dampness.

To clear lung metal, and remove mucus and dampness

For the purpose of clearing lung metal, and removing mucus and dampness I used the Cangzhi formula (see "Lung Metal chapter"). I asked the patient to cook one packet of the Cangzhi formula but to finish it over five days. The first day after taking the herbs, he felt the body was quite fresh, but after taking it for two days, he felt his lower back pain had worsened. At this point I changed the formula to warm his kidney water, and clear liver wood.

To warm kidney water and clear liver wood

For the above intention, I again used a very simple and small dosage formula.

Warm Kidney Water and Clear Liver Wood formula:

Angelica sinensis (danggui) 2g
Radix morindae officinalis (bajitian) 1g
Rhizoma curculiginis orchioides (xianmao) 1g

Ginseng (renshen)1g
Rhizoma anemarrhenae (zhimu) 1g
Cortex phellodendri chinensis (huangbai) 1g

Warm Kidney Water and Clear Liver Wood Formula in Chinese 温肾水，清肝木汤：

当归2g 巴戟天1g 仙茅1g 人参1g 知母1g 黄柏1g

The patient took one packet of the herbs and his lower back pain was significantly improved and he didn't have any uncomfortable feelings; but after taking the second packet of the herbs, he felt the body heat had worsened, so I changed to the clear liver wood, and cool blood formula again. This time I only used three herbs: Gypsum (shigao) 2g, Talcum (huashi) 2g, Glycyrrhiza (gancao) 2g .

He took one packet of the herbs, and felt the body was cooler and more comfortable, but after the second packet, the burning pain in his fingertips and scalp worsened again. So I changed to the loosening spleen soil formula above. As such, I repeatedly changed around the above four formulas, after six months he was able to take them without much adverse reactions, however, his original condition didn't improve much either.

In the following three years I gradually added more herbs and increased the dosage to his formulas until he was able to take all formulas at normal dosages without adverse reactions. By then, his general condition was much improved. The sticky and sweaty skin, the burning pains in the fingertips and scalp were much less and no longer persistently there, and his urine colour was lighter. When I had him take the Erxian formula (see the "Kidney Water" chapter), each time his sexual desire, erection, and premature ejaculation were improved, as was his nervousness. Only the skin rashes, and sticky loose bowel motions were the same, also he still couldn't take any of the formulas consecutively for more than three days without feeling uncomfortable.

I then gave him the strong Tujingpi formula for removing dampness and detoxifying poison (see page 152). After taking one packet of the Tujingpi formula, he had five episodes of watery bowel motion, but felt a lightness and cleanliness of the body that he had not ever felt. In the next two days he didn't take any herbs, but his bowel motion was formed and easy. He took another packet of the herbs then felt low in spirits, and a bit nervous, so he went to back onto the Erxian formula.

For twelve years he changed from one formula to another but eventually, apart from his hair loss, which didn't recover, all the other symptoms basically disappeared. The credit, though, must also go to the fact that during this long treatment he was able to stop using pharmaceutical drugs and no longer ate sweets.

Case Number Two

A 25-year-old man came for a consultation for having no appetite. He was very thin, could not eat much of his meals, and each time he ate something, he had to go to open his bowels almost immediately. The stool was sticky, loose and could not be cleaned out completely. Around his mouth, cheeks, and his back there were layers and layers of pimples. They were red and solid, some were joined together and had pussy points. His hands were sweaty. He was constantly tired, when he pushed himself, he would suffer lower backaches, and after having sex, he also had lower back pain. He was often thirsty, liked to drink water, but after drinking, he needed to urinate shortly after, and his urine was dark yellow with bubbles. He also did not sleep well. He had dreams every night which were of being busy or of being trapped; such as looking for someone but unable to find them, or having too many things to do and feeling overwhelmed.

Spleen soil yang damage, which hinders its permeability and ability to transform food, causes the symptoms of low appetite, and emaciation. Loss of the permeability of spleen soil prevents the yang qi of the reasoning zhi from being exercised, so his thoughts were disordered and he had dreams of being busy but with no clear way of accomplishing what needed to be done. Loss of the permeability of spleen soil blocks the water passages. As the palms are the satellites of spleen soil, water spills over from the palms, so he had sweaty hands. When kidney water heat is low, cold water in the root of kidney organ causes blood and qi congestion in his lower back, so his lower back was aching. With lack of yang qi he was tired. With kidney water heat loss, water fails to rise and he was thirsty, and without kidney water heat the water goes down but not up, so he had frequent urination. The slowed water flow causes dampness in the water passages, and the fermenting dampness creates heat, therefore his urine was dark with bubbles. With liver wood yang damage, this allows the damp poison to grow in the blood passages, and so he had pimples. With damp poison in the blood in the large intestine, his bowel motions were sticky, loose and incomplete. Treatment was to first loosen spleen soil, second to warm kidney water, and third to cleanse liver wood.

For the first step, I prescribed the Xianglian formula (see page 181) to loosen spleen soil, and rejoin the wuxing organs. The patient took three packets of the herbs, but did not have much of a reaction. Then I prescribed the Erxian formula. After one packet of the herbs, the lower back pain disappeared, and the urine was less frequent, but he felt bloating of the stomach, and passed a lot of smelly wind. His stool was stickier and more incomplete, and his pimples had become more painful. This reaction indicated that some of the warm heat from the Erxian formula could not all get through the spleen soil to reach to kidney water, and had helped the fermentation of dampness in both spleen soil and liver wood, so his stomach was bloated with a lot of smelly wind, and the pimples became more painful. I then prescribed the Xianglian formula again.

After taking three packets of Xianglian formula, the bloating and passing of wind had settled, but the lower back pain came back. I put him back to Erxian formula for three days, the back pain got better, but he had been passing wind again, although they were not as smelly as before, and his appetite had improved, which meant that the spleen soil had been loosened up. I changed the formula to Erxian Zhuxing, which was mainly to warm kidney water and on the side to clear dampness both in the spleen soil and liver wood. After taking 7 packets of the herbs, he felt every symptom was improving. But because of his busy life, later he would only take about on average five packets of the herbs a month. Four years later, he slept deeper without too many busy dreams, no excessive passing of wind, and once a day he had a formed bowel motion. He no longer had back pains, even after sex. He had good energy, good appetite, and his pimples were much improved, but after eating sugary foods or too much food with artificial preservatives and additives the pimples were sure to come back.

Erxian Zhuxing formula:

Epimedium brevicornum (yinyanghuo) 30g
Rhizoma curculiginis orchioides (xianmao) 15g
Radix morindae officinalis (bajitian) 15g
Polygala tenufola (yuanzhi) 10g
Angelica sinensis (danggui) 20g
Rhizoma anemarrhenae (zhimu) 10g

Cortex phellodendri chinensis (huangbai) 10g
Gentiana scabra (longdancao) 30g
Polygoni multiflori (yejiaoteng) 30g
Zizyphus jujube (fried) (suanzaoren) 15g
Concha margaritifera (zhenzhumu) 30g

Concha haliotidis (shijueming) 30g
Concha ostreae (muli) 30g
Ossa draconis (longgu) 30g
Olibanum (ruxiang) 5g
Myrrh (moyao) 5g
Paeoniae lactiflora (chishao) 30g
Rheum officinale (dahuang) 10g
Saposhnikovia divaricate
(fangfeng) 30g
Magnolia officinalis (houpo) 10g
Areca catechu (dafupi) 10g
Atractylodis lancea (cangzhu) 15g
Atractylodis macrocephalae (baizhu) 30g
Arisaematis rhizoma (tiannanxing) 10g

Erxian Zhuxing Formula in Chinese 二仙术星汤:

淫羊藿30g 仙茅15g 巴戟天15g 远志10g 当归20g 知母10g 黄柏10g 龙胆草30g 夜交藤30g 炒枣仁15g 珍珠母30g 石决明30g 牡蛎30g 龙骨30g 乳香5g 没药5g 赤芍30g 大黄10g 防风30g 厚朴10g 大腹皮10g 苍术15g 白术30g 天南星10g

The Erxian Zhuxing formula is the Erxian formula with the addition of Olibanum (ruxiang), Myrrh (moyao), Paeoniae lactiflora (chishao), Rheum officinale (dahuang), Saposhnikovia Divaricate (fangfeng), Magnolia officinalis (houpo), Areca catechu (dafupi), Atractylodis lancea (cangzhu), Atractylodis macrocephalae (baizhu), Arisaematis rhizoma (tiannanxing). Olibanum (ruxiang), Myrrh (moyao) are herbs to remove damp poison in the blood. Paeoniae lactiflora(chishao) and Rheum Officinale (dahuang) cool the blood, and detoxify poison. Saposhnikovia divaricate (fangfeng) removes turbidity and protects the skin. Magnolia officinalis (houpo), Areca catechu (dafupi) loosen spleen soil, free qi flow and cease bloating; Atractylodis lancea (cangzhu), Atractylodis macrocephalae (baizhu) loosen spleen soil, remove dampness and mucus. Arisaematis rhizoma (tiannanxing) dries dampness, dissolves mucus, and dispels nodules.

Case number three:

A 35-year-old woman came for help as she suffered from tightness of chest and shortness of breathe. Two years before the visit, she was admitted into hospital for having pneumonia and was treated with antibiotics for more than a month. Afterwards, she still had tightness of chest but her chest x-ray showed no problem. She also felt exhausted and without energy. She had since had much less blood quantity with her menses. She had restless sleep, was very emotional, and teary.

The yang damage of lung metal fails to isolate turbidity, which allows dampness and mucus to grow in the qi passages and causes tightness of chest and shortness of breath. In the wuxing cycle, lung metal creates kidney water. Yang damage of lung metal makes weaker kidney water, and weak kidney water stores less yang heat. Yang heat is the resource of body energy and the condition for reproduction. Deficiency of yang heat is the result of fatigue and insufficient blood flow in her menses. Kidney water heat loss causes liver wood dryness, which further causes heart fire to float, and disturbs the rest of the spirit, so she had restless sleep. Lung metal yang damage prevents the yang qi of the lofty zhi from being exercised, so the spirit was trapped and saddened, and she was teary.

The treatment was to cleanse lung metal, dissolve mucus; warm kidney water, nurture liver wood, and ground heart fire.

To cleanse lung metal I used the Qingdai Haige formula (see page 227). After taking one packet of herbs, the patient felt easier in her chest, but the next two packets of the herbs didn't make any difference to her tightness of the chest. I then changed to the Erxian formula to warm kidney water in order to raise water up to the lung metal and soften mucus. She took three packets of the herbs, and felt more energy, slept better, and her moods were more stable. Then she took another 7 days of the Erxian formula, then she began to cough out large amounts of thick mucus, and the colour was greenish yellow. This was the phenomenon of stagnant mucus being soften and excreted. At this moment I changed back to the Qingdai Haige formula to dissolve mucus and cleanse lung metal. She took 30 consecutive days of the herbs; the mucus gradually reduced and became thinner. But she felt very weak, and could not have a good night sleep. So I changed back to the Erxian formula for seven days. For two years, the patient took alternately the Qingdai Haige and Erxian formulas with occasional breaks, and she recovered form the tightness of chest, fatigue, and restless sleep symptoms. Her menses also became normal again, and her moods became stable.

Cases number four:

A 52 years old woman came for a consultation. As a child she had been sexually abused. Thereafter, she continually suffered from fear and anxiety attacks. She had been on anti-depressant drugs on and off for many years and had been admitted into mental hospital several times, and had electrical shock treatments. At the first consultation, emotionally, the patient was suffering fear, anger, panic attacks, worry, and sadness. Bodily she had a heavy and aching lower back, and was fatigued. Her body was tight and all her joints were intermittently aching. She had only 2-3 hours of sleep each night. She had a lot of stomach pains and sour reflux from the stomach. She often felt tightness of chest, expectorated mucus, and had a very unpleasant body odour.

Frightening events had damaged the yang qi of the enduring zhi of the spirit, which then failed to lead the yang qi of heaven and earth through to kidney water, and caused kidney water heat loss. At the time of the consultation, the initial cause of her spirit disturbance had long passed, but the kidney water heat damage had not recovered and obstructed the reconnection of intimacy between spirit and kidney water. Therefore the problem had been prolonged, deteriorated over time, and damaged the other wuxing organs. The yinyang disorder of wuxing organs then came back to affect the spirit and body's cooperation, so she suffered multiple emotional disorders as well as bodily pains associated with all the wuxing organs.

Kidney water heat loss causes water flow congestion, so she had a heavy and aching lower back. The deficiency of yang qi storage then made her tired. Liver wood yin damage caused body inflexibility so she suffered from tightness of the body. Liver wood yang damage causes dampness and mucus to proliferate in the blood and stagnate in the joints; so she had joint pains. Heart fire yin deficiency causes the fire not to be grounded; and the floating fire disturbs the rest of the spirit, so she could not sleep well. Spleen soil yang deficiency leads to the loss of its permeability, and prevents qi and water from flowing through. The qi blockage causes stomach ache; the water flow blockage causes dampness and water reflux. In the wuxing cycle, sour is wood and wood controls soil. The weak spleen soil leads to the over control by liver wood, so the reflux is sour. Yang damage of lung metal fails to isolate turbidity, so she had bad body odour, and spat mucus; the mucus blocks the qi passages, so she had tightness of the chest.

Emotionally, with kidney water heat damage, the yang qi of the enduring zhi fails to be carried through and then the spirit feels fear. When liver wood yin damage causes loss of flexibility, the yin qi of the striving zhi is unable to be exercised, so the striving zhi is firm but inflexible, which causes anger of the spirit. When there is heart fire yin deficiency, the yin qi of the aspiring zhi cannot be exercised, which causes the aspiring zhi to be ungrounded, and the spirit feels panic. With spleen soil yang deficiency, the spleen soil adheres but is not loose, and the yang qi of the reasoning zhi is unable to be exercised, and the reasoning zhi is mired and there is a feeling of worry. With lung metal yang damage, the lung metal fails to isolate turbidity, then the yang qi of the lofty zhi is prevented from being exerted and there are feelings of sadness.

The treatment is to re-establish the intimacy of the spirit with each of the wuxing organs. First is to warm kidney water to increase energy, stop back pain, and reunite the spirit with kidney water. Then nurture liver wood, relax body tension and provide a harmonious condition to invite the spirit's intimacy. Next to ground heart fire to invite the spirit's resettlement and have restful sleep. Then loosen spleen soil to allow qi and water to pass through, and stop stomach aches, relieve sour reflux, and promote the intimacy of spirit with spleen soil. Furthermore, cleanse lung metal to dissolve mucus, refresh body odour, and free chest tightness, as well as to attract the intimacy of the spirit with lung metal. Finally to cleanse liver wood, remove dampness, and open the meridians to stop joint pains.

To warm kidney water, nurture liver wood, and ground heart fire, I mainly used the Erxian formula. To loosen spleen soil, I mainly used the Xianglian formula. To cleanse lung metal, remove mucus and free chest tightness, I mainly used the Cangzhi formula. To remove dampness and free meridians, I mainly used the Qiteng formula.

The patient took herbs on and off for fifteen years, during this time she completely stopped all pharmaceutical drugs, and was able to look after her family and live normally.

For the Erxian formula and the formula explanations see the "Kidney Water" chapter; for Xianglian formula, see the "Spleen soil" chapter; for Cangzhi formula, see "Lung Metal" chapter; for Qiteng formula, see the "Liver Wood" chapter.

Sprains & Bruises

The clearest demonstrations of the logic of "where there is blockage, there is pain" are the cases of external injury. External injuries damage the passages of the body qi and blood and causes qi and blood stagnation and pain. The treatments are to free qi and blood flow, invigorate blood, and dissolve stagnation.

Sprains

A 9-year-old boy had sprained his left ankle and attended my clinic within an hour. The pain was localised in a small area; it was slightly swollen, with no obvious bruising. But he could not put weight on the foot; and when he tried to turn the foot outward, he felt a lot of pain.

Method of treatment:

1. I inserted six acupuncture needles tightly together just around the injury area and heated the area with a heat lamp for 30 minutes.
2. I lightly massaged the area where I found a small protruding joint and where he felt the most pain. The surrounding areas had no pain, which meant the injury was a slight joint dislocation. So it was safe to give a slight stretch. I continued to give the area a gentle massage but with light stretches. After about 10 minutes, there was a loud sound of clicking joints, and then he was able to turn his foot outward. But to protect the freshly injured area, it needed a herbal bandage.
3. The area was bandaged with egg white and powdered Fructus Gardeniae (zhizi) paste overnight and the next day changed to a new application of the paste. By the third day, the injury had completely recovered.

Powdered Fructus Gardeniae (zhizi) and egg white paste:

Fructus Gardeniae (zhizi 栀子)   Egg white 1
20g

Fructus Gardeniae (zhizi) and egg white paste in Chinese 蛋清栀子膏:

栀子20g 打细粉，鸡蛋清1个

Mix the powdered Fructus Gardeniae (zhizi) with egg white to make a paste and apply on the injured area, then wrap with a gauze bandage. **Fructus Gardeniae** (zhizi 栀子) has a bitter taste and cold yinyang nature. It goes into the lung meridian. The paste clears heat, invigorates and cools blood; stops bleeding and promotes blood flow.
Egg white binds the herbs together and adheres to the skin. Egg white warmed by body heat hardens with the herbs together to support and stabilize the injured area and enables the herbs to stay close to the injury for healing. Although it sticks to the skin, egg white will not block air to the skin, so it has no damaging effect on the skin.

Sprains often involve joint dislocations which must be corrected when there is no bone injuries or when bone injuries have recovered. I had a 70-year-old male patient who had a left collar bone broken 30 years earlier. But after the bone had healed, he still could not use his left arm. He came for a consultation because the left arm had been aching severely for more than six months. So I gave him an acupuncture treatment just on the A-shì points (pain points), followed by massage and stretching, it didn't take much time before we heard a clicking sound, and his 30-year-frozen shoulder joint was relocated, and his pain was relieved immediately and he could move the arm again.

Bruises

A 45-year-old woman came for treatment of a sprained ankle. As soon as she had the fall, she tightly clamped her hands around her ankle in an attempt to stop blood pouring out of its passage. After 10 minutes or so, the pain was eased, she bandaged the injured foot with a cloth and came to my clinic. At that time, there was no obvious bruise, and it was only slightly swollen. But the whole ankle had no strength. She could not move her foot at all, and the injured foot could not bear any weight. Lightly tapping above the injured ankle, she felt shaking pain on the foot.

The fact that the foot could not bear weight, could not move, was weak, and painful when tapped are all signs that there was bone damage. Normally, when there is bone damage, bruises will show, but because the patient stopped the blood pouring out immediately after the injury, so there was no apparent bruise.

When there is a bone injury, it cannot be massaged or stretched until the bone injury had recovered. For this case, acupuncture in conjunction with heat lamp treatment on and around the injured foot was given for 40 minutes, then the foot was bandaged with an application of the powdered Wuhuang formula.

After the acupuncture the pain was significantly reduced as the acupuncture had freed the qi stagnation. After applying the Wuhuang formula, the following day the patient's foot was quite swollen, and where the paste had been applied were purple coloured dots, which were the breaking of blood clots. The patient had stopped the blood pouring out of the blood passages, but there was still blood clots that had formed inside the blood passages congesting blood flow. The congested water and dampness in the blood passages gradually seeped out, so she had a swollen foot. After two months of daily changing bandages, the swelling completely disappeared, but occasionally the foot would swelled up when over used. On and off she pasted the herbs for a year, the foot was basically normal but felt tighter than the good side. By this time, it was safe to give massage; so she had two acupuncture and massage treatments, and the tightness was relieved. However, it was after two years before the injury was completely healed to the point that the patient could not tell which had been the injured foot.

Wuhuang formula:

Fructus gardeniae (zhizi) 50g	(huangqin) 30g
Rheum officinale (dahuang) 30g	Coptis chinensis (huanglian) 30g
Scutellaria baicalensis	Phellodendri chinensis

(huangbai) 30g   Myrrh (moyao) 20g
Olibanum (ruxiang) 20g   Curcuma longa (jianghuang) 30g

Wuhuang Formula in Chinese 五黄膏:

生栀子50g 生大黄30g 黄芩30g 黄连30g 黄柏30g 乳香20g 没药20g 姜黄30g

Fructus gardeniae (zhizi 栀子) cools blood, and frees blood flow.
Rheum officinale (dahuang 大黄) cools blood, and dissolves swelling.
Scutellaria Baicalensis (huangqin 黄芩) removes dampness, and dissolves swelling.
Coptis chinensis (huanglian 黄连) cools blood and dissolves swelling.
Phellodendri chinensis (huangbai 黄柏) removes heat stagnation and dissolves swelling.
Olibanum (ruxiang 乳香) invigorates blood, and dissolves swelling.
Myrrh (moyao 没药) invigorates blood, breaks down old stagnant blood, and dissolves swelling.
Curcuma longa (jianghuang 姜黄) breaks down old stagnant blood, dissolves swelling, and frees qi flow.

All the herbs dissolve swelling, Fructus gardeniae (zhizi), Rheum officinale (dahuang), Scutellaria baicalensis (huangqin), Coptis chinensis (huanglian), Phellodendri chinensis (huangbai) are used to cool blood and stop bleeding, they also free blood flow. Olibanum (ruxiang), Myrrh (moyao), and Curcuma longa (jianghuang) invigorate blood, break down old stagnant blood to relieve pain.

The paste preparation:

Grind the herbs into powder, take 80g of the powder, use 2 egg white to form a slightly runny paste. Apply the paste with a 1cm thickness all over the front and back of the ankle; then bandage with a cloth. The paste has two purposes; one is to invigorate blood, stop bleeding, dissolve stagnant blood, and stop pain; second is to stabilize and protect the injured ligaments and bones.

Currently, Western medical treatments for ankle sprains use ice packs to stop bleeding and ease pain. But after a sprain, the bleeding happens quickly and stops quickly as blood clots up. By the time the ice pack is applied, the spilled blood has become clotted. Using ice packs can temporarily ease some pain, but it hardens the clot and prevents the body to absorb it later on. Thus, the clot stretches the ligament surrounding the joint, making it loose, and failing to protect and stabilize the joint. Then sprains recur over and over. Such cases would then need frequent and long term acupuncture and massage to recover.

A 49-year-old woman came for a consultation after she had a car accident a week earlier. After the accident, she felt a constant deep sharp pain in her stomach, but couldn't pinpoint the spot. There was no damage or bruises on her skin. She had a biomedical examination and was found to be all clear. But where there is pain, then there must be stagnation. A qi passage blockage would induce sharp pain; a blood passage blockage causes persistent pain in a fixed position. The treatment was to invigorate blood, dissolve blood stagnation, and free qi passages. I used the Honghua formula.

After taking three packets of the herbs, her pain was reduced, but a large bruise appeared covering half of her abdomen and back. She was shocked and worried as to whether the herbs had caused broken blood vessels. But if it were the herbs that caused massive abdominal bleeding, she would have had dizziness, fatigue and other symptoms, and the pain would not reduce. On the other hand, the herbs do not have the effects of haemolysis to cause bruises. The term huoxue 活血 in traditional Chinese healing is now interpreted as breaking blood cells like biomedicine, but it is in fact to invigorate blood functionalities. So the bruises were the old stagnant blood clots being dispersed. Therefore I prescribed the same herbs for another week. When she returned for a follow up consultation, the bruises were mostly gone and the pain in the stomach had been completely removed.

Honghua formula:

Carthamus tinctorius (Honghua) 30g
Panax Pseudoginseng (powdered) (sanqifen) 15g
Olibanum (ruxiang) 10g
Myrrh (moyao) 10g

Charred Typha angustifolia (puhuangtan) 10g

Ligusticum wallichii (chuanxiong) 15g

Toosendan fructus (chuanlianzi)

5g

Curcuma longa (jianghuang) 15g

Paeoniae alba (baishao) 20g

Angelica sinensis (danggui)20g

Honghua Formula in Chinese 红花汤:

红花30g 三七粉15g 乳香10g 没药10g 蒲黄炭10川芎15g 川楝子5g 姜黄15g 白芍20g 当归20g

Carthamus Tinctorius (honghua 红花) has a pungent taste, and warm yinyang nature. It goes into the liver and heart meridians. It invigorates blood, opens meridians, removes stagnant blood, creates new blood, calms the foetus, and removes a dead foetus.

Panax Pseudoginseng (powdered) (sanqifen 三七粉) removes stagnant blood, and creates new blood.

Olibanum (ruxiang 乳香) invigorates blood, dissolves swelling.

Myrrh (moyao 没药) invigorates blood, breaks down stagnant blood, and dissolves swellings.

Charred Typha Angustifolia (puhuangtan 蒲黄炭) removes stagnant blood, stops bleeding.

Ligusticum wallichii (chuanxiong 川芎) opens qi passages.

Toosendan fructus (chuanlianzi 川楝子) opens qi passages.

Curcuma longa (jianghuang 姜黄) breaks down stagnant blood, dissolves swellings, and opens qi passages.

Paeoniae Alba (baishao 白芍) opens blood passages, smooths blood flow, and dissolves swelling.

Angelica Sinensis (danggui 当归) harmonizes the wuxing organs, invigorates and nurtures blood.

In the formula, Carthamus tinctorius (Honghua), powdered Pseudoginseng (sanqi), Olibanum (ruxiang), Myrrh (moyao), charred Typha Angustifolia (puhuangtan) are used to invigorate blood and remove stagnant blood. Ligusticum wallichii (chuanxiong), Toosendan fructus (chuanlianzi), Curcuma longa (jianghuang) are used to open qi passages, Paeoniae alba (baishao) is used to smooth and free blood flow, and Angelica sinensis (danggui) is used to harmonize the wuxing organs to promote recovery.

Quick Guide

Yinyang nature of spirit, body, signs of illness, & principles for treatment

Wuxing organs	Liver wood	Heart fire	Spleen soil	Lung metal	Kidney water
Spirit Zhi	Striving	Aspiring	Reasoning	Lofty	Enduring
Spirit Yin Zhi	Supple	Prudent	Thoughtful	Affable	Imperturbable
Spirit Yang Zhi	Straight	Ardent	Orderly	Dignified	Excited
Spirit Yin deficient	Angry	Panicky	Bored	Isolated	Manic
Spirit Yang deficient	Timid	Downcast	Doubting	Sad	Fearful
Nature of wuxing organs	Yang	Yang	Yin	Yin	Yin
Yin role	Flexible	Grounded	Adhering	Gathering	Stationary
Yang role	Erecting	Floating	Loosening	Separating	Moving
Passage	Blood	Spirit	Food	Qi	Water
Healthy wuxing organ	Upright, flexible, stores blood, removes stagnation, cleans body	Lively, steady, stores the spirit, moves & calms body	Bearing, transforming, connects wuxing organs, nourishes body	Gathers moisture & qi; separates turbid & fresh; refreshes body	Stores water & heat; provides strength; supports growth, fertility; moistens body

Yinyang nature of spirit, body, signs of illness, & principles for treatment, cont.

Wuxing organs	Liver wood	Heart fire	Spleen soil	Lung metal	Kidney water
Yin deficient illness	Blood heat, tight body	Restless	Unable to receive; loss of appetite	Fever, dry throat, short of breath	Lack of body fluid, dark urine
Yang deficient illness	Dampness & mucus in the blood	Lethargic	Loss of permeability & digestion problems	Body unfresh; tight chest	Fertility, growth, energy, water flow problems
Pulse (normal)	Erect & flexible	Bouncing evenly	Full & light	Bouncing steadily	Bouncing smoothly
Pulse (yin deficient)	Tight	Floating	Empty	Rapid	Astringent
Pulse (yang deficient)	Floppy	Sunken	Heavy	Hesitant	Slippery
Tongue (normal)	Pinkish	Tender texture	Thin coating	Moist	Smooth
Tongue (yin deficient)	Deep red	Firm, thick	patchy coating, peeled off	dry & cracked	thin & small
Tongue (yang deficient)	Dark	bloated & empty	thick & greasy	covered with sticky saliva	big & floppy
Skin (normal yinyang order)	Smooth without bumps, not discoloured	Shines	Pores open & close freely	Crisp, fresh	Elastic
Skin (yin deficient)	Deep red	Shines with floating light	Sweaty	Dry	Rough

Yinyang nature of spirit, body, signs of illness, & principles for treatment, cont.

Wuxing organs	Liver wood	Heart fire	Spleen soil	Lung metal	Kidney water
Skin (yang deficient)	Dark, jaundiced, rashes, sores	Dull	Unable to perspire	Damp and sticky	Inelastic
Treating yin deficiency	Clear heat, cool blood	Ground heart fire into kidney water	Moisten & enrich soil	Clear heat, detoxify poison	Create new water, clear heat, detoxify poison
Treating yang deficiency	Clear dampness, detoxify poison, invigorates blood	Strengthen yang heat, ground heart fire	Loosen spleen soil	Clear dampness, dissolve mucus	Warm kidney water, ground heart fire into kidney water

Methods for decoction preparation & drinking

For herbal decoctions, it is better to use a clay pot to boil the herbs. A stainless steel pot may also be used, however, metal pots evaporate water more quickly so extra water is usually needed to provide an adequate/extra time for cooking. The methods described below are for clay pot cooking instructions. Apart from some of the special herbal preparation methods that have been described in the chapters, the general cooking instructions are as follows.

Formulas that contain the Erxian formula

Formulas that contain or which are based on the Erxian herbs require a longer cooking time than other formulas as there are many root herbs and shells that need extended cooking to ensure all the properties of the herbs are extracted. Also some of the herbs need longer cooking to remit their overpowering yinyang nature. The method for cooking is as follows:

Place the herbs into a clay pot, add 2 litres of cold water, and bring to boil on a high heat, then reduce the heat down to medium and continue boiling for around 2 hours to reduce the liquid down to 250 ml. Strain the liquid into a jug or large jar, and add another 500 ml of cold water to the herbs in the pot, and boil again on high heat for 20 minutes to reduce the liquid down to 250 ml. Pour out the liquid into the same jar as the first lot of cooked herbs. Altogether there should be 500ml or two cups of herbs to drink. If after cooking there is too much liquid left, continue cooking to reduce it down to 250 ml. If the liquid is insufficient, then add more water and bring to boil to get back to 250ml.

Smaller formulas

Formulas such as Xianglian are relatively smaller packages, so they do not need as much water as large formulas. The cooking method is as follows:
Place the herbs into a clay pot, add 1 litre of cold water, and bring to boil on a high heat, then reduce the heat down to medium and continue boiling for 1 hour to reduce the liquid down to 250ml. Strain the liquid into a big jar, and add another 400 ml of cold water into the pot and boil it down to 250 ml in 20 minutes. Mix the two decoctions together in the jar.

Large formulas

Large formulas such as Tubie Diyu, and Cangzhi are prepared the same way as the smaller formulas such as the Xianglian formula, but need an extra 500 ml of water for the first cooking, and to maintain boiling for 1 hour to get 250ml of liquid left. In the second cooking, add 400 ml of cold water and boil down to 250ml of liquid in around 20 minutes; then mix the two preparations together.

Formulas that have aconitum carmichaeli

Any formulas with aconitum carmichaeli (fuzi 附子, caowu 草乌) must be boiled for at least two hours in order to render harmless any poisonous effects. Such formulas include Erxian Fugui, Erxian Fugui Dahuang, Erxian Wutou Yuxu, Erxian Xionghuang, and Qiteng.

Taking the decoction

Drink one cup (250 ml) of the concoction each time, twice a day. If the herbs were cooked at night, drink one at night and another one next morning. If the weather is cold, the decoction can be left at room temperature for around 24 hours. If the weather is warm or hot, place the decoction in the refrigerator, but before drinking, warm it up to at least room temperature. Sometimes people leave their decoction for more than two days, in such cases, it should be brought to boil and then cool down before drinking. Do not use the microwave to warm the decoction as it damages the nature of the herbs.

Glossary

aspiring zhi the yang of the aspiring zhi of the spirit is ardent, the yin of the aspiring zhi is prudent, so a person has desire but also reserve.

blood (血 xue) is the aggregation of the yinyang essences of the wuxing organs. Blood clears decay, removes congestion, and keeps the body clean .

dampness (湿 shi) is unfresh water. When water flow becomes impeded and doesn't flow freely, dampness occurs.

enduring zhi the yin of enduring zhi of the spirit is calm, the yang is excited, so a person is confident, decisive and calm.

heart fire yin keeps the spirit resting in its house, and makes the body calm.

heart fire yang keep the spirit awake and makes the body active.

heaven and earth heaven is above us, earth is beneath us, in others words, the universe.

jingluo (经络) the passages through which the body connects with heaven and earth.

jingmai (经脉) the main routes of the body which connect with heaven and earth along which yinyang qi flows.

kidney water yang moves water to prevent water retention and facilitates reproduction and growth, and provides energy to the body.

kidney water yin moistens the body and reserves body heat.

liver wood yin sustains the suppleness, and flexibility of the body.

liver wood yang sustains the straightness and firmness of the body.

lofty zhi the yin of the lofty zhi of the spirit gathers spirits together, the yang of the lofty zhi filters the gathered spirits and keeps ones alike together, so a person is friendly but dignified.

lung metal yang separates turbid and clean qi and expels body wastes and retains the clean, and keeps the body fresh.

lung metal yin gathers moisture and qi from heaven and earth, and the internal body, so the body is moist and full.

luomai (络脉) a network of passages that connect jingmai to each other.

mucus (痰 tan) congealed dampness.

qi (气) is the measure of the quality of yin and yang. Often translated in English as energy, force, breath, air.

reasoning zhi the yin of the reasoning zhi of the spirit is lingering, the yang of the reasoning zhi is sorting, so a person can think before acting.

spleen soil yang spleen soil yang has a permeable and loosening nature, which lets the wuxing organs to pass through, and transforms and transports food.

spleen soil yin spleen soil yin has an adhesive nature, which holds wuxing organs together and bears food.

striving zhi the yang of the striving zhi of the spirit is firm, the yin of the striving zhi is flexible, so a person is firm but gentle.

turbid and turbidity (浊气), refers to wastes, unclean fluids, and unclear qi.

wind (风 feng) is rough or unsmooth qi flow in the body.

wuxing the cycle of dynamic transformation between wood, fire, soil, metal and water. Wu (五) means five, and xing (行) means movement. Wuxing is often translated into English as five elements, or five phases .

yang (阳) the bright side of a mountain, the base of all things and phenomena that are bright, upward moving and active by nature. The sun, a bright day, mobility, hot, rising, fluctuating, loose, separating, upright and opposing are yang. The spirit is yang.

yin (阴) the dark side of a mountain. All things and phenomena that are dark, downward moving and passive by nature, e.g the moon, a dark night, stillness, cold, sinking, stability, adhering, gathering, soft and resisting are yin. The body is yin.

zhi (志) means will, or ambition. The qualities of the spirit.

Index of Treatments

Index of Formulas

Index of Herbs

CPSIA information can be obtained
at www.ICGtesting.com
Printed in the USA
LVHW021535110221
679071LV00010B/1001